CANCER HEALING ODYSSEY

Natural, organic, whole food
is a divine blessing...
a gift of Heaven and Earth...
the seed of our growth
in Health, Peace,
Goodness and Beauty.

Let us work to create Health
for ourselves and
our families,
and among all People
on planet Earth.

Let us eat slowly
in Gratitude and Friendship,
so that in this very hour
the Kingdom of Heaven
may exist among us.

Peace be with you.

Cancer Healing Odyssey

Sarto Schickel

PAXDIETA BOOKS
PHILADELPHIA

This book presents information based on the unique personal viewpoint
and opinions of the author. It is not intended to be a substitute for diagnosis
and treatment by a physician or other professional healthcare provider.

The author and publisher are not responsible for any adverse effects the
reader may experience from the use of any information contained in this book.
In addition, they can not be held responsible for any errors or omissions that
may be contained in this book.

In the event you have a health matter that requires medical advice,
the author and publisher urge you to seek out and consult
with a competent healthcare professional.

This book outlines one person's use of conventional medicine
in association with various alternative therapies.
It is not a guide to the Gerson Therapy. Anyone interested in the Gerson Therapy is
encouraged to contact The Gerson Institute in San Diego, California.
Anyone interested in the macrobiotic philosophy and diet is encouraged
to contact the Kushi Institute in Becket, Massachusetts.

Mention of certain individuals, organizations or companies in this book
does not imply endorsement by the author or publisher, nor does mention
of such individuals, organizations or companies imply that they endorse
this book, its author, or the publisher.

Published By:

PAXDIETA BOOKS, INC.

4622 Osage Avenue
Philadelphia, PA 19143
CancerHealingOdyssey.com

Cancer Healing Odyssey is available online and at bookstores. It is also available for
special promotions, conferences and events. For details call: 215 476-4949.

Library of Congress Control Number: 2011915844
ISBN-13:   978-0-615-54000-9
ISBN-10:   0615540007

Book design and editing by: Kim Metzgar
Cover design by: John Gummere
Cover photo by: Jacques Schickel

FIRST EDITION—Second Printing 2012
Printed and Manufactured in the United States of America

For Sun Hee
my beautiful wife

for my mother
Marnie
whose example
taught me
love
patience
peace of mind
and
generosity

&

for my daughters
Arianna
and Julianna
who make every day
alive with joy

Contents

Chapters

Appendices

Wisdom

Theological-Philosophical-Practical Wisdom which never
loses sight of the Totality—the Wholeness of Life and Truth:

"God is love, and he who abides in love abides in God, and God...in him."
—FIRST LETTER OF JOHN 4:16

*"Love is love. It is the power of powers. 'Tis why we live.
'Tis our last refuge, our first hope, our unsullied and simplest joy."*
—LOUIS SULLIVAN

*"Whenever I lift my mind and heart to God (Love),
miracles happen within me."*
—NORBERT H. SCHICKEL, JR.

*"To know God, to recall nature, to acknowledge Wholeness
is the highest wisdom to which a human can aspire."*
*"The world of life is governed by the law of God:
the body and the land are not two."*

"Saints and wise men have long advised, 'Return to Nature.'
*....Yet the method that makes a return to nature possible is so very simple.
There is no other way than by making ourselves, our organisms, one with her.
We must eat natural foods."*
—GEORGE OHSAWA

9

"Let food be thy medicine and thy medicine be thy food."
—HIPPOCRATES

*"I am more than ever convinced that biochemistry and metabolic science
will be victorious in healing degenerative disease, including cancer if the whole
body or the whole metabolism will be attacked and not the symptoms."*

*"I repeat: In general, the recovery from a malignancy means
the restoration of the whole body from a kind of degeneration."*
*"We do know that a healing apparatus is present and functions in a healthy
body—and we learned, in addition, by means of this treatment that it can be
reactivated if the body can be sufficiently detoxified
(in degenerative diseases and cancer)."*

"It must be natural food, grown in a natural way."
—MAX GERSON, M.D.

*"The healthy, happy man has understood that to live a joyful life, no matter
where on this earth, he must first of all make himself one with his environment.
He must eat, drink, and behave in a manner that does not
alienate him from the orderly, simple truth of nature."*

*"Blood circulates, we move, sleep, eat, digest, the brain
thinks, we speak—all miracles.
As long as that which makes these things occur—the power of God or Life—
is moving within us, we are alive and can cure sickness."*

"True health is that which you yourself have created out of illness."
—GEORGE OHSAWA

Acknowledgments

(A message from Sarto Schickel and Sun Hee Lee)

We would like to thank not only those who helped with the creation of this book, but also those who helped us survive the ordeal of cancer diagnosis and treatment. We discovered that a stage IV cancer diagnosis not only affects the person who is ill. In addition, it affects the spouse, children, immediate family and extended family. Further, it affects the school and church community. In our case, all of these parties showed tremendous kindness and understanding of the crisis which came upon us.

Sun Hee has been blessed with three very talented and dedicated conventional doctors at a Philadelphia area hospital. In addition, she has been blessed by wonderful alternative doctors, especially Dr. Hernandez of the Gerson clinic in Mexico. The dedicated staff at the Gerson Institute in San Diego was also most kind and helpful during the application and follow-up process.

We thank Charlotte Gerson, daughter of the late Dr. Max Gerson and founder of the Gerson Institute, for her tremendous insight and generosity of spirit. We thank Howard Straus for his encouragement to consider writing a book, and for *his* inspiring and excellent biography of Dr. Gerson entitled: *Dr. Max Gerson—Healing the Hopeless.*

We thank Sarto's late aunt Mary and uncle—William Schickel—a patient of Dr. Gerson from 1952, for the inspiring example of how to face a health crisis as a couple, and how to defeat advanced cancer using Gerson Therapy.

During the most difficult first year after diagnosis, numerous members of the Lee and Chung families have been exceptional in their kindness including: Wonja, Chun-Jun, Jeong Hoon, Won Hoon, Kyung Hee, David, Jeff, and Danny.

We thank our long time friends: Miss Cho, Julie, Agnes and Orhan, Tamae, Susie, Okkwon and Ken, Anne and Jean, Linda and Ken, Susan and Rafael, Jeremy and Katia, as well as David and Charlotte, for all of their many kindnesses. Thanks to photographer John Woodin for the preparation of a beautiful video of the Healing Benefit Concert. Thanks to Nancy Drye for the gift of hope in a tiny bottle. Thanks to Mike Drake for his endless patience printing early drafts.

Many thanks to macrobiotic friends in Philadelphia who have encouraged us in this book project: especially Stephen Glickman who sparked its beginning, and Kerry Palanjian and Sis Mamolen for many useful editing suggestions. Thanks to Howard Waxman, owner of natural foods store Essene, for providing an oasis of health in Philadelphia. We appreciate the lineage of macrobiotic teachers who have influenced us including: Sagen Ishizuka, George Ohsawa, Michio and Aveline Kushi, Geraldine and Stanley Walker, Denny and Susan Waxman, and Christina and Robert Pirello. Thanks to Virginia Harper, author of *Controlling Crohn's Disease—The Natural Way,* and Sarah Dickinson Murray for reading and commenting on the working drafts.

Schickel family members have also shown incredible kindness, and we especially thank Sarto's mother Marnie, uncle Lou, as well as Anderson, Schickel and Haine cousins. For kindness at every turn we also thank: Marti, Nimr, Bill, Trina, Tom, Young Mi, Agnes, John, William, Pauline, Norb, Benitta, Bruno, Amy, Jacques, Abe, Kathy, Ceci, Sue, and Raissa. We thank Kay and Mark in a special way, for encouraging us to write this book, and for a special brand of solidarity. We thank Ruth for being with us in the first few days after the diagnosis.

Our friend Okkwon Kim was instrumental in organizing a Healing Benefit Concert which allowed us to make the trip to the Gerson Clinic in Mexico. We thank all the musicians who performed including the incomparable Sung-Ji Kim, as well as Catherine Pyun, David Aker, Bihn Park, Kevin Louie, Ryan Louie and our daughter Arianna. Special thanks to David Shunskis and the staff at Trinity Memorial Church who made it all possible.

Members of Sun Hee's Korean Church—Emmanuel Church in Philadelphia—offered amazing support in many different ways: by providing meals after the surgery period and later, by coming to pray and visit at our home. Members too numerous to name attended the Healing Benefit Concert, to help make it an event of substance and spirit. We give sincere thanks to all who helped organize and support the concert, and to those who attended. A very special thanks to Yikwon

Kim and Paul Lee for their help, and Pastor Park for his eloquent and uplifting prayers at the Healing Benefit Concert.

We also express profound thanks to Pascale Davidson of the French International School and David Felsen of Friends Central School, who have shown great kindness and sensitivity to our daughters during this challenging period.

All of this incredible kindness—poured out from heaven and earth— is appreciated beyond measure. This book is *the return on investment of this loving kindness.* We hope it can help to save the lives of women and men from around the world—who are inspired by Sun Hee's *healing odyssey,* utilizing both conventional and alternative medicine.

This is the story of Sun Hee's recovery—as told by her devoted husband. With gratitude to those who assisted Sun Hee, and with blessings to all who may find this humble book.

Sarto and Sun Hee

Note to the Reader
For the sake of confidentiality, the names of the doctors in this story have been changed:

—Dr. Ryan was Sun Hee's surgeon.

—Dr. Allen was the assistant surgeon.

—Dr. Chetry was the associate doctor.

—Dr. Hernandez was the Gerson Clinic doctor.

Preface

This book is a personal story written as hope and inspiration for all those who have been diagnosed with cancer and are looking to combine conventional and alternative treatments, to increase the likelihood of success in healing their illness.

When my wife Sun Hee was diagnosed with stage IV ovarian cancer she was in a state of total shock and despair. She had a large ovarian mass in the abdominal cavity and the cancer had spread to the chest cavity—where she had a fluid build-up called a pleural effusion. On September 28, 2007, two days after her inital doctor visit, Sun Hee had a portion of the fluid removed from the chest cavity. This provided some relief and made it easier for her to breathe. This reduced the pleural fluid by about two inches as shown on the x-ray taken immediately after the procedure.

The very next day on September 29, 2007 Sun Hee began an alternative nutritional and detoxification therapy. Her health improved dramatically and significantly in these first two weeks while she was waiting for surgery. In fact, her pleural effusion reduced by an additional 1.375 inches in just 10 days. A sequence of four x-rays shown in Chapter 4 document the complete disappearance of the pleural effusion—a result of Sun Hee's use of conventional and alternative approaches.

On October 15, 2007, Sun Hee had abdominal surgery to remove the primary ovarian tumor and survived a complicated recovery room crisis. She continued her nutritional and detoxification therapy for the six weeks after surgery. She then continued an adjusted alternative nutritional program while receiving a total of eight chemotherapy infusions of carboplatin and taxol over the next seven months.

When her doctor recommended twelve more *maintenance* chemotherapy treatments, Sun Hee decided it was time to try another approach. By good fortune some of Sun Hee's good friends organized a Healing Benefit Concert which allowed us to go to an alternative health clinic in Mexico in July 2008 for 10 days.

Sun Hee made dramatic progress at the clinic, losing her chemo-caused jaundiced appearance in just eight days. She learned a special food and juicing therapy that allowed her body to receive ideal human nutrition on an hourly basis. She also learned about detoxification methods and supplementation.

Subsequent to leaving the clinic Sun Hee has made excellent progress. After six months back home Sun Hee went through a huge healing reaction—which had been predicted by the staff at the clinic six months in advance. Now, over four years after her diagnosis, Sun Hee is feeling healthy with normal CA-125 levels (the last at 26 vs

3,745 originally at diagnosis—on a scale with 0 to 35 being normal). The pleural effusion is no longer indicated on the chest x-ray. Sun Hee plans to continue her nutritional and detoxification therapy for another six months until her blood work is more fully rebuilt and the healing process is complete.

Significantly, Sun Hee's results appear to be better than perhaps 99% of other cases of ovarian cancer stage IV, where a large malignant pleural effusion is involved. According to my research, medical science has not yet cured any cases of ovarian cancer with a malignant pleural effusion.

This is a cause for concern—and it is a rather unnerving statistic—even when we see that Sun Hee is doing so well. Despite this worry, Sun Hee is a living example of what progress can be achieved when alternative nutritional and detoxification therapy is combined with conventional medical treatments.

This is a very personal story of Sun Hee's healing odyssey, combining alternative and conventional treatments. We hope that it can:

(1) Inspire you to be proactive in your own healing.
(2) Inform you by direct example how Sun Hee
      achieved her results, through use of alternative and
      conventional medicine.
(3) Lead you to your own unique path to healing.

We hope the miracle of healing that Sun Hee has received—by the work of her doctors (both conventional and alternative) and by her own efforts, together with those of her family (who helped with the organic vegetarian food and juices in the kitchen)—can also be yours. This combined approach is work intensive but a great journey of growth and love. The most critical thing is to begin.

The logic for embracing an alternative nutritional and detoxification program is simple. Regardless of what essential treatments one may choose from the field of conventional medicine—one must still eat and drink something—so why not eat and drink the most ideal food and drink that one can to help rebuild the body's immune system. This can help to fight the cancer—from the inside out—to achieve authentic healing.

Introduction

When we researched ovarian cancer and malignant pleural effusions we found shocking data summarized in this statement below:

"The diagnosis of a malignant pleural effusion signifies a poor prognosis because it is usually a manifestation of far-advanced disease. In a meta-analysis of 417 patients with malignant pleural effusions, the median survival was 4 months. Eighty percent of patients were alive at 1 month, 54% at 3 months, 31% at 6 months and 13% at 1 year following a diagnosis of a malignant pleural effusion. Patients with gastrointestinal tract tumors, lung cancer, and ovarian cancer had a median survival of (less than) 4 months, whereas those with breast cancer and lymphoma had a median survival of (greater than) 4 months."

(Source: *Seminars in Respiratory and Critical Care Medicine* 22(6):607-615, Copyright 2001 Thieme Medical Publishers)

At present we find that Sun Hee is out over four years from her original diagnosis. Her pleural effusion is no longer indicated on x-ray. Her last CA-125 test is in the normal range. Why is Sun Hee's outcome so dramatically different from the cases that are described in the above quotation? Quite possibly, we may know the answer.

The key to the success that we found for Sun Hee is to *begin right away with alternative diet and detox*—from day one—and to blend with great care conventional and alternative approaches. At the end of this book, I expand on this theme with a chapter entitled, *Conclusion: A Path to Healing In Ten Steps*. The process of finding the right combination of conventional and alternative approaches is critical for someone suffering a serious cancer.

Relying only on the cancer killing and removal powers of conventional medicine, with its chemotherapy, radiation and surgery, is not logical. One must also rely on the regenerative and healing power of a helpful alternative diet—with its vegetarian meals, juices, detoxification and supplementation—as is found in the Gerson Therapy. In my view, this combined approach makes true healing from a serious cancer condition possible, and more likely.

The reasons why few people attempt this type of integrated approach are complex. One must note that two world-views seem to exist side by side. One possible explanation may be that very few health practitioners are conversant in both the conventional medical model and in the alternative models, such as the macrobiotic diet or the Gerson Therapy.

Some will say there is a vast conspiracy by the medical establishment to reject alternative therapies that can essentially be carried out at home in one's own kitchen. There may be some truth to this or it may be that we live in an age of increasing specialization; and the medical training of today focuses more or less exclusively on such specialized ways. In that context, home-based alternative therapies such as the Gerson Therapy or macrobiotic diet may seem quaint, and perhaps unscientific—since there has not been an expensive million dollar randomized double-blind clinical trial to prove effectiveness.

Another criticism leveled at alternative or integrative healing stories is that they are anecdotal but not real scientific evidence. We challenge this interpretation as not logical. For example, when I found my irritable bowel issues were gone in a week on the macrobiotic diet—what more evidence was needed? That was enough scientific evidence for me to know that I was heading in a good direction.

When Sun Hee found that her terrible cough was gone in a week on a modified Gerson program—and the fluid in her chest dropped by 1.375 inches in ten days—what more scientific evidence was needed that this was a very beneficial direction? We are so grateful that we knew about the Gerson approach—because this allowed us to implement this powerful nutritional and detoxification method beginning the first day after the shocking diagnosis of stage IV ovarian cancer was delivered to us.

But how was it possible that Sun Hee's cough went away so quickly and how was it possible that the fluid level dropped so much in only ten days? This has to do with internal healing which is true healing.

Let me elaborate with an example with which we are all familiar. When a person breaks their arm, the doctor may reset the arm into proper position with a brace or cast, but the *healing process* is not something that the doctor does. The healing process happens on a cellular level as the broken bones knit themselves back together.

Because the healing process is inherent to a healthy body—but fails in an unhealthy body—the focus of the Gerson Therapy is to make the body healthy again, as quickly as possible, by carefully calibrated nutrition and detoxification. Then, the hope is that the more healthy body's own healing power kicks-in and fights to destory the cancer. This was Sun Hee's goal as she embraced conventional and alternative medicine to heal from stage IV ovarian cancer.

1

Personal History and Diagnosis

My wife Sun Hee Lee was born in Taegu, South Korea, into a family with two sisters and two brothers. She attended elementary and middle school in Taegu in the years after the Korean War. During High School she lived with her older sister in Seoul, in order to attend Ehwa attached High School. Upon graduating, Sun Hee matriculated at Ehwa Women's University and later Ehwa Graduate School where she studied music composition. In her available spare time Sun Hee enjoyed playing piano and cello.

After completing her university studies in Korea, Sun Hee traveled to the United States where she studied English at Temple University. At Drexel University she received an MBA. In the early 1980s Sun Hee and I met while we were both living at International House of Philadelphia. We dated for several years and were married in Bala Cynwyd in 1990; then began life together in University City, Philadelphia. I received a Bachelor of Science degree from Cornell University and later a Master of Architecture degree at the University of Pennsylvania. We adopted two children, both born in Korea. Arianna and Julianna bring us great joy and happiness. Arianna is a talented violinist; and Julianna is a talented scholar who dreams of becoming a writer or an artist.

We have the greatest family and friends; and live in a supportive and beautiful neighborhood. This has helped us to get through the many challenges of the last few years beginning with the shocking news of September 26, 2007. Sun Hee had developed a terrible cough, one that was shocking when heard. It was the kind of cough that turned heads in alarm. We thought and hoped it was simply a case of very bad bronchitis. In late September 2007, Sun Hee visited a doctor in Philadelphia who diagnosed stage IV ovarian cancer with spreading to the chest cavity.

On September 26, 2007 a chest x-ray was done and the written report stated:

> *"Impression: PA and lateral views of the chest show a large pleural effusion with atelectasis. This raises concern for a mass. A CT scan of the chest is recommended. The left lung is clear and the visualized aerated right upper lung field is clear."*

The next day, on September 27th, a CT scan of the abdomen and chest was done and the report stated:

> *"Impression: Large right pleural effusion with shift of the mediastinum to the right and marked atelectasis in the right middle lobe and lower right lobe. This is most likely related to*

metastatic disease to the pleura. Large midline cystic and solid
mass most likely ovarian in origin but the exact site is difficult
to determine."

The CT scan confirmed a large primary tumor in the abdominal cavity. There was a large pleural effusion—fluid built up in the chest cavity— creating pressure on the lungs. On the right side one lobe of the lung was partially collapsed, and another had suffered near complete collapse. Initially the question was whether the fluid had cancer cells in it—whether it was a pleural effusion, or a malignant pleural effusion. The pleural fluid filled the chest cavity outside the lungs, 7/8ths of the way up on the right side.

On September 28, 2007, about 1.4 litres of pleural fluid was drawn out after insertion of a long needle through Sun Hee's back. A follow-up x-ray was taken shortly thereafter. According to the cytology report, the pleural fluid was found to contain cancer cells. The report stated in part:

> *"CYTOLOGIC INTERPRETATION AND DIAGNOSIS:*
> *FINAL INTERPRETATION:*
> *(NON-GYNECOLOGIC)*
> *Adenocarcinoma present, see note.*
> *NOTE: The patient's previous ovarian carcinoma was not*
> *available for review, but the morphology of the tumor cells*
> *could be compatible with an ovarian primary.*
> *Clinical correlation recommended."*

Metastasis had already occurred. Ovarian cancer spread to the liver or the pleural cavity is classified as Stage IV—terminal cancer, with essentially no cured cases on record. Our research showed that 80% to 85% of these patients die within one year. In addition to this tragic news, we also received a shocking report on the blood test called CA-125, the generally recognized ovarian cancer tumor marker. Sun Hee's CA-125 blood test result was 3,745, with normal being 0 to 35. The news was both shocking and emotionally devastating. With two young children to raise, our family faced a very uncertain future. Many patients with ovarian cancer, coupled with a large pleural effusion (fluid built up in the chest cavity between the lung and the wall of the chest cavity) and acute cough, live only a few months. We were in a crisis mode. Everything seemed to be on the table—even life itself.

2

Emotional Challenge

In the beginning we shed many tears. Each conversation with a close friend or relative brought more tears. Beautiful, wonderful friends stopped by which brought more tears, but also some solace as well. Church members visited and prayed which was deeply appreciated. It was helpful but also brought more tears. We remembered that Christ also faced a death sentence—and yet lived out the meaning of his short time remaining on earth with great nobility and for the greater good of humanity. A profound and shocking realization suddenly arrived that health, hope, *and life* can so easily slip away.

Research on the Internet was very enlightening but not reassuring. We finally found one conventional medical case on record, allegedly cured, for stage IV ovarian cancer wherein the patient had had a malignant pleural effusion. This was not 1% cured—but only one single individual in all of medical history! This case had been complicated, with the cancer spreading to the brain after chemotherapy and the need for brain surgery at that point. Five years later they were saying this lady was cancer free. This seemed to be the one and only case medical science had ever cured, where a malignant pleural effusion was involved. Ovarian cancer with the malignant pleural effusion certainly appeared to be 99.99% fatal.

It was both shocking and devastating, and brought on a great sense of helplessness, hopelessness and depression. When we got the telephone call, with the bad news of the positive cytology report on the pleural effusion, we were sitting together at the long table in our dining room. We had been expecting the call and had pen and paper ready for taking notes. The doctor said he was, "Sorry to report that the cytology report taken from the pleural fluid sample shows that the cancer has spread to the chest cavity, and is likely ovarian in origin." Sun Hee was completely overcome—crying uncontrollably and almost unable to breathe. I told the doctor to hold the line, then put down the phone while I tried to calm Sun Hee down. Fortunately Sun Hee did not pass out. We quickly learned that a stage IV cancer diagnosis hits like *ten tons of bricks*.

That evening the cough seemed to get worse. Knowing it was cancer changed the game and Sun Hee now became very aware of the crisis in her body. The swelling in her abdomen was not just a middle aged belly—it was *the tumor*. The cough was not terrible bronchitis—it was *approaching death*. That night I woke up in the middle of the night— shaken to the core with a shocking dream. In this dream Sun Hee was in the bathroom coughing up volumes of blood from her lungs into the toilet, when she suddenly fell back and died in my arms on the bathroom floor. It was such a shocking dream that I did not tell Sun

Hee anything about this dream until the writing of this book began over two years later. How quickly the nature of our lives, dreams and thoughts had changed.

At this time I called Charlotte Gerson (who I had spoken with before in efforts to help other friends and relatives) and emailed her Sun Hee's medical records to get her informal feedback. Charlotte called with great concern saying that it was a very advanced case—with atelectasis—which is a partially collapsed lung. She did not know whether Sun Hee would be accepted by the Gerson Clinic in Mexico, if that was what we wanted. But Charlotte did encourage us to have Sun Hee begin the Gerson Therapy at home to see if Sun Hee responded.

I did not tell Sun Hee about this pessimistic outlook by Charlotte for fear of sending her over the edge and into despondency. However, this one phone call sent me into a great depression, which I tried to hide from Sun Hee. I had always viewed the Gerson Therapy as something that could help a "hopeless or terminal" case. Now Charlotte seemed to be saying it may be too late, even with the Gerson Therapy, given Sun Hee's advanced condition with the pleural effusion and collapsed lung.

During this early time after diagnosis I always remained calm and stalwart when around Sun Hee, giving her constant encouragement and projecting a positive outlook. While driving and talking in the car with Arianna and Julianna on the way to school, I was often on the edge of tears but managed to keep composed. When alone by myself in the car, it was much harder.

The day after the conversation with Charlotte—after dropping off Arianna and Julianna at school—I pulled out of the school driveway and was overcome with emotion, crying uncontrollably, and finding myself gasping for breath. Fearing for a possible auto accident as I drove down Highland Avenue, I pulled over the mini-van and got out to take a walk to get fresh air. The waves of emotion continued unabated as I walked and within thirty feet I was overcome—falling to the ground struggling to breathe normally. On my hands and knees I stayed there on a homeowner's grassy lawn, next to the sidewalk, trying to calm down and catch my breath.

A lady driving by stopped her SUV and came over to see what was the matter, perhaps wondering if I had suffered a heart attack. I blurted out to her that, "My wife is dying of ovarian cancer." We spoke briefly together and I began to calm down. She offered her cell phone number in case I needed someone to talk to, which was declined as not needed. I noticed that the lady had a son in her car wearing a yarmulke. Then I realized that this Good Samaritan was in fact a modern orthodox Jewish woman. Remembering Bible readings about the Good Samaritan, I sensed a strong connection to Biblical times, and was grateful and comforted by her stopping.

Reflecting on this later, I realized the power of hope. When I began to lose my sense of hope—due to my interpretation of the phone call with Charlotte—then I had become overwhelmed with powerful emotions and the feeling that the situation was impossible. I was thinking that Sun Hee would die and our family, as presently constituted, would be destroyed. This thought was simply unbearable.

There was one other Good Samaritan woman who showed up at this time. My sister Ruth drove up from Washington with her daughter Monet, to lend support, as soon as she heard about Sun Hee's diagnosis. Having had her own brush with a serious health issue, Ruth was very aware that the first week after diagnosis is the toughest mentally, when the patient and the family must come to terms with the bad news delivered by the doctor. In fact, Ruth was with us on September 29, 2007, the very first day that we started the modified Gerson Therapy, a day after Sun Hee's definitive diagnosis. It was Ruth, always a devoted sister and sister-in-law, who helped us with the first Gerson juices, and who helped me to keep Sun Hee's spirits up in the first few dark days.

3

The Secret—The Trinity of Natural Healing

In the chaos and pain of those first few hours, after learning of the stage IV ovarian cancer diagnosis, we searched for mental clarity and a positive direction. We recalled that we knew of a few brave individuals—who had dared to go against the conventional medical dogma of despair and hopelessness, when it came to stage IV cancer. They had chosen a different way, and had found a unique, alternative pathway to recover their health.

We thought of Anthony Satillaro M.D., of Philadelphia, whose book I had read in 1984. In his book Dr. Satillaro described how he had just buried his father—and was himself suffering from stage IV cancer—when, on his way home from his father's funeral, he picked up two hitchhikers. They told him about the macrobiotic diet; and how it could improve his health, so that his own body could cure the cancer. Satillaro was President of Methodist Hospital in Philadelphia at the time.

Despite his high rank, Satillaro's desperation allowed him to listen to the improbable story of the two young hippies who were so certain the macrobiotic diet could help him recover from cancer. He drove them to 4th and South Streets—which is located exactly between two historic residential areas called Queen Village and Society Hill—and followed them into a natural foods store called Essene, looking for Denny Waxman, a macrobiotic counselor.

Getting into the macrobiotic diet under Denny's guidance, Dr. Satillaro made a full and dramatic recovery, and lived for about a decade before getting sick again and finally passing away. Dr. Satillaro wrote a book titled: *Recalled By Life*, co-authored by Tom Monte. It was written up in a six page article in LIFE Magazine in August 1982, showing dramatic before and after full-body scans. They showed how Dr. Satillaro had witnessed multiple tumors—located in diverse places all over his body—disappear under the healing influence of a macrobiotic diet. The cover of this issue of LIFE featured Marilyn Monroe, twenty years after her death in 1962. This impressive little book introduced me to macrobiotics in 1984. At that time, I had been suffering from irritable bowel syndrome. By adopting the macrobiotic diet, I found relief of my symptoms in less than a week. This was a remarkably quick result and it made a profound impression on me.

We also remembered my uncle, William Schickel, who found in *Prevention Magazine* a cancer therapy created by Dr. Max Gerson. Dr. Gerson was born in Europe in 1881 and died in New York in 1959. My uncle Bill consulted Max Gerson M.D. in New York City in 1952—at Gerson's office at 815 Park Avenue—and then began the Gerson Therapy thereafter. With the diligent support of his young wife Mary,

Bill was able to implement the Gerson Therapy at his farmstead in Loveland, Ohio. Within a few weeks he was feeling much better, and within two years his advanced retroperitoneal lymphosarcoma had apparently vanished.

In 1958 Dr. Gerson published his classic book, *A Cancer Therapy— Results of Fifty Cases*, a year before his own death. The book lays out the theory and practice of the Gerson Therapy and contains detailed medical records on fifty patients. My uncle is listed in the book as Mr. W.S., case #18. He was thirty two years old in 1952 when he met Dr. Gerson. He had three children at the time. Bill Schickel lived another fifty seven years as his family expanded to eleven children and countless grandchildren. Mary Schickel died in 2007. Bill died in July 2009, one month before his 90th birthday.

After Mary died, Bill wrote a moving tribute to Mary in a small and beautiful volume entitled: *Mary Frei Schickel—What a Woman!* In this book he discusses their use of the Gerson Therapy. He also wrote a two page article that was published in the *Gerson Healing Newsletter*. It described his experience of consulting with Dr. Gerson, and how he recovered with the guidance of this good doctor, and by the work of his devoted wife Mary. Bill and Mary both appear, and Bill was interviewed, in the 2006 documentary, *Dying to Have Known*, a movie about the Gerson therapy by cinematographer Stephen Kroschel.

With the tremendous example set by Dr. Satillaro and Bill Schickel, we were determined to use alternative medicine as a complement to conventional medicine. We began discussing which approach or combination to use. Sun Hee has always had a lot of faith in the medical establishment, and I not so much, believing that true healing must be inwardly generated—primarily through diet, detoxification, and an optimistic creative outlook. Sun Hee wanted to go forward with surgery, which I thought was a good use of conventional medicine. Before her diagnosis, I had read a booklet published by Charlotte Gerson (Dr. Max Gerson's daughter) telling the dramatic stories of numerous recovered ovarian cancer patients. All had initial surgery and then, in most cases, skipped chemotherapy—opting instead to go directly into the Gerson Therapy. Therefore, I was not enthusiastic about chemotherapy. However, Sun Hee—after considering all her options, and after talking with her family in Korea—decided chemotherapy after surgery was the necessary next step. She felt she could use the chemotherapy for its cancer-killing abilities, and then rebuild by detoxifying the chemo out of her body using Gerson Therapy.

I discovered that in these very hard decisions, only the patient can decide. The opinions and wishes of the spouse are secondary. There is some evidence that if a patient believes chemotherapy will be helpful and that the side effects will be mild—that will be the likely result. However, if the patient feels the chemotherapy will not be beneficial, and the side effects will be horrible—that will be the likely result. This speaks to the issue of the mind of the patient and how it interacts with the therapy choice, whether it be conventional or alternative.

In her inspiring book, *A Time to Heal*, Beata Bishop writes about the emerging field of psychoneuroimmunology or PNI. She points to research that shows that one's essential belief system and thinking can greatly affect the immune system. In short—belief becomes biology. This brings to mind a well known quote from Werner Erhard which expresses this same truth: "As we speak, not only are our words in a state of birth, but also *the very thing* about which we are talking."

This then is my view of the secret of natural healing for cancer—the *Trinity of Natural Healing*—which is embraced in slightly different ways in both Gerson and macrobiotic approaches:

> TRUTH: Positive thinking, personal responsibility—living within the natural order.
> GOODNESS*:* Abundant nutrition—pure water, organic food and juices, supplements.
> BEAUTY*:* Detoxification of organs, tissues and cells—creating a clean, beautiful body.

It was this *healing knowledge* that Hippocrates found, that Dr. Max Gerson and George Ohsawa rediscovered, that Dr. Satillaro and Bill Schickel utilized, and that the vast majority of cancer patients—sadly—never find, or find too late. One of the purposes of this book is for *this secret*, which has been known for over two thousand years, to be more available to all who are ill. In fact, one shocking reality about modern cancer treatment is that it largely ignores this *golden triangle, this Trinity of Natural Healing*. Most cancer patients are never told that *careful nutritional change may save their life*, that they can use methods like coffee enemas *to detoxify their body*—and the culture of despair and hopelessness associated with the cancer industry tends to kill any *positive outlook for success*, by making it an article of faith that cancer is "incurable."

In place of the *Trinity of Natural Healing*—positive thinking, abundant nutrition and detoxification—the cancer patient is often given only the trinity of modern oncological medical care—surgery, chemotherapy and radiation. By ignoring three quarters of what the cancer patient needs, is it any wonder that positive results from modern cancer treatment are in the main, so elusive? (See Appendix IV for further discussion.)

In place of traditional natural healing—which focuses on nutrition, detoxification, and positive thinking (on what the patient can do for himself)—modern medicine focuses instead on what the doctor can do, while utilizing very expensive procedures and medicines. This singular focus by the mainstream medical doctors has helped create the alternative movement which has arisen to fill the vacuum. From conventional doctors we often heard, "Be sure to eat a lot of protein" as the typical dietary advice, with no advice given on detoxification methods; and the advice to eat a lot of protein is quite possibly wrong for a cancer patient.

In fact, macrobiotic diet relies on a low protein diet for a cancer patient. The macrobiotic diet is considered a grain-based diet—utilizing brown rice, barley, millet, and oats in the main, supplemented with vegetables, beans, tofu, tempeh, sea vegetables, miso soup, and limited fruits. Depending upon the specific circumstances, some fish may be added. A macrobiotic counselor will typically customize a dietary program for each client depending upon the issues involved. Detox is by special baths and body scrubs along with special teas and soups. Body work such as Shiatsu is encouraged.

In a similar manner, the Gerson diet also relies on both a low protein and a low fat diet. Oil in cooking, and salt in any way, is forbidden. The emphasis is on oatmeal and fruit for breakfast along with a glass of juice. For lunch and dinner the focus is on potatoes, occasional brown rice, vegetables, salads, fruits, plain nonfat yogurt, a special vegetable soup and a glass of juice. The Gerson diet is simple. Detox is by coffee enemas. Yoga and other harmonious modalities are encouraged. As explained later, Gerson Therapy also uses many daily vegetable juices as well as numerous supplements.

When a macrobiotic or Gerson patient goes into a regular grocery store, he or she must avoid nearly everything in the store, as it is mostly packaged and processed food products and drink, except for the fresh produce section and grain aisle. Ideally all produce purchased should be organically grown. A good theme for the cancer patient could be expressed this way: *"Eat natural and organic food—not industrialized and chemicalized food products."* This brings to mind the statement of an African American lady, about 120, the daughter of a slave, who was asked about her philosophy of nutrition. She simply said: *"I eat only that which grows from the ground."* This wise woman was a person who had not lost touch with nature—plants, sun, soil, water and wind—or with common sense.

4

Beginning the Gerson
Therapy at Home

Since surgery was in two weeks, we got busy implementing a modified Gerson Therapy for this first two week period which meant: (1) vegetarian food, (2) vegetable juices, (3) coffee enemas. At this time we did not use the various supplements that are the 4th component of the Gerson Therapy. The first day after Sun Hee's diagnosis, we started the demanding Gerson Therapy with nine special organic home-pressed vegetable juices each day, and three vegetarian meals made with organic ingredients and no salt or oil. Sun Hee took three 15-minute retention coffee enemas daily, to help move the bowels and to detoxify the liver, as is the Gerson way. In this initial period, Sun Hee took three carrot juices, three green juices, and three carrot-apple juices daily—all homemade—which were consumed immediately.

Many people misunderstand the purpose of the coffee enema in the Gerson Therapy. Dr. Gerson found that the caffeine gets absorbed by the hemorrhoidal veins in the rectal-colon area. It then travels via the portal vein to the liver, where it dilates the bile ducts. In this manner, the liver is more easily able to discharge its toxic products into the intestinal tract, as the bile flow is increased. For the Gerson patient, the coffee enema is incredibly important to do in combination with taking the juices. The juices drive toxins and debris from the cells in the body to the liver, which can be overwhelmed without the relief provided by the coffee enemas. Generally a 3-to-1 rule is observed. If nine eight-ounce juices are taken daily, then three enemas would be used each day.

In the first few days after the definitive diagnosis of ovarian cancer with a malignant pleural effusion—after the fluid was drawn down on September 28th—neither Sun Hee nor I could sleep. Knowing what the cough was all about, it was very hard to ignore it as we had previously, since it was worsening. The act of lying down to sleep caused the pleural fluid to move around which set off coughing bouts. We might sleep for perhaps fifteen minutes and then there would be a coughing bout. Neither Sun Hee nor I got more than two total hours of sleep each night. On the third night I said: "Sun Hee, tonight I will sleep in another room *so I can't hear the cough*—otherwise I will be unable to have any strength to help you during the day." Sun Hee understood and agreed.

Fortunately, progress using the modified Gerson Therapy was almost immediate. After a few days the cough was lighter with Sun Hee feeling a bit better. This alone was a huge relief. Each day that the cough was lighter gave us inspiration and motivation to apply the Gerson Therapy, which is very difficult and work-intensive. It is also rather expensive and relentless. After six days the daytime cough was gone. This was a huge milestone which gave us a great sense of hope. After eight days the nighttime cough was gone. These very fast results were stunning.

Inspired by these results, our conviction grew that the combination of juices, detoxification, and organic vegetarian food was helping. After ten days another x-ray was taken on October 9th. It looked nothing like the x-ray taken after a small portion of the fluid had been drawn down on September 28th. (Four x-ray plates follow.) Comparing the x-rays dated 9/28 and 10/9, you can see that the fluid in the right chest cavity showed a quite remarkable decrease in pleural fluid, by about 1.375 inches in only ten days. With this x-ray in hand, Sun Hee came out of her shell emotionally. She began to express some positive thoughts saying: "Will we be able to afford all the carrots and greens needed for two years on the Gerson Therapy?" That statement showed a significant psychic shift, as Sun Hee was now thinking ahead by a few years, rather than thinking she might be dead in a few months. Her mind was on a positive track.

We were also so busy making juices and carrying out the program that we had little time for depression. The physicality and pro-active nature of the modified Gerson program was therapeutic, and indeed quite uplifting for the mind and the body. Without it, the depression of the first few days may never have lifted.

See Appendix III to view eleven pages of daily schedule sheets, with notes, showing how we implemented the modified Gerson Therapy in the first eleven days. At the bottom you can see hand-written notation of Sun Hee's improving condition. We consider this an eleven-day miracle that set the stage for Sun Hee's ongoing good results. The pleural fluid dropped approximately 1.375 inches during the ten day modified Gerson Therapy period—9/29/07 to 10/9/07. This is an unheard of result in the annals of cancer medicine. (See x-rays.)

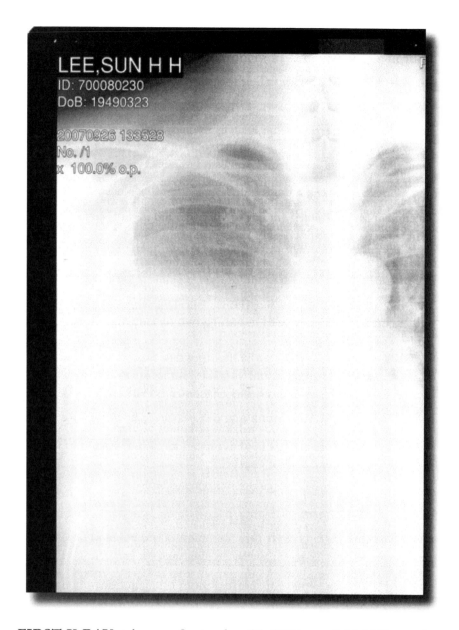

LEE,SUN H H
ID: 700080230
DoB: 19490323

20070926 133528
No. /1
x 100.0% o.p.

FIRST X-RAY: taken on September 26, 2007—at Initial Diagnosis. This shows a very large right pleural effusion. White area shows the level of fluid built up in the chest cavity.

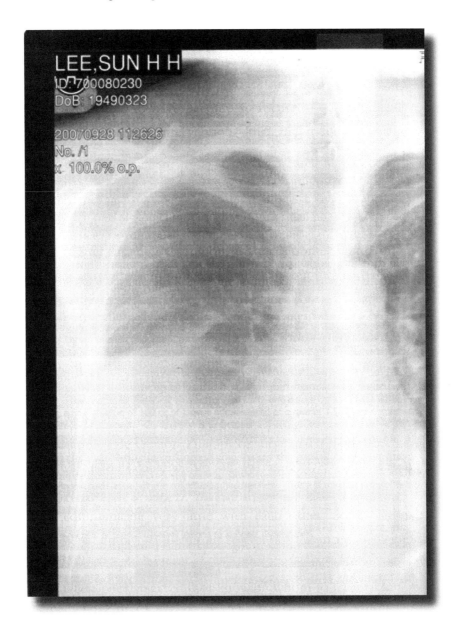

LEE,SUN H H
ID: 700080230
DoB: 19490323

20070928 112626
No. /1
x 100.0% o.p.

SECOND X-RAY: taken on September 28, 2007—after 1400 mL of fluid was drawn out. This shows a quite significant decrease of 2 inches in the pleural fluid as a result of the needle draw-down (thoracentesis).

THIRD X-RAY: taken on October 9, 2007—after 10 days on modified Gerson Therapy. This shows an additional and quite significant 1.375 inch decrease in the pleural fluid since the x-ray of September 28th, 2007.

FOURTH X-RAY: taken on June 16, 2008—after completion of nine months of alternative diet therapy with seven months of chemotherapy. "The prior large right pleural effusion is no longer identified." (Report: p. 48)

Patient name: LEE, SUN H **Sex:** F **Date of birth:** ▓▓▓▓▓▓▓

Mrn: 00725531-8   **Accession number:** 4672530   **Primary Acn:** 4672530

Scheduled date: 2008.06.16 15:05   **Completed date:** 2008.06.16 15:21

Report Date: 2008.06.16 16:57   **Department Code:** CHEST

Referring Physician: ▓▓▓▓▓▓▓▓▓▓ MD

Exam: CPAL/chest 2 views   **Exam status:** Final

Comments: BXBS

History:

Diagnosis: PLEURAL EFFUSION

Diagnostic Report

Impression: No active disease seen in the chest.

Comment:

PA and lateral radiographs of the chest are compared with 10/17/07.

The prior large right pleural effusion is no longer identified.

The lungs are clear. The heart and mediastinum are normal. No pleural effusions seen on the current examination.

Radiologists:
Responsible providers: ▓▓▓▓▓▓▓▓▓▓▓
Contributing providers: ▓▓▓▓▓▓▓▓▓▓▓

http://oasis▓▓▓▓▓▓▓▓fm/MrnReportsDisplay/report.cgi?ris_exam_id=4672530&pid...   2/3/2009

FOURTH X-RAY REPORT: completed June 16, 2008—and provided to Sun Hee by her doctor on February 3, 2009.

The disappearance of Sun Hee's pleural effusion is a point of great pride. For nearly all other stage IV ovarian cancer patients who have pleural effusions—*the pleural effusions do not disappear.* They typically reaccumulate and must be managed by additional thoracentesis procedures, or even by the injection of talc into the chest cavity, to try to block the fluid from being produced by the cells which line the wall of the chest cavity. Nowhere in our research did we find cases where stage IV ovarian cancer patients had the pleural effusion completely disappear, and then not reaccumulate.

PLEURAL EFFUSION DISAPPEARS

The method by which the pleural effusion disappeared from Sun Hee's chest cavity is a good illustration of the principle of utilizing both conventional and alternative medicine.

FIRST: Sun Hee had a thoracentesis procedure on 9/28/07 and after an x-ray was taken showing a 2 inch drop in the pleural fluid. *(Result of conventional medicine.)*

SECOND: Sun Hee then went on a modified Gerson Therapy for 10 days and had an x-ray on 10/9/07, which showed approximately a 1.375 inch drop in pleural fluid. *(Result of alternative medicine.)* At this point there was only 2.375 inches of pleural fluid left in the chest cavity and one has to wonder if it too would have been gone in about one more month on the modified Gerson Therapy. Next, Sun Hee had surgery—which made the pleural effusion worse on the right side, and caused an effusion on the left side.

THIRD: After surgery on 10/15/07, Sun Hee did partial Gerson

Therapy for six weeks, then macrobiotic diet and chemotherapy for seven months. On 6/16/08 an x-ray was taken showing no pleural effusion on either the left or right side. (*Result of conventional and alternative medicine.*)

9/26/07: 5.75 inches of pleural fluid as measured from the bottom of the chest x-ray, on the day of first diagnosis.

9/28/07: 3.75 inches of pleural fluid as measured from bottom of chest x-ray, after thoracentesis. (*Result of conventional medicine.*)

10/9/07: 2.375 inches of pleural fluid as measured from bottom of chest x-ray, after ten days on modified Gerson Therapy. (*Result of alternative medicine.*)

6/16/08: 0 inches of pleural fluid as measured from bottom of chest x-ray, after seven months of chemotherapy and macrobiotic diet. (*Result of conventional and alternative medicine combined effect.*)

5

Surgery and Recovery Room Crisis

S urgery was scheduled for October 15th, 2007, at a Philadelphia area hospital. Dr. Ryan was to be the principal surgeon. He came highly recommended by another doctor Sun Hee knew, so we had a good feeling that it would all go well.

As we got closer to the surgery date, Sun Hee eased off the modified Gerson food and juicing program, and the enemas. She had not been taking the Gerson supplements up to this point. Sun Hee began to eat more normal food for a few days prior to surgery. I had been taking measurements of Sun Hee's abdominal dimension for several days and it was shrinking somewhat. The evening before surgery, Sun Hee took the hospital required milky-white liquid called magnesium citrate. The next morning, before heading to the hospital, I took an abdominal measurement—it had grown considerably and the abdomen was clearly swollen again. It was rather shocking that with only one cup of this foreign substance, the body would react so negatively and so quickly.

We arranged for our daughters, Arianna and Julianna, to stay with our good friends Anne and Jean. Their daughter Mia was in the same class with Arianna at school. This was necessary as Sun Hee was likely to stay in the hospital for up to five days. I needed to stay at the hospital with her, for support and personal assistance.

We arrived early at the hospital and parked in a convenient garage. We walked across a pedestrian sky-bridge and began an elaborate check-in procedure that began with a great deal of additional paperwork. Finally, Sun Hee was taken in for pre-op procedures. I was wanting to see her once that was done, for a brief visit before she went into surgery. With the help of our friend Linda, I was able to find my way to see Sun Hee, as she lay on the moveable bed, just before she was taken to the operating room. It was at this meeting that one of the assistant doctors told me that the CA-125 test on October 9th was 3,824, up 2.1 percent from the original test taken on September 26, 2007, when it was at 3,745. This was very disappointing to me, as I had hoped that the result would show a lower number, due to the ten days on the modified Gerson Therapy. Only later did we learn that the CA-125 often goes up, before it comes down, when on the Gerson Therapy. The CA-125 ovarian tumor marker blood test has a normal range of 0 to 35.

Once in the operating room Sun Hee was soon sedated and surgery commenced. The next thing Sun Hee remembers is being in the recovery room, coming to, and having a visit from Dr. Ryan. He said the surgery went very well and that he managed to get all the cancer he could see in the abdominal cavity. Meanwhile, I was holed up in the family waiting room when I got a call from Dr. Ryan. He said the surgery went very well, and that things inside the abdominal cavity looked much better than expected. There was a primary tumor that was taken out—but the other spreading they thought was there, based on the CT scan of late September, was not found at all. This was a surprising finding. I wondered to myself if this disappearance of minor bits of cancer, at other sites within the abdominal cavity, could be due to the modified Gerson Therapy used during the two week period from September 29th to October 14th.

So then began a wait of nearly four hours, with my sister Ceci in the family waiting room, and never getting permission to go to the recovery room. I kept inquiring as to what was going on, and was constantly told nothing of any substance. At first I was not too worried, but as time marched on I became increasingly concerned. Finally I had to use pretty aggressive tactics of demanding, again and again, to have permission to go to the recovery room. Later, I demanded to know where the recovery room was and explained that I would go there with or without permission. Only then did I finally get a call from Dr. Allen, who was supervising the recovery effort. She said there were some recovery complications. She would be down in a few minutes to meet with me and explain it all. Ceci had left by this time. Now, Sun Hee's friend Miss Cho was with me as we waited to get this important report from the assistant doctor.

When Dr. Allen arrived she explained that there had been significant internal bleeding in the abdominal cavity, which was unusual and that only happens in a small percentage of cases. She explained that a surgical clip may not have closed a severed blood vessel completely, or there could be another unknown cause. They had added four units of blood to stabilize Sun Hee. I was grateful the tumor was gone, but now realized that Sun Hee had *a belly full of blood* instead. The doctors were debating whether to take Sun Hee back into the operating room, to open her up and fix what was wrong, or whether to wait it out, to see if the bleeding would stop of its own accord. They had been giving her various medicines to bring up her blood pressure, which had dropped very low, and to bring down her pulse, which was running very high at 120 beats per minute. She was in a fragile and life threatening condition.

On the way up to the recovery room I asked Dr. Allen, "On a scale of 1-to-10 how big a crisis is this?" Dr. Allen said it was perhaps a seven, so I knew it was quite serious. Once in the recovery room, I found Sun Hee covered from head to toe on the surgical bed, with a vinyl shower cap over her hair. She was very groggy but still could speak, though rather weakly. She recognized me and was relieved to see me.

First, I planted a kiss on Sun Hee's forehead, and then placed my left hand on her forehead—as I had seen my mother do so many times, with sick brothers or sisters. With my right hand I held Sun Hee's right hand. After just a few moments, I glanced up at the monitor, and saw the pulse rate begin to move—120, 119, 118, 117, 116—over the course of just eight seconds. Very interesting, I thought. Keeping up this hands-on-presence, I watched further as the pulse continued to drop—115, 114, 113, 112, 111, 110, 109—and it just continued on down to 100, 99, 98, 97, and then still further until it reached 88. All of this happened in just a matter of five minutes.

After fifteen minutes in this position, I left Sun Hee's side and went over to talk to Dr. Allen. She was sitting nearby at a computer terminal reviewing Sun Hee's vital signs and other data. Dr. Allen shared some of the details from the surgery. When they opened up the abdominal cavity things inside looked much better than they had expected, based on the CT scan taken earlier. The spreading of the cancer they expected could not be found, and the main tumor seemed smaller and less problematic than expected.

They had begun to wonder if Sun Hee only had a large benign cyst, and not a cancerous tumor. So they took a sample of the ovarian tumor—held up the surgery—and sent it to the lab to get biopsy results. They were thinking that if it was not cancerous then they would not have to do a total hysterectomy, but would only remove the tumor. Dr. Allen then explained that the biopsy report came back positive for cancer. So they then proceeded to remove the tumor, the uterus, and in fact gave Sun Hee the full debulking routine, as is typical for serious ovarian cancer cases.

Later, I learned that while removing the tumor, which was fluid filled, it was accidentally punctured, and the fluid spread throughout the abdominal cavity. No doubt the doctors washed out the abdominal cavity as best they could. But the possibility of spreading, with new seeding of tumors in the abdominal cavity, was now a significantly increased risk—due to the accidental spilling of this fluid. Such a puncture is obviously not desirable, but it apparently does happen in a small percentage of cases, despite the best efforts of the doctors.

Dr. Allen further explained that Sun Hee was the very first patient she and Dr. Ryan had ever encountered, wherein the cancer had spread to the chest cavity but not to any other locations—such as onto organs in the abdominal cavity, or onto the wall of the abdominal cavity itself. Then I began to think to myself: "Was it possible that two weeks on the Gerson Therapy had cleaned up the spreading of the cancer to the other locations, that the original CT scan seemed to indicate was present?" And thinking further: "If the pleural fluid had decreased by 1.375 inches in only ten days under the influence of the modified Gerson Therapy, was it also possible that in just two weeks the Gerson Therapy had caused the disappearance of the expected spreading within the abdominal cavity?" It was a dazzling possibility.

I did not know for certain the answer to these intriguing questions. At that time we did not discuss anything about the Gerson Therapy with Dr. Allen, as per Sun Hee's request. The lymph node biopsy report later showed that two of six lymph nodes which were removed had cancer. This was another serious issue but not a surprise, given that we knew already that cancer had spread to the chest cavity. The biopsy report on the pleural fluid which was drawn on 9/28/07 was positive for cancer, as described in Chapter 1. This, combined with the biopsy report the day of the abdominal surgery, left no doubt that Sun Hee had stage IV cancer. The abdominal surgery biopsy report of 10/15/07 states in part:

"FINAL DIAGNOSIS:
1. Left ovary and tube, 582.7 gm, salpingo-oophorectomy;
Clear cell adenocarcinoma, ovary, 18.5 cm, see note.

5. Left aortic lymph nodes, biopsy:
Metastatic adenocarcinoma involving two of six lymph nodes
(2/6) with focus of adenocarcinoma involving adjacent vessel."

While we were speaking, I asked whether Dr. Allen had seen the x-ray taken on October 9th, and she said she had. She stated that the reduction of the pleural fluid, compared to the earlier x-ray on September 28th was, "Very unusual and not something I have seen before." With Dr. Allen I did not speak about the Gerson Therapy, but I believe strongly that this reduction—which happened before surgery and chemo—could only be a result of the modified Gerson Therapy program. It was a moment of inner celebration for me, as I felt this was clear evidence of the benefits of the Gerson Therapy, and clear evidence that I was encouraging Sun Hee in a good direction. I then recalled seeing a Gerson documentary movie in which a patient, with Extra-Ovarian Primary Peritoneal Carcinoma, had found her abdominal ascites decreasing significantly, after only twenty four hours on the Gerson Therapy. We were putting two and two together, and it certainly spoke strongly of the benefit of Gerson Therapy.

After this brief x-ray discussion, Dr. Allen and I both looked up at the monitor to the right of Sun Hee's bed and noticed the pulse rate had gone back up to nearly 116. Dr. Allen then said, "You better get back over there as you really have an amazing effect on your wife's pulse." Again, I went over and again placed my hands on Sun Hee's head, and held her hand. I then watched as Sun Hee's pulse came back down again, to the 88 to 92 range, during the next three minutes.

I then began to wonder whether the same effect could have been accomplished by the nurses who were attending Sun Hee. I wondered: "Has modern medicine lost the simple human touch?" I now had powerful, real-time, graphic, computer-illustrated evidence of what I always knew—that there is much healing power in basic human contact, especially in the *healing hand.*

The recovery room nurses and Dr. Allen worked very skillfully, and with great dedication, to salvage what was a difficult recovery room situation. Thankfully, they had success. Shortly after the pulse rate came down, the bleeding seemed to slow, and Sun Hee's blood pressure improved. The worst seemed to be over, though Sun Hee was still in a fragile state in the intensive care unit.

6

Five Days in the Hospital

After release from the recovery room, Sun Hee spent two days in the intensive care unit, where there was considerable staff attention to her vital signs and all of her needs. She was hooked up to a whole host of tubes, wires and monitoring devices. Sun Hee's feet, legs, thighs and abdomen were swollen. She was still experiencing shortness of breath, as she had an abdomen full of blood. This prevented the diaphragm from allowing the lungs to expand easily. Her blood pressure was low but improving. Her pulse rate was high but improving. The fluids they gave her by IV seemed to bring on much of the swelling, or maybe it was simply the trauma of the surgery. One was a saline solution, another was for nutrition. Others were for delivery of medicines. At one point the nurse added a fluid drip with potassium, when these levels were found to be low. They were all foreign substances, not the things a body normally consumes; but, one does not question much when one is in the ICU. The doctors and nurses hold the patient's life in their hands.

As a devoted spouse, I was there as constant watch to see if anything looked amiss. If a light started blinking on the monitor, I notified the nurse at the station to come and check it. Being a constant companion and support for Sun Hee was just what any ICU patient needed. Our friend Linda, who worked at the hospital, would drop by at least one or two times each day. It was very helpful to have a trusted friend to talk with, and to use as a sounding board. The Korean minister, Pastor Park, came for a visit as did our good friend Agnes and my sister Ceci.

Each morning the doctors would begin their rounds early by turning on all the lights, which roused us from our slumber. Dr. Allen came in right at 7 a.m. with one or two assistants. She removed the dressings on the incision, cleaned the area, and changed the dressing. The incision was vertical, both above and below the *belly button*, about eight inches long. In the cleaning process, she would often press slightly, to force blood collecting in the crevices of the healing wound to come out. She also examined the abdomen, in general, for swelling and fluid. As she would press on one side, the other side would swell up and push out. This showed that there was still a lot of blood inside, as a result of the recovery room bleeding crisis. Over time, we were assured, this blood would be reabsorbed by the body and all would return to normal.

Dr. Allen, a Fellow at the hospital, was the best doctor in the world as far as we were concerned. She was highly intelligent and demonstrated exceptional empathy with her patient. Her personal demeanor was one of an elevated person. She was impeccably polite. At 8 a.m. Dr. Ryan and one of his assistants would come in for a brief visit. Dr. Ryan had a sterling reputation in the field. He was very polite and soft spoken, though he usually spoke few words. He struck us as a person of great experience and sincere integrity.

We wondered if he chose not to get close to the patients and the family members in order to keep a professional distance, or perhaps to protect himself emotionally in the event the patient died. We surmised that since he had worked in the field of ovarian cancer for some time, it must be very difficult emotionally—since most of the advanced patients died, and generally sooner rather than later. Sun Hee was very fond of Dr. Ryan and had implicit trust in his ability to help her accomplish her recovery goals.

During the first few days we did not have any chance to see Arianna and Julianna, who seemed to be having fun staying with friend Mia and her family. I spoke to the girls a few times and assured them that *Umma* was doing well and not to worry. After two long days in the ICU, Sun Hee was finally taken to a regular room in the hospital. She had not eaten at all in the ICU, but soon she was able to have some clear liquids which was a relief. Her legs, thighs, and abdomen were still swollen, but her vital signs were more stable at this point in time.

Wednesday, Thursday, and Friday nights were spent in the regular room, where Sun Hee was attached to less equipment. After two days she was able to use the bathroom. I was on hand all day and night to assist Sun Hee, when called upon for help. It was very difficult and painful for Sun Hee to get out of the bed and into a standing position with the walker. After using the bathroom it was also a big deal getting her back into the bed. The nurses were experts at this and could adjust her position in the bed by moving a small sheet under her, with each nurse grabbing one side of the sheet—and giving it the heave-ho! The nurses were universally upbeat and professional. I slept in a pullout chair by the bed each night and got about four hours of sleep. Given the amount of ongoing interruptions each day and night by orderlies, nurses and doctors, it was hard for either Sun Hee or me to get proper sleep. At some point during our stay, Pastor Park came again and prayed for Sun Hee, which was much appreciated. On Friday afternoon, Anne brought Arianna and Julianna to the Hospital. They were so happy to see their *Umma*, it was a sight to see. Their energy was bouncing off the walls, and there was much chatter and excitement. Linda continued to visit each day, as did Miss Cho.

During the first day in the regular room, Sun Hee was encouraged to sit up. With help she was able to stand and move to the bathroom, then around the room. Each day was progressively better. By the end of our stay at the hospital Sun Hee was able to take walks in the hallway outside the room. This felt good as one sensed progress. We were both anxious to get home as soon as possible. Finally, on Saturday morning, we were told by Dr. Allen at the 7 a.m. visit that we could go home. Later this was delayed, as there was a last minute order to have a CT scan to check for pulmonary blood clots. Sun Hee and I were not pleased.

This test required a solemn trip into the bowels of the Hospital where all the doors seemed to be marked with poison or radiation signs. It was the least happy memory of our stay at the hospital. Forever the medical skeptic, I wondered if this CT scan was really needed, or if it was medical overkill. On reflection, I decided, the doctors were simply being cautious and being certain there was no problem. Still, I did not like seeing Sun Hee being exposed to chemical dyes and radiation. A friend had told me that one CT scan is equal to 137 x-rays.

7

First Six Weeks After Surgery

Coming home late in the day on Saturday was a real milestone. We collected our belongings as a staff member ordered a wheel chair. We said goodbye to the staff members who were there, feeling very grateful for these professional men and women—and the work they did each day. We took the elevator down to the second level, where I pushed Sun Hee in her wheel chair across the sky-bridge toward the parking garage. Next, we paid our parking fee and took the elevator to the rooftop parking level. It was mid-afternoon—but felt like morning! It was a day of great happiness as we felt that step one in the recovery process—surgery—was now complete.

My sister Kay was on hand to help with the homecoming. It was a huge relief for Sun Hee and me to be back under our own roof with our daughters. Though treated beautifully by Anne and Jean, they had still been most anxious about the possible loss of their Mother—in the event something went wrong in surgery. Arianna later told us that she had fun during the day, but cried every night before she fell asleep while Sun Hee was in the Hospital.

It felt odd but very liberating to again drive down Spruce Street, as we headed west to the Garden Court section of University City—a neighborhood that is just west of Center City Philadelphia. Arriving at home, we parked and made our way slowly up some steps and toward the entry door. Kay opened the door. There was great rejoicing with Arianna and Julianna seeming to bounce off the walls. Each step was a challenge. Going up steps was easier than going down, so Sun Hee stayed on the second floor for the next two weeks.

Once at home, we began a limited and modified Gerson Therapy. We started with three juices each day and three vegetarian meals, with no enemas since Sun Hee was so sore and healing the large incision. There was still much swelling in her feet, legs, thigh, and abdomen. We continued this pattern for the next five days. On October 25th, we returned to the Hospital to meet Dr Ryan for a post-surgery visit. Dr. Ryan said he had taken some tests of Sun Hee's blood samples and found that her blood had poor clotting ability. He asked whether Sun Hee had taken any supplements in the few weeks before surgery. Sun Hee replied accurately that she had not used any supplements.

At that meeting Dr. Ryan said the wound was healing well and that he would like to start chemotherapy in three weeks. Sun Hee said that, "We are going to another hospital to get a second opinion regarding chemotherapy." Dr. Ryan said that was fine, and printed out some of the records we asked for, so we could share them with the other oncologist. That evening Sun Hee informed me that she wanted to live 10 or 20 more years; and she wondered if we could afford all the carrots and greens needed for the next two years of Gerson Therapy. This positive projection by Sun Hee was quite a change from her attitude before surgery, when she wondered if she would live to Christmas. Two months later, on Christmas day, we took video while opening presents with Sun Hee, as we were worried it would be be our last Christmas together as a family.

CALL TO EVELYN

Around this time, I called the Gerson Institute and was given the phone number of Evelyn, whose story had been published in the Gerson Healing Newsletter. We called to England and were most impressed by what she said. She had had stage IV ovarian cancer with some tumors on the liver and some near the bowel, with her CA-125 level near 300. She had ovarian cancer surgery in January 1995 and after that the CA-125 was down to about 190. She had radiation in February. By September the cancer came back.

Her son then encouraged her to go to the Gerson Clinic in Mexico, but she was so frightened she chose chemotherapy instead, due to alternative therapies being virtually unknown at that time. At the end of six chemotherapy treatments, applied between October to April, doctors gave her a guarded prognosis—saying her cancer would come back, as the liver tumors were still there though somewhat reduced in size. After these six chemotherapy treatments her CA-125 was about 50. Normal range is 0 to 35. The doctors suggested still more chemotherapy, but Evelyn felt it was time for a new approach, and applied for permission to go to the Gerson Clinic in Mexico.

In June, Evelyn went to Mexico. By October her CA-125 was below 31, the bowel and liver tumors practically gone. Much to her credit, Evelyn stayed on the Gerson Therapy for a total of three years, to be sure her body was fully healed. Even today, over 15 years later, Evelyn quite often has pain in her feet when walking, and in bed at night, which she attributes to neuropathy caused by chemotherapy. Though she is no longer on the complete Gerson Therapy, Evelyn indicated she still takes one double-sized green juice and one double-sized carrot-apple juice every day. She eats organic and vegetarian meals. Over 15 years later, Evelyn said her scans continue to be normal.

Evelyn's story gave me great hope that Sun Hee might be able to go directly to the Gerson clinic as a first resort, reserving chemotherapy as a last resort. But Sun Hee interpreted the story of Evelyn differently. She reasoned that since Evelyn had done chemotherapy, and then Gerson Therapy, to defeat a stage IV ovarian cancer diagnosis, that this was to be her approach as well. Evelyn's story solidified Sun Hee's desire to do chemotherapy and then Gerson therapy, in an integrative approach.

Luckily, Evelyn and my wife were able to learn about and embrace the Gerson Therapy, for use in a complementary way with conventional medicine, before it was too late. So many millions of others have gone to their graves, never even being aware that dietary programs such as Gerson Therapy may have helped to save their lives. Gerson family members believe—and there is evidence to support it—that the Gerson Therapy has been actively suppressed for the past sixty years, in an attempt to discourage patients from trying this natural and beneficial dietary and detoxification therapy. This seems to me to be classic "silo thinking"—the belief that the only legitimate approach is one a certain group owns, practices or is knowledgeable about. The medical profession has been stuck in the "chemo silo" for some time—since 1942 to be quite precise.

THE VERY FIRST CHEMO PATIENT IN 1942

The very first chemo patient in the world was Mr. J.D. at Yale University in 1942. He was in the terminal stages of lymphosarcoma. He was given a chemotherapy called nitrogen mustard, which had been derived from a lethal gas used in the trenches of World War I. Within a few days, his tumors began to get softer and over a few months disappeared. Shortly thereafter, he died. This one failed case inspired and led to the multi-billion dollar chemotherapy industry. Though the patient died, the research scientists then believed they had proof that cancer could be treated with chemicals, according to David S. Fischer, M.D., clinical professor of medicine. (*Yale Medicine 2005* article by John Curtis) Such reasoning, based on a failed case, seems a real stretch to me.

In 1952, another patient was in the terminal stages of lymphosarcoma. He was Mr. W. S. who is Case #18 in Dr. Gerson's book: *A Cancer Therapy—Results of Fifty Cases*. On the Gerson Therapy he made a full recovery and lived 57 more years until the summer of 2009, when he died one month before age 90. That patient's case (like vitually all of the Gerson cases) has been largely ignored by the medical profession. Mr. W.S. was my uncle Bill (William Schickel). A few years before he died, Bill wrote about his own case in an eloquent and moving article in the Gerson Healing Newsletter; and he appeared in the excellent Stephen Kroschel documentary film, *Dying to Have Known,* in 2006.

It is ironic and perhaps telling that the very first chemotherapy case, Mr. J.D., (a failed case) was the foundation upon which was built such an enormous and controversial industry. It is also ironic that *the case that the establishment rejected may become the cornerstone* of a new day of cancer treatment, in the holistic and integrative era to come. This new era is being built without any substantial funding, by patients and their families who have seen and witnessed cancer being healed with their own eyes. Case by case, the evidence is emerging that cancer can be healed by addressing the problem in an integrative way— combining conventional medical diagnosis and critically needed medical intervention, together with holistic nutrition, detoxification and a positive mental framework.

These cases (such as my uncle's, Sun Hee's and Evelyn's) are coming out to the public without any significant backing by the medical establishment, or even by the media establishment. Today, in our new internet era, successful ideas and therapies cannot be so easily suppressed or swept under the rug. This is why there is now more interest than ever in approaches like the Gerson Therapy, macrobiotic diet, and other healthy and holistic modalities.

It is worth noting that antibiotics also came on the scene around 1942. It was an era of great belief that the cure for any disease would be a pharmaceutical *magic bullet* of some kind, prescribed by a medical doctor and backed up by scientific studies. The notion of prevention was little discussed in 1942. The notion of healing serious disease by holistic and dietary therapy was considered quackery.

Please note that a positive mental framework does enhance the immune system, but this is only one of the benefits. The greatest benefit is that it allows a sick person to believe they can get well; and this allows them to embrace the day by day tasks which are required for an approach such as the Gerson Therapy. The patient, who simply does not believe that Gerson Therapy will make any difference, will never be able to muster the energy to follow the demanding Gerson program. And if such a patient does not follow the program, the beneficial biochemical changes will not occur in the body.

Simple changes are profound. For example, a Gerson patient tends to become much more alkaline due to consumption of the vegetable juices. Cancer then begins to recede rather quickly, in many cases. One lady I know, Lillian by name, found that her breast tumor changed from hard to soft in six days on a Gerson juicing program. If that had happened with a chemotherapy agent, it would have stimulated millions in research. With carrot and green juice as the active agents, seemingly little or no interest is shown by medical researchers, as there are no apparent backers available to finance such research.

8

Meeting with Macrobiotic Counselor

About one month after surgery, Dr. Ryan was pushing for chemotherapy to begin. I was very concerned whether it was the best next step, so I arranged to get a second opinion at a suburban hospital where the oncologist recommendation was the same—to have chemotherapy with carboplatin and taxol. This was considered the gold standard of conventional ovarian cancer follow-up after surgery.

We now had two opinions from the conventional side; we then proceeded to get two from the alternative side. First, I arranged a consultation with Denny Waxman, a well known macrobiotic counselor in Philadelphia. We had first learned about Denny from reading Dr. Satillaro's book, *Recalled by Life*, as mentioned earlier. Denny had studied with Michio Kushi starting back in the late 1960s. He had a reputation as someone who had helped achieve miraculous results with some patients, guiding them in their use of organic macrobiotic diet, by the careful application of the yin and yang balancing principle—focusing on foods considered more balanced such as grains and vegetables, and avoiding more yang foods such as meat, as well as more yin foods such as sugar.

We visited with Denny at his home in the Queen Village area of Philadelphia. When we arrived his assistant had Sun Hee fill out some forms. Denny then came into the room and greeted us very warmly. I had known Denny for many years so it was great to see him. He talked with Sun Hee and asked a lot of questions. He then asked Sun Hee to remove her shoes and socks. Next he did his physical examination which consisted of looking at Sun Hee's arms and hands, face and eyes, feet, and the lower portion of her legs. Denny examined them visually at first looking for colorations that may indicate cancer present in the body, and then held his hand over certain areas to examine *chi (energy) flow* via the energy meridians. When he had finished, he asked Sun Hee to put on her socks and shoes, and then we all sat down again at the conference table.

Denny said that by his analysis, the cancer at this point was very inactive. It appeared that the modified Gerson diet was being very helpful. He did not have any objection to Sun Hee continuing the Gerson diet, or beginning the macrobiotic diet. Denny preferred the macrobiotic diet, but respected Gerson Therapy, which he considered more on the *yin* side of the spectrum with its extensive use of raw vegetable/fruit juices. He pointed out that the one common thing, among all of the better known healing diets, is that they are typically *plant-based* diets emphasizing organically grown food.

Denny felt that Sun Hee should either choose the Gerson diet or the macrobiotic diet and not try to mix the two together—as they each had their own constellation of elements which may not work together if they were mixed. Charlotte Gerson had made a similar recommendation— that we follow the Gerson Therapy strictly without mixing in other items from the macrobiotic diet. Denny then proceeded to go through twenty or more pages of detailed macrobiotic recommendations for diet and lifestyle, marking each page to adjust for the particular things he felt Sun Hee needed.

Lastly, Sun Hee asked Denny about whether chemotherapy was a good idea. Denny said that in some cases chemotherapy could knock the cancer back and give the patient more time to live—and thus more time in which to implement health improving changes such as the macrobiotic diet. But chemotherapy was also damaging to the entire body as well, especially the bone marrow. Only Sun Hee would be able to know what was the right thing to do.

CALL TO SAMANTHA

We asked Denny if he knew of any ovarian cancer patients who had done well using the macrobiotic diet. Unlike the conventional doctors who had not given us any names of patients, Denny reached for his cell phone and searched for fifteen seconds, coming up with the name of Samantha (not her real name). We later called Samantha and found that she had originally had stage II ovarian cancer and had a CA-125 around 400. This dropped to less than 15 after surgery and three chemotherapy infusions. After three treatments her doctor said it was best to stop, "So we do not weaken you too much."

Samantha then applied the macrobiotic diet. She was advised by Michio Kushi that during the first year on the diet, after chemotherapy, there would be a point where the CA-125 would go up out of the normal range and then back down. Samantha saw that this happened exactly as Michio predicted. Samantha is now out 16 or more years from diagnosis, still in remission, and still on the macrobiotic diet. The visit with Denny was uplifting and hopeful. We did not know it yet, but Sun Hee was to have a similar healing reaction, wherein her CA-125 would spike up and then come back down. This happened six months after her trip to the Gerson Clinic in Mexico as will be described later.

9

Integrative Medicine Department at Jefferson

On November 11, 2007 we had a meeting with Dr. Anthony J. Bazzan, M.D., at the Jefferson Myrna-Brind Center for Integrative Medicine in Philadelphia. He had with him one of his students from Thomas Jefferson University. Dr. Bazzan was very personable and very open to hearing about what we had been doing, both conventionally and with alternative diets. He seemed to be positive about most aspects of macrobiotic diet and Gerson Therapy. However, he was concerned about so much carrot juice with the Gerson program, as he felt it had excessive natural sugars, which might cause cancer growth. I had discussed this same issue with Charlotte Gerson by phone on one occasion. She dismissed this concern as a non-issue, as regards using carrot juice in the context of the *complete* Gerson Therapy.

Dr. Bazzan was optimistic and hopeful for Sun Hee's recovery. He listened to her breathing from the back side with a stethoscope. He showed me how to listen comparatively, first to the normal left side, and then the right. On the left, I listened near the top and could hear normal breathing. Moving down to a middle position, and then a lower position, the breathing continued to be normal. Then Dr. Bazzan guided me to listen to the right side of the body, again from the back. At the top position the breathing sounded normal. In the middle position one could hear breathing, but it was not entirely normal—this was the partially collapsed lobe. In the lower position one could not hear any breathing at all—this was the almost completely collapsed right lower lobe.

Dr. Bazzan explained that in this way one can monitor the pleural effusion inexpensively without the constant need for x-rays and CT scans, though at certain intervals these tests would still be recommended. I later got a stethoscope for use at home and would, every two weeks or so, listen to Sun Hee's breathing. Over a period of several months, I was able to hear continuous improvement. After several months of improvement, I heard a rather strange ticking sound, which went away after a few weeks. We surmised that it might possibly be the sound of the lung re-expanding and returning to normal.

At the end of our meeting, Dr. Bazzan recommended blood tests for Sun Hee, and indicated that after their review he would develop a proposed integrative program. It would likely include intravenous Vitamin C which they have found to be very helpful as either a complement to, or in some cases an alternative to, conventional chemotherapy. We did the battery of blood tests a day later along with a CA-125 test, which we had requested.

In the end, we did not choose the intravenous Vitamin C therapy. We felt that the Gerson Therapy—which included abundant levels of vitamin C and virtually all other vitamins, naturally found in carrot juice and green juice—was the way for Sun Hee to move forward. However, we appreciated and respected Dr. Bazzan's integrative approach that he and his colleagues have implemented for many patients. Integrative medicine, if it were to more fully embrace alternative therapies like the macrobiotic diet and Gerson Therapy, will in my opinion, have greater success and broader acceptance.

OUR OWN INTEGRATIVE PROGRAM

It is ironic that though we did not use the medicine (intravenous vitamin C) offered by the Department of Integrative Medicine at Jefferson, our overall approach was an integrative one, as we combined conventional cancer care (surgery and some chemotherapy) with Gerson and macrobiotic dietary programs. In essence, we invented our own integrative program—a program that made sense to us, and that in the end appears to have succeeded very well.

Sun Hee did not ever consider relying solely on conventional cancer care, as the statistics seemed to indicate that the result would almost certainly be death. Sun Hee was uncomfortable to go *only alternative* as some have done, since her case was advanced at stage IV. She was, therefore, determined to avail herself of the benefits of modern medicine also. She never doubted whether surgery and chemotherapy were the necessary first steps. And, as described in Chapter 4, Sun Hee already had used a modified Gerson Therapy in the first two weeks before surgery—and had seen amazing benefits. Thus, her own integrative program was taking shape.

As a result of assisting Sun Hee with her own integrative approach, I have have had the opportunity to reflect on what are the *essential elements* of such an integrative approach. The *Integrative Healing Paradigm* description and diagram, in Appendix IV at the end of this book, summarizes my thinking on this important subject. The recipes Sun Hee used in her recovery process are described in Appendix V which is entitled: *Paxdieta Healing Recipes.*

10

CA-125 Saga Begins

CA-125 means Cancer Antigen 125, with a normal range of 0 to 35. This is a blood test that is an ovarian cancer tumor marker. Sun Hee's original CA-125 test on September 26, 2007 was 3,745. Her November 12, 2007 CA-125 test at Jefferson came back at a value of 366, which was down from the pre-surgery value of 3,824 taken on October 9th. This was a 90.5 percent decrease. It was definitely due to the surgery, and perhaps secondarily due to the modified Gerson Therapy program Sun Hee had been following for the previous six weeks. Such a dramatic decrease shows the benefit of surgery.

In any event, the big 90.5 percent drop a month after surgery was great news. As any ovarian cancer patient knows, CA-125 tests *bring both hope and despair*. Though not a perfect indicator of the presence of cancer, the CA-125 test is, nonetheless, a general indicator of the amount of cancer present. It is also used to monitor the effectiveness of chemotherapy, or other therapies, after surgery. Sun Hee and

I followed these CA-125 tests with great interest and pride as they continued to drop.

On November 26th, 2007 Sun Hee had another CA-125 test at the Hospital. Thus, exactly two weeks had elapsed since the Jefferson test on November 12th. This new CA-125 test came in at 321, or a 12.5 percent drop from the 366 test result just two weeks earlier. Was this drop a continuing result of the surgery that had happened 40 days earlier—or was it the result of the modified and partial Gerson Therapy Sun Hee had been following carefully since the October 15th surgery?

I tended to give credit to the Gerson Therapy, since that was the only thing that we had followed in the last two weeks. In that time there had been neither surgery nor chemotherapy, so it seemed likely that the Gerson Therapy was being effective. This was a very critical question because I had hoped Sun Hee could defeat her cancer with Gerson Therapy, and not have to suffer the well known side effects of chemotherapy. To get an informal second opinion at this point, I talked with an oncologist friend from Kentucky who is very respected in his field. The question I posed to him was whether there was an immediate urgency to begin chemotherapy—or whether it would be okay to delay it for a few weeks, with testing for CA-125 again at that point, hoping for a drop in levels. The doctor responded by saying that either going ahead with chemotherapy or delaying by two weeks would be fine.

His reasoning was that if chemotheray ultimately proved to be effective, it was just as likely to work two weeks later. And there was no rush to get the chemotherapy started in order to prevent metastasis, as metastasis had already occurred. My doctor friend reasoned that, "The horse has already left the barn." The cancer was already in both the lymph nodes and in the pleural cavity, thus fully metastasized and stage IV.

Since the CA-125 levels had dropped 12.5 percent in two weeks, it was entirely plausible they would continue to drop under the Gerson diet program. He said it was also possible that the 12.5 percent drop was not significant because CA-125 values can often move up and down within a range. Thus, a 12.5 percent drop, by itself, indicates nothing definitive. What one is looking for, he explained, is for a continuing pattern that is downward. That would show that the therapy, whether conventional or alternative, is in fact working.

At this point I strongly urged Sun Hee to delay chemotherapy, while continuing the Gerson diet with a new test of the CA-125 in two weeks. My feeling was that if the CA-125 continued to drop, it was a sign that the immune system had kicked in and was now killing the remaining cancer cells naturally. That was the ultimate goal—to be able to fully recover without the devastating effects of chemotherapy. Ultimately and obviously however, it was Sun Hee's life and her decision to make. I had no choice but to accept her decision and give her support. Eventually I made a last ditch effort, and begged for even one more week after which the CA-125 test could again be taken. It was not to be. Sun Hee's mind was made up.

What follows on the next page is a summary of all blood test results to date, including the CA-125 ovarian cancer tumor marker.

Summary of Blood Test Results for Sun Hee Lee

Blood Test	CA-125	WBC	RBC	Platelets	Hemoglobin	ANC
Range	(0-35)	(4-11)	(3.8-5.3)	(150-400)	(12-16)	(1.8-7.5)
9/24/07	**3745**	8	3.94	353	12.2	6.1
10/9/07	**3824**	9.6	3.82	396	12.2	
10/15/07				-----Surgery at Hospital		
11/12/07	**366**			---CA-125 Test at Jefferson		
11/26/07	**321**	7.9	3.61	297	12.1	5.9
11/29/07				1st Chemo Treatment: Carboplatin and Taxol		
12/10/07		2.9	3.24	202	11	1.1
12/24/07	**186**	7.4	3.63	252	12.3	5.5
12/27/07				2nd Chemo: Carboplatin and Taxol, (Neulasta)		
1/7/08		22.8	3.11	138	10.6	20.7
1/14/08	**135**	10.1	3.13	252	10.6	8.3
1/17/08				3rd Chemo Treatment: Carboplatin and Taxol		
1/28/08		2.6	2.45	185	8.5	1.1
2/4/08	**70**	2.3	2.57	87	9	0.6
2/12/08	**63**	3.8	2.64	129	9.6	2.5
2/14/08				4th Chemo Treatment: Carboplatin and Taxol		
2/25/08		1.8	2.34	162	8.8	
3/3/08	**44**	2.2	2.23	108	8.7	0.9
3/10/08	**44**	2.8	2.41	120	9.1	1.5
3/13/08				5th Chemo: Carboplatin and Taxol, (Neulasta)		
3/24/08		15.6	2.38	121	9.1	13.1
3/31/08	**41**	5.7	2.23	112	8.5	3.9
4/3/08				6th Chemo: Carboplatin and Taxol, (Aranesp & Neulasta)		
4/14/08		12	2.51	93	9.5	10.2
4/21/08	**37**	5.5	2.74	91	10.6	3.9
4/28/08	**32**	3.9	2.64	94	10.2	2.5
5/5/08	**26**	3	2.84	127	10.8	1.7
5/8/08				7th Chemo: Carboplatin and Taxol, (Neulasta)		
5/19/08		9.8	2.52	69	9.9	7.9
6/2/08	**30**	3.7	2.47	185	9.6	2
6/5/08				8th Chemo: Carboplatin and Taxol, (Neulasta)		
6/16/08		12.9	2.23	110	8.7	10.8

Blood Test	CA-125	WBC	RBC	Platelets	Hemoglobin	ANC
6/23/08	**24**	5.7	2.3	85	8.8	4
6/30/08	**30**	3.1	2.26	110	8.9	
7/7/08 Gerson Mexico Clinic		4.2	2.59	113	10.1	
7/14/08 Gerson Mexico Clinic	3		2.65	127	10.2	
8/20/08	**24.9**	3.1	2.88	172	10.9	1.6
9/24/08	**21.7**	3.4	2.99	179	11.1	1.9
10/22/08	**17.6**	3.5	2.88	192	10.7	2.2
12/22/08	**35.2=HR**	2.9	3.16	179	11.5	1.5
1/27/09	**51.5=HR**	3.5	3.15	214	11.4	2.1
3/26/09	**27.3**	3.7	3.09	194	11.1	2.2
6/11/09	**26.8**	3.7	3.31	221	11.9	2.1

HR = Healing Reaction (see chapters 18 and 19 for discussion)

No blood testing was done after the 6/11/2009 test, due to financial constraints and a finding that *not testing* brought Sun Hee *greater peace of mind*. While the scientist in me regrets this, the last year and a half of *going on faith* has been much more peaceful for Sun Hee.

11

Chemotherapy Starts—Tense Words with Dr. Chetry

Sun Hee chose to begin chemotherapy on November 29th, 2007. We drove to the Hospital and parked in the hospital garage. It was early morning and the sun was shining. As we walked across the sky-bridge, I noted that Sun Hee looked good, she seemed so strong now. It had been six weeks since her surgery. Her body had demonstrated amazing healing power. She had healed her abdominal incision in miraculous fashion. Her energy was now vibrant. I only wanted one more week, to see if Sun Hee's own healing power would continue to eat up and destroy the cancer, as it appeared to be doing under her partial Gerson Therapy.

If she chose this way and it worked, Sun Hee would not have to take damaging chemotherapy, which we knew would kill cancer cells, but would also devastate her bone marrow and its ability to produce new blood cells. Her doctors, of course, never mentioned bone marrow damage to Sun Hee in conversation, but I'm sure it was on the paperwork she ultimately had to sign before taking chemotherapy. Sun Hee was walking fast across the sky-bridge because she did not want to be late for her pre-chemo appointment with Dr. Ryan.

At 8 a.m. we arrived for her pre-chemo physical exam, not with Dr. Ryan, but his associate Dr. Chetry. During this visit, I explained about the vegetarian diet and detoxification program Sun Hee had been doing the last two months, and that we had tested the CA-125 at Jefferson, when we went for a second opinion. The result had come in at 366 at Jefferson. *"What was the recent CA-125 test here?"* Sun Hee asked Dr. Chetry. The doctor looked in the patient book and indicated it was 321. I spoke up noting that a drop from the earlier test of 366, to the current test of 321, was about a 12% drop in two weeks. I asked Dr. Chetry: *"Would it not make sense to delay the chemo for two weeks, and test again, to see if the CA-125 could reduce naturally—as it has come down 12% in two weeks, under the diet and detoxification therapy Sun Hee has been following?"*

Dr. Chetry responded curtly by stating, *"There is no medical evidence that carrot juice and coffee enemas can cure cancer."* She then turned to Sun Hee and said: *"You don't have to have chemo if you don't want to, but you don't want the tumor to regrow do you?"* This statement expressed Dr. Chetry's conviction that chemotherapy was the only logical next step, and to avoid it was to guarantee the tumor would re-grow. To me, it felt like a bold attempt to scare Sun Hee into taking the chemotherapy with fear and intimidation tactics. Sun Hee was convinced by Dr. Chetry's statement, and it kept her in line and on the chemo track. I had failed to gain for Sun Hee even a one week reprieve. We had no doubt that Dr. Chetry genuinely believed in the chemotherapy approach, and that she was sincerely doing what she felt was best for her patient.

Next I asked Dr. Chetry: *"If the CA-125 is coming down as shown by the recent tests, could the cancer be regrowing at the same time?"* I had asked my oncologist friend from Kentucky this same question the night before, and had received the reply that: *"It would be very weird for the CA-125 to be dropping while the cancer is regrowing. I have never seen that."* Dr. Chetry seemed genuinely flummoxed by my question and hesitated in answering for a few seconds; then she stammered something to the effect that: *"Well, it could happen in some cases."* Dr. Chetry was very clearly irritated by what she no doubt viewed as a challenge to her authority. She then left the room abruptly and closed the door rather strongly, perhaps as a way to express her frustration at my questions. Sun Hee was caught in the middle between a zealous husband and a zealous doctor.

I was greatly disappointed that Dr. Chetry left so quickly because I had one last question, which was: *"Can you show us the medical evidence that chemo can cure stage IV ovarian cancer?"* It was an important question and I felt that I already knew the answer—that there was, in fact, no medical evidence that chemo can cure stage IV ovarian cancer—it can only delay death by some weeks, months, or years. It does not truly cure the cancer condition or its fundamental root cause.

Dr. Ryan had already told us that chemotherapy could in many cases knock the cancer into remission—but that it usually comes back in about 90% of cases within a year. Hence no cure. When it comes back, as it always seems to, more chemotherapy is generally administered which usually works less well than the first series. This process can then continue a third time with perhaps another type of chemotherapy, and again and again...until death. This is why an ovarian cancer diagnosis is so devastating. I was determined to find a different result for Sun

Hee, and had hoped for her to avoid chemotherapy altogether, as the seven ladies in the Gerson booklet had done. It was not my decision, however, and Sun Hee was charting her own course. It was her life at stake and she obviously had to make her own decisions in the matter.

Five minutes later one of the assistants asked us to come into a small office where they asked Sun Hee to sign several sheets of paper declaring that the chosen chemotherapy could cause all sorts of horrible side effects, including hair loss, bleeding, neuropathy, and many other things, and even death—and that, in effect, if any of these things happened the hospitals and doctors were not responsible. Sun Hee dutifully signed the papers and we proceeded to the chemo room on the Hospital's upper floor.

During Sun Hee's first chemotherapy treatment, I found myself in a state of great conflict and anxiety. Chemotherapy went contrary to all of my beliefs in more natural ways to recover health. It was therefore, very hard to watch my wife being *partially poisoned*, as I viewed it. Obviously Sun Hee felt much differently and, like the ideal patient she was, trusted implicitly that the doctor would not be giving this treatment if it was not the best way.

Sun Hee said that I was so unhelpful during the first chemotherapy session, that we mutually agreed that I would not be present for the chemotherapy sessions after that. For the next seven treatments, I would drop off Sun Hee in the morning, then go home and prepare some healthy food and drink for her. I would deliver the food around noon and then return to pick her up around 3 p.m.

The chemotherapy was carboplatin and taxol. One was adminstered and then the other. The whole process took about four hours, as the medicine was dripped into her veins. In some cases, the following day, Sun Hee would return for an injection to boost her white blood count. It was called Neulasta and is noted on the Summary of Blood Test Results chart in Chapter 10.

Sun Hee did not lose her hair on schedule as the nurses had predicted. She eventually lost it, but the loss was very gradual and much later than had been indicated. Perhaps this was due to her innate strength, or due to the high quality food and drink with which we were fortifying her system. Unlike some patients who embrace the process by cutting off all their hair, Sun Hee hung onto her hair as long as possible, and wore a hat starting after the fourth chemotherapy session.

12

Chemotherapy & Macrobiotic Diet

During the chemotherapy period, from November 29th, 2007, through July 6th, 2008, Sun Hee used a combination of macrobiotic diet and a limited juicing program inspired by the Gerson approach. She used no coffee enemas and no supplements. Sun Hee consumed three vegetable juices per day and had three hearty vegetarian meals, inspired by both the macrobiotic and Gerson traditions.

Sun Hee, therefore, did not follow the basic Gerson Therapy during this seven month period. Gerson Therapy is very specific and definitely does not include miso soup, fish, and daily use of brown rice—which are all elements we used from macrobiotic tradition. The vegetable dishes that Sun Hee used however, would have easily fit within either the macrobiotic or the Gerson guidelines—as they were generally steamed and cooked without salt and oil.

Sun Hee's modified macrobiotic program (during chemotherapy) is shown below:

JUICES

One green juice, one carrot juice and one carrot-apple juice (2/3 carrot, 1/3 apple) each day—taken mid-morning, mid-afternoon and in the evening. Each juice was about 8 ounces in size. We used only organic ingredients.

BREAKFAST

Oatmeal and fruit such as a pear or apple for breakfast, with Kukicha tea. Some days we had oatmeal and miso soup for breakfast.

LUNCH

Brown rice, raw green salad, two cooked vegetables, potato or yam, Hippocrates special soup 3x per week and miso soup 3 times per week. Kukicha tea after each meal.

DINNER

Brown rice, salad with many ingredients, two cooked vegetables, potato or yam, Hippocrates' special soup 3 times per week and miso soup 3 times per week. White meat fish or salmon, or bean dish or tofu—about 2 times per week total. Kukicha tea after each meal.

OTHER SOUPS

Sun Hee also occasionally used some Korean dishes such as Pine Nut Soup or Wakame seaweed soup.

BREAD

Sun Hee also had a small amount (one or two slices per day), of high quality organic multi-grain bread, or 100 percent rye bread, usually toasted and plain.

SNACKS

Sun Hee ate modest amounts of many common types of fruit such as: grape, apple, pear, orange, kiwi, cherry, plum, cantaloupe, honeydew, papaya and mango. Also included were certain typical Korean fruits such as Asian pear and persimmon, as well as pomegranate (originally from Iran). Generally, Sun Hee ate fruit between meals as a snack, or after meals as dessert.

DRESSING

Sun Hee used olive oil and vinegar on salads (apple cider vinegar, brown rice vinegar or balsamic vinegar).

OIL and SALT

No oil was used in cooking. No salt was used except what was in the miso soup.

ORGANIC

Sun Hee generally only used organic foods—which are grown without chemical fertilizers and pesticides.

FORBIDDEN FOODS

Canned food, processed food, meat, seafood, eggs, cheese, butter, milk, soy milk, chips, commercial breads, pastries, pasta, ice cream, candy, coffee, alcohol, soft drinks, salt, MSG, sugar, jam, nuts and nut butters.

VEGETABLES

Used regularly—asparagus, broccoli, beets and beet tops, brussel sprouts, bok choy, carrot, cauliflower, chard, cabbage (red and white), daikon, kale, lettuce (romaine and red leaf), onion, parsnip, potato, pepper (green and red), spinach, scallion, squash (many types), tomato, watercress and yam.

GREEN JUICE

Sun Hee made her green juice from romaine and red leaf lettuce, chard, watercress, beet tops, green pepper, green apple and red cabbage.

PORRIDGE

A favorite dish made from left over brown rice involves adding a certain amount of spring water to a pot 1/3 full of the brown rice. Bring it to a boil and add in succession: chopped onion, carrot, cabbage, bok choy, broccoli, and cauliflower—cooking at a modest boil for 10 to 15 minutes. Then simmer on low for 20 to 40 minutes. At the end add miso—by first dissolving the miso paste into some of the liquid in a separate bowl, and then by adding it back to the pot—simmering on low for five minutes, stirring gently. One needs to experiment with the right amount of water as well as the right amount of miso. In fact, each time we make this dish it is different. If we use less rice and too much water it can be more like soup. If we use more rice and less water, it comes out more like porridge. It is a very hearty dish that is especially good in fall, winter and spring. If it tastes salty, then too much miso was used.

ENEMAS

None were used during the chemotherapy period. In Charlotte Gerson's book, *Healing the Gerson Way*, I recall she suggested one coffee enema daily during the chemotherapy period, along with three juices per day, for someone on a partial and limited Gerson Therapy. Sun Hee asked Dr. Ryan about coffee enemas during the chemotherapy period. He suggested it was not a good idea, though he did not say why he felt this way, and I sensed he probably was unfamiliar with coffee enemas.

Therefore for the entire chemotherapy period, Sun Hee did not use any coffee enemas. Whether this was the right way to go, we will never know. We do know that at the end of the chemotherapy period, Sun Hee became rather yellow. It is very likely she would have benefitted from the detoxification provided by the coffee enemas. Sun Hee chose not to use the full Gerson Therapy during the chemotherapy period, in large part because Charlotte Gerson does not recommend it. We agreed and felt it would be impossible to implement when one is severely weakened with cytotoxic chemotherapy and other drugs. It is hard to do nine hours of work each day when laid up in bed.

Due to the damaging effect of chemotherapy, Sun Hee felt a need for some fish, beans and tofu as well as miso soup. These foods are not on the Gerson Therapy, but are on a typical macrobiotic diet. Sun Hee also wanted regular use of brown rice which is used in the Gerson Therapy only once per week.

TRAUMA FROM CHEMOTHERAPY

During the seven month chemotherapy period, Sun Hee suffered many side effects such as exhaustion, hair loss, tingling in her hands and feet, leg heaviness between ankle and knee, occasional black and blue spots on the legs, chest pains, nausea, and general heaviness in the chest region. After taking chemotherapy, which consisted of Carboplatin and Taxol, Sun Hee was usually okay for a day and a half. Then she would suddenly feel very weak and need to stay in bed for about a full week. She would literally beg me to bring her the Gerson juices and macrobiotic food, as they were always helpful in reviving her energy.

Each chemotherapy treatment was devastating physically and emotionally. When we dropped off Sun Hee near the hospital, on the way to our children's school, she would stand on the sidewalk waving and crying. Getting chemotherapy was obviously very devastating for her. Julianna our youngest, who is usually very strong emotionally, would often cry as well when we drove away after dropping off Sun Hee. Intuitively Julianna knew this was *a serious and dangerous business*, so to speak. As the chemotherapy period continued, we carefully monitored the CA-125 level each time and saw steady progress. But we also saw rather devastating effects on the red and white blood cell counts which dropped dramatically. See the blood test summary chart in Chapter 10 for a summary of all blood tests to date. After six treatments, Sun Hee felt she had had enough chemotherapy.

Therefore, Sun Hee began a process of delay in late April 2008, hoping to avoid treatment number 7. After a few weeks of delay, she got a call from Dr. Ryan's office. The assistant spent ten minutes on the phone, putting on considerable pressure, but Sun Hee held her ground, and refused to have any more chemotherapy. A half hour later, one of the doctors called, and spent another ten minutes exerting even more pressure by saying, "It is a very aggresive cancer and it will come back unless you take the final two chemotherapy treatments." Then she acknowledged that it would recur in any case, but that Sun Hee would have a longer remission if she had the treatments.

After getting these two phone calls in quick succession, Sun Hee went from being happy and optimistic to being severely depressed and withdrawn. She looked shell-shocked, just like she had looked when she was first diagnosed. After these calls Sun Hee's will to resist more chemotherapy (which she had been firmly committed to) dissolved, and fear took over. We discussed it and Sun Hee knew of my strong objection to any more chemotherapy. At that point, I took a long walk for over an hour as I wanted Sun Hee to be able to make her decision in peace, without pressure from her husband. After all, it was her life. I knew the only good decision would be the one that Sun Hee made. When I got back home I found that Sun Hee had capitulated, and called back, agreeing to the doctor's demand. I was not happy with the pressure the doctors were putting on Sun Hee. It is one thing to make a clear and professional recommendation, it is another to exert undue pressure. As much as I disagreed with the *chemo, chemo and more chemo approach*, I do not doubt that Sun Hee's doctors were sincere in their belief that more chemotherapy was the very best thing to be done. However, I strongly disagreed with their approach, which seems to lead to such generally poor overall results.

The last two chemotherapy treatments seemed to make Sun Hee very weak. When I saw her lying in bed, the life force seemed drained from her face. She had the look to me, in those times, of approaching death. When Sun Hee was finally done with treatment number eight on June 5th, 2008, she had blood work done on June 11th. One of the doctors congratulated Sun Hee on finally completing chemotherapy. It was a good feeling for Sun Hee to be finally done with the chemotherapy ordeal.

On June 16th, Sun Hee had an appointment with Dr. Ryan. In this appointment Dr. Ryan indicated he wanted Sun Hee to have 12 additional chemotherapy treatments which he called *maintenance chemotherapy*. Sun Hee asked if they were really necessary. Dr. Ryan responded that Sun Hee had a very aggressive type of stage IV ovarian cancer and that they were needed to keep the cancer from regrowing. He did acknowledge though, as he had always said before, that eventually the cancer would come back, even if more chemo was used. Sun Hee asked what would come after the maintenance chemotherapy. He then indicated that they would keep giving chemotherapy until the body could no longer take it. Sun Hee was in a state of shock at his proposal and said she would think about it.

After the meeting with Dr. Ryan, Sun Hee remembered she wanted to get a chest x-ray. She spoke to a nurse and requested a chest x-ray indicating she had felt some sensations in the chest region and was worried. In addition she wanted the chest x-ray plates for our trip to the Gerson Clinic. The staff at Dr. Ryan's office did not seem inclined to give her the x-ray and Sun Hee kept waiting for it. After a 45 minute wait, they arranged for the x-ray, which was accomplished in another part of the building. Sun Hee waited and got the film sheet of the completed x-ray as she had done with the previous three x-rays. All four x-rays are included in Chapter 4 where you can see Sun Hee's progress.

It is interesting to note that after getting the June 16, 2008 x-ray, Sun Hee found that her doctors did not push for maintenance chemotherapy anymore. They left her alone for the next six months. I wondered then, and still do today, whether they left her alone because they had seen the dazzling x-rays of June 16, 2008, which seemed to my eye to show no pleural effusions at all. Perhaps they realized that with a very clean report on the pleural effusion, and the chest region in general, there was no more justification for maintenance chemotherapy.

At that point, in early July 2008, Sun Hee and I were busy with preparation for going to the Gerson Clinic in Mexico. It was strange indeed, that although the x-ray report from June 16th, 2008 turned out to be a very good and clean report, her doctor never sent her the written report. In fact, she never received a copy of it from her doctor, until nearly eight months later, when she requested it in person, and received it from Dr. Ryan in an office visit on February 3, 2009. A man of few words, he said as he handed it to Sun Hee, "It's clear."

13

Healing Benefit Concert

In late April 2008, I answered a call from Okkwon, a long-time family friend. Okkwon was asking about how things were going with Sun Hee's health. I indicated that Sun Hee wanted to go to the Gerson Clinic in July, but that it may be impossible due to the high cost. Okkwon said, "Why don't we organize a fundraiser?" The discussion then turned to various options. We finally settled on the idea of a Healing Benefit Concert. Next, I discussed it with Sun Hee. She was very unhappy and upset. She felt it was an imposition on others and would not have any part of it. A few days later Okkwon called Sun Hee and they discussed it. Finally, Sun Hee showed some signs of receptivity. It would be held in a very beautiful place—Trinity Church. Our children's piano teacher was the Music Director there. He made all the arrangements with the Church. We would have a group of wonderful classical musicians. It would be a beautiful event.

Okkwon then invited a group of Korean friends, including well known singer Sung-Ji Kim, for a planning party at our home. One person said it was a great idea. Another said only 10 or 15 people will come out for a classical concert. Okkwon kept focused and said: "Lets set a date and draw up the letter of invitation." Okkwon later made her first draft of the invitation letter, which looked very good, and with a few adjustments, it was ready to go out to family, friends, and church members.

Sung-Ji Kim, a vocal graduate of the Curtis Institute of Music, would be the principal performer. Our daughter Arianna would play violin. Korean Church member Catherine Pyun would play oboe. Other friends from near and far would sing or play other stringed instruments. It was coming together. One day Arianna took the invitation to her school to explain why she must miss another school event happening at the same time. Kathy, an administrator, spoke to me the next day. She said that she and the head of the school had seen the invitation. They wanted to send it home in the Wednesday note, so each family in the school would receive one. I was very surprised and touched by this gesture of solidarity. The concert was coming together. Energy was building. The concern people had for Sun Hee was real and they wanted to help. The concert was the way. It was the equivalent of an Amish barn raising. In this case Sun Hee's very life was being "raised" to a new level of hope and expectation. The communal voice was speaking, that Sun Hee was important; that this family was important.

Several members of Sun Hee's Korean Church were anxious to build support at the church. An advance copy of the musical program being prepared by my brother-in-law Mark Saur was provided. The Korean church members, who had been so faithful in praying for Sun Hee, and bringing over the special mushroom water and certain Korean foods after the surgery were now preparing to support the Healing Benefit Concert. The pastor would come to Trinity Church and offer prayers as part of the event. Numerous friends and family members offered to bring food. Notable among them were my friends, Susan and Rafael, who prepared several dishes and brought them on the train from New York City to Philadelphia. Several women from the Korean church prepared large food platters with fruit.

June 1st was the date of the Healing Benefit Concert. It was sunny and pleasant, a perfect day. A large crowd of people attended and filled the Trinity Church. The Healing Benefit Concert was an artistic and fundraising success. An audio-video recording of this concert may be

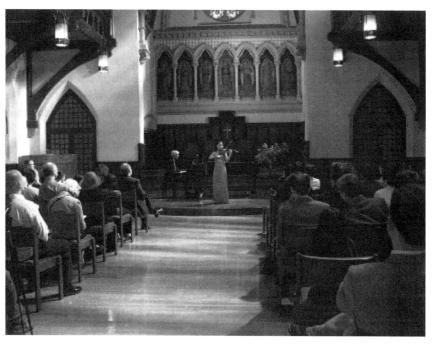

Our daughter Arianna (age 13) performing at the Healing Benefit Concert, Trinity Church in Philadelphia, on June 1, 2008. Sun Hee is on left in large hat.

available on DVD in the future. The blessings of heaven seemed to shower down upon Sun Hee in her time of need. Significant funds were donated, making Sun Hee's trip to the Gerson clinic possible.

Sung-Ji Kim's performance was a triumph—a work of art that could stand against any great soprano in the world. It was a great honor to have a person of her artistic stature (www.sungjikim.com). Arianna, in a long gown, played the Bruch violin concerto, 3rd movement with dazzling verve and energy. Bihn Park, a young cellist, wowed the audience with unaccompanied Bach. Our neighbor David Aker, a Jewish cantor, sang several beautiful Hebrew songs and then added a light touch with a Gershwin tune. Kevin and Ryan Louie, who played viola and violin, and Catherine Pyun, who played her haunting oboe—rounded out the concert with beautiful and stunning performances.

The concert was a success on many levels. It was a great statement of love and support for Sun Hee on an emotional and spiritual level. Her family and friends were at her back, in a big way, with an attendance of over two hundred. It allowed us to get Sun Hee to Mexico—to have her ten day sojourn at the Gerson clinic—to begin the next leg of her healing odyssey.

When we finally arrived at the clinic in Mexico, we met another patient from Canada whose friends had organized a massive benefit concert with an attendance of 2,500 people. It was most impressive the way family and friends would come out in support of a stage IV cancer patient. It is also interesting that this Canadian patient and Sun Hee seemed to be among the most dedicated of all of the patients at the Gerson clinic.

When we returned from the clinic in Mexico, Sun Hee tried to convey what she had been going through with her diagnosis and also her feeling about the Concert. This passage below summarizes some of her thoughts:

"When I first learned that I had ovarian cancer, I was overwhelmed and I tried to hide, feeling ashamed. I asked my husband not to tell anyone, including my family and friends. I thought I would die soon and I was very depressed.

But thankfully my husband called my family in Korea and our best friend Okkwon, and also spoke with our friend Yikwon when he visited. Very soon I received calls from my family in Korea and Okkwon. Then a delegation visited from Emmanuel Church, which brought so much comfort to me. Pastor Park came that day and the whole group prayed for my recovery. After that so many members of Emmanuel Church brought food over and flowers. Slowly, I began to feel somewhat more optimistic.

I have pursued conventional treatment and a special dietary therapy created by Dr. Max Gerson, which has saved many hundreds of advanced cancer patients. My dream had been to go to the Gerson Clinic near San Diego after completion of the surgery and chemotherapy. Because it is not covered by insurance and due to financial constraints, it seemed impossible.

Then Okkwon got involved and organized the beautiful Benefit Concert and made this dream a reality. Recently I returned from

10 days at the Gerson Clinic and already there are signs of improvement as a result.

The Healing Benefit Concert was truly a gift from God for me. The love and support I felt—the healing power of God's love that came through the presence of so many friends and family— and the power of the beautiful music was just overwhelming. It was a huge boost for me in every way. When Pastor Park prayed for me, I felt the presence and power of the Holy Spirit in that room, and in my heart. With so much kindness and love, I feel I must now make a full recovery, by the grace of God, for the sake of my children, and through the benefit of my conventional and alternative therapies."

Okkwon Kim, Julianna, Sun Hee and Arianna after the Concert

14

Trip Into Mexico—Two Ovarian Cases

The Benefit Concert was held on June 1, 2008. Sun Hee still had one more chemo treatment scheduled for June 5th. Sun Hee was obviously still wearing her hat as she was totally bald from the chemotherapy. Before her final two chemotherapy treatments, Sun Hee had resisted her doctor's orders with attempts at delay. In the end she had taken them after being convinced by her doctors of their necessity. However, they no longer had any beneficial effect on the CA-125. They clearly weakened Sun Hee and made her recovery via Gerson Therapy a longer process. In particular, the last two chemotherapy treatments had made Sun Hee *liver toxic,* and she now had a rather yellowish cast on her hands and face. It was not a good sign. Sun Hee could not wait to get to Mexico and begin the full Gerson Therapy under the Gerson-trained Mexican doctors who have helped so many people over the years.

With the help of a generous brother, we had two round-trip airline tickets from Philadelphia to San Diego. With the proceeds from the Benefit Concert and a gift from a most kind sister, Sun Hee was able to afford the fees at the Gerson Mexico clinic. A few days before we left for San Diego, in early July 2008, my sister Kay and brother-in-law Mark came to pick up Arianna and Julianna, and drove them to upstate New York for a large Schickel family reunion. We knew they would have the time of their lives with so many wonderful aunts, uncles, and cousins. They would also get to see my Mother—their *Grannie*—whom they dearly love.

Sun Hee and I flew to San Diego and spent one night at a small motel not far from the airport. We met Sun Hee's cousin and her husband who came by for a brief visit. They had been dealing with a cancer issue in their family, so we had much to talk about. In the morning we rose early so we could meet our escort Judy Jacobson, who would drive us into Mexico. Judy had a large and comfortable white van, and we loaded our suitcases and climbed in. Joining us was another cancer patient and her son, who had also spent the night at the motel. It was ironic but this other Gerson patient also had ovarian cancer. Suja (not her real name) could not speak English, but her son Valerian (not his real name) spoke English perfectly. We began to share with each other about the struggles of dealing with ovarian cancer.

Suja had had surgery and then chemotherapy yielding a short remission. The cancer returned and she was then given more chemotherapy and received an even shorter remission. When the cancer returned again, her doctors then administered even more chemotherapy which provided no value. Three years out from her diagnosis, she had an abdomen full of ascites—fluid caused by the cancer which is often a sign of approaching death—and was in obvious discomfort and distress. She had the look of a suffering person, of great dignity and humanity, who was hanging onto the last shreds of hope.

Her son was her constant and loyal support. Both were soft spoken and very elegant people. Suja made a valiant effort, but while at the clinic she made little or no progress. And after she returned home she passed away within a month and a half. The fluid had not reduced at all during the stay at the clinic. Her body, having had three years of almost constant chemotherapy, had no bounce left. It simply did not respond to the presence of high quality and abundant nutrition. The cancer and the chemotherapy had destroyed the life in this elegant, serene, and suffering woman.

By comparison, Sun Hee was in relatively better shape, though only nine months into her own saga. She had no abdominal ascites and no pleural fluid at this point. Her recent CA-125 was at 30 and it was possible she was in remission. Was Sun Hee's remission to be a short one, followed by more chemotherapy and then more...until death? She was yellowish in complexion. Had the cancer spread to the liver? Sun Hee was going to the Gerson clinic to rebuild her body and her immune system in order to prevent a recurrence—which is what almost all women with this condition would experience within a year of completing the first chemotherapy.

As I engaged in conversation with Suja and Valerian I observed the way she held her abdomen with one hand, so obviously full of the dreaded ascites fluid. I felt very sad and frustrated. Then I recalled the way that Sun Hee's pleural fluid (in her chest cavity) had dropped by 1.375 inches in ten days on the modified Gerson Therapy, and the way her cough went away within a week. My thought was: *"All patients should have access to the Gerson approach—from day one—and not only as a last ditch effort, after they have literally been destroyed by three years of chemotherapy."*

On that ride into Mexico I made a promise to myself, that if Sun Hee continued to do well on the path she had chosen, combining alternative and conventional medicine from day one, and made a full recovery—I would write a book to share the story of her success with others who are suffering, in order to bring true and authentic healing to a larger group of cancer patients.

The contrast between Sun Hee and Suja had yet to fully play out and I did not know for sure where it would lead, but they clearly had chosen two different pathways. Suja chose to fight cancer with surgery and chemo only for the first three years, as her oncologists no doubt had advised. Sun Hee chose a modified Gerson Therapy from day one, along with surgery and a more limited use of chemotherapy. We did not know, and still do not know the final outcome, but it was very clear to me and to Sun Hee that she had derived huge benefits from beginning the modified Gerson Therapy on September 29, 2007. She was lucky indeed to be able to start the modified Gerson Therapy the day following her definitive diagnosis of metastasis—when the cytology report on the pleural fluid sample (drawn out on September 28, 2007) confirmed that adenocarcinoma was present, and could be compatible with an ovarian primary.

Beginning the Gerson Therapy on day one was only possible for Sun Hee because I was educated and knowledgeable—and because I was the nephew of William Schickel. I was personally familiar with my uncle's own healing story under Dr. Gerson's guidance in 1952. My bookcase already contained a copy of Dr. Gerson's book, *A Cancer Therapy— Results of Fifty Cases*. If Sun Hee had been married to someone not familiar with Gerson Therapy, her story would very likely be identical to the story of Suja, with her three years of chemotherapy, but no true healing. Why is this? I reason that the vast majority of patients seem to listen primarily, and perhaps only, to their conventional oncologists. The oncologists certainly never discuss Gerson Therapy, macrobiotic diet, or any alternative method. When asked they typically say "Alternatives don't work" and "Now is not the time for alternatives" as Dr. Ryan had said to us.

Why do the doctors respond in this way? No doubt it is because of their training and education. There is little research done on anything except pharmaceutical drugs because the costs of research are so massive. In the absence of a large-scale study published in a peer-reviewed journal, doctors are simply not comfortable recommending alternatives to the standard methods, which usually involve some combination of surgery, chemotherapy and radiation. Only in more recent years do we see the seeds of change, with the establishment of *departments of integrative medicine* at major hospitals. For the vast majority of cancer patients, however, effective integrative care is still not an available and viable option at mainstream hospitals. This will not change until the oncologists embrace integrative approaches, which may be a long time—as it takes decades for ingrained practices in medicine to change.

15

The Gerson
Clinic Experience

The drive from San Diego to the Mexican border was about thirty minutes. It then took another fifteen minutes to arrive at the Gerson Clinic. Although one can simply drive across the border going into Mexico without stopping—getting back into the U.S. is a much longer process—Judy, our driver, stopped and parked the van near the Mexican border office. She went into a customs building to apply for a special permit for our group of patients and family members. She assured us this was necessary so we did not have any challenges during our stay at the clinic or on our coming back into the United States.

Once on the Mexican side of the border the scenery changed dramatically. We seemed to drive south for only a brief time, then turned toward the west and drove along the Mexican side of the border. On our right we could see the seemingly endless wall, and in some cases a double set of walls, that had been built in the San Diego-

Tijuana corridor. To the left we saw very tiny and very poor homes, perched precariously on the hillsides. Eventually this rural scenery gave way to a more suburban and then to a more urban environment, as we approached the outskirts of the Tijuana region. We reached a turn off to the right and headed west for an urban enclave built along the Pacific ocean.

After driving several blocks in a built-up downtown area, we turned right and after a block right again—then drove up to a tall white masonry wall with a large grey steel gate. Judy beeped the van horn and the staff of the Gerson Clinic opened the gate. Judy pulled the van into a beautiful Mexican courtyard. We were warmly greeted by Juan, an administrator, and other staff members. We were shown to our room and the schedule for the first day was described to us. We were to report for an initial meeting with the doctor in about 30 minutes. We then pulled together Sun Hee's medical records for the meeting.

We met Dr. Pablo Hernandez, a middle-aged Mexican doctor who was to be our primary doctor while at the clinic and afterward for followup. Dr. Hernandez was very friendly and polite. He asked many questions and details as he typed into his computer—taking down the details of Sun Hee's case. This took about 45 minutes. We then went to an adjoining room for a brief physical exam. Dr. Hernandez was very positive about Sun Hee's progress and prospects. Two other doctors, whom we also met over the course of our stay, were also very positive and encouraging to Sun Hee.

Then Dr. Hernandez pulled out a special form and began prescribing the beginning Gerson Therapy program for Sun Hee, which consisted of vegetables juices, food, supplements, and coffee enemas. She began with only six juices and two coffee enemas. This was about 1/2 of what a normal Gerson patient receives. Sun Hee was not a normal Gerson patient. She was a patient who had been *pretreated* with chemotherapy. She would therefore receive less juices and enemas than the full Gerson Therapy; otherwise, she would detoxify too quickly, which could be very difficult and painful, producing a feeling like she was on chemotherapy again, while re-experiencing the various side-effects of chemotherapy.

Dr. Hernandez explained that the juices drive toxicity out of the body's cells—including chemotherapy that is stored in the body's tissues. These toxins are processed by the liver, and its waste is deposited into the digestive system via the bile duct, where it can be reabsorbed while passing through the small intestine. In this way the chemotherapy gets back into circulation in the body, and the patient may feel as though they are on chemotherapy again. The Gerson program is reduced to produce less effect on the patient. Thus, the detoxification process for patients pretreated with chemotherapy must be done more slowly. The program Dr. Hernandez prepared included many vitamins and dietary supplements, as well as a daily injection of crude liver extract and vitamin B12.

At this initial meeting we showed Dr. Hernandez four x-rays showing Sun Hee's progress in reducing the pleural effusion. Dr. Hernandez was very happy to see that such huge progress had already been made prior to coming to the clinic. He talked with great animation and enthusiasm as he viewed these x-rays—feeling they were strong evidence for the benefit Sun Hee had already received, from the modified Gerson

Therapy she had used. In this regard, Sun Hee was rather unusual. Most of the other patients were just starting alternative diet therapy for the first time at the clinic.

Sun Hee arrived after having been on alternative diet therapy for a full nine months—first for two months on a modified or partial Gerson Therapy in October and November, and then for seven months on a macrobiotic diet with strong Gerson influence added in. Now Sun Hee was anxious to start the full Gerson Therapy—which she believed would be quite helpful in detoxing the chemotherapy still left in her body—and in rebuilding her damaged immune system. After our meeting with Dr. Hernandez, we enjoyed a delicious lunch in the dining room, with a view overlooking an outdoor courtyard and pool. Stainless steel trays of vegetarian foods were arranged on two buffet tables at the end and on one side of the dining room. We entered the room, greeted a few of the other patients and their companions, then selected our food. Each day there was Hippocrates special soup—a creamy soup made from celery root, leek, onion, potato, and tomato, along with a bit of garlic and parsley. It was cooked for one and a half hours on a low flame, and then put through a food mill which made it very creamy. This was used twice daily on the Gerson diet.

We also filled a plate with salad—with many ingredients—including romaine, red leaf, onion, cabbage, and green and red peppers. We used flax oil dressing, with no vinegar, as is common for Gerson patients. Apple cider vinegar is often used separately, as a dressing on cooked vegetables. We filled a second plate with baked potato, beets, broccoli, and a corn and string bean combination. There was plain nonfat yogurt for those patients whose guidelines permitted it. Included also was a glass of carrot-apple juice in a plastic cup with a number written on the top. The number was the room number of each patient. For dessert we had one or two slices of plain, saltless, 100 percent rye toasted bread, which was surprisingly delicious.

Lunch and dinner in this Gerson world had a similar pattern, with the primary differences being in the choice of vegetable dishes and the occasional use of brown rice, in lieu of baked or steamed potatoes. We discovered some wonderful combinations. If one had yogurt over steamed beets, it was divine. The same was true if one placed yogurt over a steamed yam or sweet potato. Even yogurt over boiled potato, seemed to make the potato more interesting. There always was plenty to eat. There were also pears and other fruit available for dessert, along with various healthy muffins that the kitchen staff prepared. One could have chamomile or peppermint tea, if one desired it. Overall, we found the lunch and dinner meals were very satisfying.

Breakfast was more simple, and consisted of fresh squeezed orange juice, wonderful creamy oatmeal, plain or with choice of plump raisins, dates, apricots, or applesauce. There was a sumptuous fruit plate that could be assembled from the array of mangos, pears, peaches, plums, and bananas that were laid out on the buffet. For dessert there was always that amazing piece of toasted rye bread with a touch of honey.

The other unforgettable part of our meals was the conversation with the patients, who seemed to come from all over the world. Patients and companions were very friendly and open with each other, about their health conditions and how they were doing. Some strong bonds were developed. The humanity of it all was striking. All nine patients except one seemed to have stage IV cancer.

Of the eight cancer patients, Sun Hee seemed to be doing the best on the Gerson Therapy. What is her secret? Diligence for one. In the next two years, she refused to travel anywhere for an overnight stay, in order not to disturb her Gerson Therapy. She wants to be in her own kitchen making her food and juices, and applying the detoxification program like clockwork. Perhaps it is her Asian work ethic or her classical music training, but she realizes that something great can only be built up from *correct daily practice*. In this case, it is her daily practice of the Gerson Therapy.

Of all the patients at the Clinic in Mexico, only Sun Hee had been using a modified or partial Gerson Therapy, or macrobiotic diet, from the very first day after her diagnosis. She used this before and after surgery, then through the chemotherapy period, which in total had lasted nine months. None of the other patients had experienced this huge benefit. Obviously, Sun Hee was extremely lucky to have known about the Gerson Therapy and macrobiotic diet, so she could begin these alternative approaches when she was first diagnosed.

These alternative approaches that Sun Hee used in the first nine months—before going to the clinic—helped to build her immune system to fight the cancer. It also assisted her successful recovery from surgery and chemotherapy with less side effects. The story of Suja, told earlier, is a stark reminder of how fortunate we were to have found the Gerson Therapy from day one—and not after three years on nearly continuous chemotherapy.

Every month after the 10 day stay at the clinic, and later every three months, Sun Hee did blood testing, after which we had a phone consultation with Dr. Hernandez. Shortly after these phone calls, we would receive an updated Hourly Schedule via email. A sample of a revised Hourly Schedule, which Sun Hee received from Dr. Hernandez in December 2008, is found at the end of this chapter. As it was designed for a specific patient, this chart is not representative of the standard Gerson Therapy program which you can find in Dr. Gerson's book, *A Cancer Therapy—Results of Fifty Cases,* in Charlotte Gerson's book *Healing the Gerson Way*, or in the *Gerson Therapy Handbook* published by the Gerson Institute.

DISCLAIMER: The patient program shown on the next page is placed here for educational purposes, so the reader understands the type of communication that Sun Hee received from Dr. Hernandez. It is not intended for actual use by the reader. If you, or a loved one, have been diagnosed with a serious illness, the author and publisher advise you to contact your doctor for proper diagnosis and treatment. We also encourage you to contact the Gerson Institute or the Kushi Institute if you desire to learn about the potential complementary benefits of the Gerson Therapy or Macrobiotic Diet, respectively.

Hourly Schedule

BNC Name: MRS. SUN HEE LEE   Start Date: DECEMBER/24/2008

Diet	Breakfast 8:00 - 9:00 am					Lunch 1:00 - 2:00 pm					Dinner 6:00 - 7:00 pm		
Time	8:00	9:00	9:30	10:00	11:00	12:00	1:00	2:00	3:00	4:00	5:00	6:00	7:00
JUICES 8 of 10 oz	Orange	Green		Apple carrot	Carrot		Apple carrot	Green			Apple carrot	Apple carrot	
Flaxs Seed oil tbsp	Take the COQ-10 with the FLAX SEED.					half						half	
Acidol capsules		2	Take before meals.				2					2	
Potassium compound sol. Teaspoon in juices	1	1		1		1	1	1			1	1	
Lugol sol. 2 % drops	1						1					1	
Thyroid grains = 1/2 tb of novotiral = 50 mcg						or 50 mcg synthroid							
Vit D-3 1,000 IU per day with magnesium, no						calcium.							
Pancreatine 325 mg		3	take after MEALS.				3				3	3	
Physical activity		Exercise simple:				walking, tai chi, wii					fitness =comput.game		
Niacin 50 mg	1			1			1				1	1	1
Liver capsules					3	Helps ANEMIA.			3		3	Take with tea.	
Coq-10 (60 mg)		2	TAKE WITH MEALS				2	Take with Flax seed oil.			2		
INFLAZIME		3	Take before MEALS.				3				3		
Imugen (colostrum)		3	Get your suplements from the ISH				3	company= good suplements			3		
Selenium	ONE	(Take one with breakfast and one with dinner.)									one		
Milk thistle 250 mg		2	Take with MEALS.				2	Helps liver function + choles			2		
Meditation and relaxation are very and most important every day of life like breathing and thinking= dreams													

Note: "No Medications." appears as vertical text in the 11:00 column and again in the 3:00/4:00 columns.

		Gerson diet	
B-12 injection aply daily after breakfast IM.	b-12 = 0.1 cc + Liver Ext. = 2.9 cc IM.		Follow the program to the letter because it works this way.
Coffee enemas	3 a day: 7 am, 12 pm, 7 pm (I wanted 4/5)		
Castor oil treatment	NOT YET	Rye bread	Continue having 2 a day.
NEXT LAB: JAN/19/08	CBC W/DIFFERENTIAL, COMPLETE METABOLIC PANEL W/LIPID PROFILE, TSH + T-4, UA.	Protein	Continue with organic plain yogur

REST IS VERY IMPORTANT, CALL OR E-MAIL IF YOU   non-fat plain yogurt 4 oz twice a
NEED TO OK. KEEP UP THE GOOD WORK.   day= 8 am + 6 pm.
CONTINUE FOLLOWING THE GERSON THERAPY THEY WAY IT IS INSTRUCTED 100 % = IT WORKS
PLEASE DON'T SHOWER IN FLUORIDE WATER (THIS IS REALY IMPORTANT I HOPE YOU UNDEF
STAND THE IMPORTANCE AND NOT BATH IN FLUORIDE WATER = SILENT POISON).
NEW LAB WORK IN JAN/19/2009 AND LATER IN JANUANRY FEB/09 CAT SCAN.

REST IS VERY IMPORTANT,
I HOPE YOU HAVE SOMEONE TO
HELP YOU WITH JUICING + COO-
KING?.   MERRY CHRISTMAS.
MD Signature.

SUN HEE'S UPDATED GERSON PROGRAM: provided by Dr. Hernandez on December 24, 2008. Dr. Hernandez generally provided an updated program every one to three months—after blood tests results were shared with him.

16

Meeting with Charlotte Gerson

Charlotte Gerson visited the Gerson Clinic on various occasions. We had arrived at the Clinic on a Tuesday. Therefore, we were not surprised to see Mrs. Gerson walking about the Clinic on Wednesday morning. At 10 a.m. she came to our room. It was a happy occasion. We had exchanged several calls and emails over many months, and now were face to face with the great lady herself—the founder of the Gerson Institute, best selling author of *Healing The Gerson Way*, and the daughter of the great Max Gerson, M.D. It was Charlotte who almost single-handedly had carried forward the work of her famous father after his death in 1959. The amazing and wonderful story of Dr. Gerson and the Gerson Therapy is told in exquisite detail by Howard Straus in his book: *Dr. Max Gerson, Healing the Hopeless.* I believe his book is profoundly important.

Considering she is not a doctor or a nurse, Charlotte has the ultimate bedside manner, as she gives each patient optimism, hope, and an education! Education is the ultimate purpose of Charlotte's life—to teach people around the world about the benefits that can arise when the body's own immune system comes roaring back to life, by implementing the Gerson Therapy. Charlotte paid careful attention to the clinic patients, giving important pointers about pitfalls to avoid while on the Gerson Therapy.

After listening intently to Sun Hee for some five minutes, Charlotte came out with a very important warning:

> *"The first thing I want to tell you Sun Hee, is that in about 5 or 6 months you will have a big healing reaction. I call it the six-month chemo healing reaction. At that time it will feel like you are on chemo again...because after six months there is a tremendous activity from the liver, discharging the chemo that has been stored in tissues and cells. I'm warning you now, that your blood work will suddenly become very abnormal. The liver enzyme counts will shoot way up and your CA-125 result will also likely go up. Don't become alarmed, as they will come back down in a few months. After that the healing process will continue with a less strong but continuous series of healing reactions every 4 to 6 weeks."*

Almost exactly six months later, we found that Charlotte's words were truly prophetic, as four liver enzymes went up dramatically on the December 22, 2008 blood test. Two liver enzymes were in a normal range around 40 IU/L and suddenly shot up to nearly 240. Then, on the next test, they came right back down. It was so shocking and dramatic, that we created the graphic in Chapter 18 to illustrate this healing reaction.

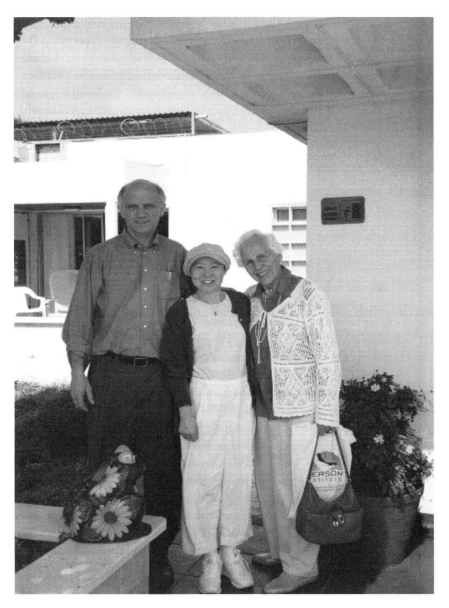

With Charlotte Gerson on July 15, 2008, after 9 days at Gerson Clinic. Sun Hee by then had lost the yellowish coloration on her face which had accumulated during chemotherapy.

How was this woman, who was not a doctor, able to so accurately predict such a reaction? Experience is the answer. Charlotte started helping her famous father when she was a teenager, and has been involved with the application of the Gerson Therapy nearly her entire life. Now at age 88, she is a beacon of light and hope for millions who have failed to find healing in the conventional medical world. She looks like a very healthy person in her 70s but speaks with the energy and conviction of someone in her mid 60s.

After her lecture at the Clinic, we asked Charlotte how many juices she likes to drink each day. She smiled and said, "As many as I can get my hands on." We noted that the Clinic staff seemed to be bringing her juices on a very regular schedule. Charlotte was implementing one of the Gerson concepts—the amazing nutritional benefit that one gets from the carrot-apple juice and the Gerson green juice, as well as all aspects of Gerson Therapy. But she warned that heavy juicing must always be accompanied by the coffee enema, so there is a balance in roughly a 3-to-1 ratio—with one coffee enema applied daily, for every three juices consumed by the patient.

The food and juices help to make up for a lifetime of nutritional *deficiency*, which along with *toxicity*, are two significant causes of cancer developing to begin with, according to Dr. Max Gerson. Remember these key words: deficiency and toxicity. To correct these problems and heal cancer, Dr. Gerson introduced the mineral and vitamin rich Gerson diet and juicing program. In addition, the Gerson program includes numerous supplements, as well as the coffee enemas which facilitate detoxification of the liver. The entire Gerson therapy is described as beautiful in the book *Healing the Gerson Way*, by Charlotte Gerson.

Charlotte had also predicted that the CA-125 test result would likely spike in about 5 or 6 months after the clinic visit. In this she was precisely correct. Sun Hee's CA-125 was 30 on June 30, 2008, before she entered the Gerson clinic. One month after the clinic stay in Mexico, it had dropped to 24.9, on August 20th. A month later it was 21.7. The next month it was 17.6. Sun Hee was very happy. However, on the December 22, 2008 blood test, it shot up to 35.2, and a month later to 51.5. Sun Hee became very depressed and unhappy. But in fact, this was part of the six-month chemo healing reaction that Charlotte had predicted. Two months later, in March 2009, the CA-125 dropped to 27.3 and then in June 2009 it was steady at 26.8. We hoped this meant that the big six-month chemo healing reaction was over, and that Sun Hee was now on a steady course, with the CA-125 in the normal range. These CA-125 results are summarized in a chart found in Chapter 10.

During a visit with Charlotte, Dr. Hernandez listened quietly and spoke little. It was clear that when Charlotte was in the room, this was her time for patient education. The success or failure of a Gerson patient depends on how well the patient is educated, how dedicated they are to the therapy, and how much help they have from a spouse or other companion. It is all very easy at the clinic in Mexico. One is treated like a rock star. The juices are made hourly and the kitchen staff delivers them to the patient personally—wherever the patient is—whether they are in their room, at pool side, in the community room or in the garden. When patients return home, only then the reality of this work-intensive therapy becomes self evident.

We wished that we could bring back home the beautiful and endlessly kind kitchen staff, who were very much loved by all the patients. These beautiful ladies, who worked so hard from morning to night, seemed to be nothing less than *the hand of God* for the patients at the clinic.

I became so fascinated with the benefits of carrot juice that I prepared a chart comparing the nutritional content of carrot juice versus coffee and tea. This chart follows at the end of this chapter. If you study this chart, you can see that carrot juice is loaded with large quantities of liquid, bio-available natural vitamins and minerals. By drinking carrot juice, carrot-apple juice and green juice, instead of water, coffee or tea, a Gerson patient derives huge nutritional benefits. These vitamins and minerals are in an easy to digest liquid form, and are 100 percent natural and organic. By consuming the juices every hour, they give the Gerson cancer patient a massive advantage for healing, as they are distributed to the tissues and cells in the body in a nearly continuous manner.

COMPARISON OF NUTRITION IN:
CARROT JUICE vs COFFEE vs TEA

FOOD	Carrot Juice	Coffee	Tea
% Calories from Carbs	90	41	100
% Calories from Fats	3	17	0
% Calories from Protein	7	42	0
Quantity	**5 cups**	**5 cups**	**5 cups**
Dietary Fiber % Daily Value	40	0	0
Protein % Daily Value	20	5	0
Cholesterol % Daily Value	0	0	0

VITAMINS

Vitamin A % Daily Value	**4515**	0	0
Vitamin C % DV	**165**	0	0
Vitamin D % DV	**—**	—	—
Vitamin E % DV	**70**	0	—
Vitamin K % DV	**230**	0	—
Thiamin % DV	**70**	10	0
Riboflavin % DV	**40**	55	0
Niacin % DV	**25**	10	0
Vitamin B6 %DV	**130**	0	0
Folate % DV	**10**	5	0
Vitamin B12 % DV	**0**	0	0
Pantothenic Acid % DV	**25**	30	0

MINERALS

Calcium % Daily Value	**30**	0	0
Iron % DV	**30**	0	0
Magnesium %DV	**40**	10	0
Phosphorous %DV	**50**	5	0
Potassium % DV	**100**	**15**	**0**
Sodium % DV	**15**	0	0
Zinc % DV	**15**	0	0
Copper % DV	**25**	0	0
Manganese % DV	**75**	15	3
Selenium % DV	**10**	0	0
Completeness Score	**70/100**	18/100	9/100

This analysis is based on information from the Web Site: www.nutritiondata.com. The symbol "—" indicates missing or incomplete value.

A critical key to healing chronic degenerative diseases is nutrition in the form of natural sources of vitamins, minerals, fiber, protein, carbs and fats. The comparison above shows what benefit comes from substitution of five cups of coffee or tea, with five cups of carrot juice! Take note of the critical mineral potassium. To facilitate healing, the interior of the cells in the body need to be low in sodium and high in potassium, according to Dr. Max Gerson. The main point here is that carrot juice is a liquid, abundant and richly nutritious food—that can foster healing by flooding the deficient cells, tissues and organs of the body with much needed vitamins and minerals, including potassium. At the same time, carrot juice is only 3 percent fat, has 7 percent protein, and has zero cholesterol.

It's best to use only organically grown carrots! We make our juices fresh at home each time and consume them right away. Dr. Norman Walker who invented the Norwalk Juicer, lived to be about 100 years old. Drinking carrot juice can be considered a supplemental form of health insurance, in that its consumption may help to insure one's health and longevity.

17

Full Gerson Therapy
After Mexican Trip

When we returned from our ten day Mexican sojourn, Sun Hee was determined to follow the Gerson Therapy 100 percent faithfully, and she delivered on this promise. Sun Hee was so devoted to her Gerson Therapy, that she refused to travel anywhere for an overnight stay, for the next year and a half. When Christmas of 2008 arrived, six months after the Clinic experience, Sun Hee refused to travel to visit my extended family, a five hour trip. So I took the trip with Arianna and Julianna. Sun Hee seemed very happy to be doing her therapy at home, enjoying some time by herself. For me to be alone at Christmas would have been a very sad time indeed, but Sun Hee was very content to be at home, preparing her daily juices, "coffee breaks" and the Gerson meals. This program was her fate and her choice, and she was embracing it in a good spirit. Today, in 2011, Sun Hee can say that she is certainly in the top performing group—of those who had been diagnosed with a similar stage IV ovarian cancer—because she is not only alive, but she is doing well and living a normal life, over four years after her diagnosis.

Upon returning home, the Gerson program Dr. Hernandez prescribed was implemented. It was a reduced program because Sun Hee had taken chemotherapy, and Dr. Hernandez said she now must be detoxified slowly. It consisted of six (rather than 12) daily juices, along with two (rather than four) coffee enemas, and those at 1/2 strength. In addition, it included the Gerson vegetarian food, numerous supplements, as well as the daily injection of crude liver extract and vitamin B12.

Keeping up with the juices was the hardest part. It was relentless. To wash vegetables, set up the machine, do the juicing, drink the juice, and clean up the machine, took about 20 minutes each time. Doing this six times daily meant, essentially, two hours per day devoted to juicing. When more juices were added later, it took a full three hours. The procedure for the coffee enemas was to boil the designated amount of coffee (we used 1/2 of the normal three rounded tablespoons of coffee per 32 ounces of distilled or purified water) for three minutes, simmer it on low for 15 minutes, then wait till it cooled to body temperature.

Sun Hee would then pour it through a cloth to separate out the coffee grinds. Next, she poured the coffee equally into several glass jars which were stored in the refrigerator. When ready to apply the enema, the contents of one of the glass jars would be warmed up to body temperature just prior to use. The details of the coffee enema preparation and procedure are described in *Healing the Gerson Way*, by Charlotte Gerson. For a patient on the more full Gerson program, with at least four enemas daily, the total time in preparation, application, and cleanup of the enemas, might average about three hours per day. Though it is a 15-minute retention enema, if one includes the preparation and cleanup time, each enema takes about 45 minutes.

Breakfast preparation and cleanup takes at least 1/2 hour while lunch and dinner take about 1 1/2 hours each. With the juicing at three hours, enemas at three hours, and the meals at three hours, a nine hour daily committment is needed. This is why it is nearly impossible to work and do Gerson Therapy at the same time. Supplements are consumed at meals and between meals, some 40 pills per day. Nine hours per day does not include the shopping time needed to replenish the mountain of greens, carrots, apples and other vegetables the diet requires. The most difficult part of the Gerson Therapy is the cost which runs about $1,500 per month. This cost breaks down as follows: organic food for eating and juices (together with other food supplies such as flax oil and organic coffee) = $30/day x 30 = $900/month; supplements = $340/month; blood tests = $200/month; and a new phone consultation with Dr. Hernandez after the blood tests results are known = $60/month.

With Dr. Hernandez receiving only a small fee, is it any wonder the oncologists have not embraced Gerson Therapy! This is a very sad and serious issue. By contrast, each chemotherapy treatment administered to Sun Hee at the Hospital, along with a single injection the next day, carried a price tag of almost $12,000 each time. Sun Hee took eight treatments over six months: 8 x $12,000 = $96,000 for chemotherapy. Many rounds of maintenance chemotherapy, which Sun Hee rejected in favor of the Gerson Therapy, would have cost between $100,000 and $200,000. Surgery had already cost about $44,000. Using conventional therapies only, Sun Hee's treatments would likely have cost about

$340,000, with death the most likely eventual end result.

Instead, Sun Hee accepted the surgery at $44,000 and the first round of chemotherapy treatments at $96,000. She then shifted to Gerson Therapy for 30 months x $1,500 per month = $45,000. The total price comes in at $185,000 with the end result being a dramatic recovery with longer life, and perhaps eventually a true cure (defined as five years out from diagnosis and cancer free). Comparing $185,000 vs $340,000, we see a 45 percent decrease in cancer care costs, by embracing the Gerson Therapy for Sun Hee, instead of the additional chemotherapy suggested by the doctors. It is my belief that by combining conventional and alternative medicine, society can achieve lower health care costs, lower health insurance, and better outcomes, leading to longer and healthier lives.

Keeping up with the costs of the Gerson Therapy—which are not covered by insurance—combined with Sun Hee not working, meant that we experienced considerable financial difficulty. Only due to the kind generosity of those attending the Benefit Concert, and many different family members and friends, were we able to survive this period while staying on the Gerson program.

Even with this help, we had to skip blood testing for Sun Hee many months and supplements sometimes ran out. It seems a Gerson patient needs to be either very frugal, modestly wealthy, or have many generous friends and relatives. For many people this kind of diet may simply be out of reach, due to finances and the lack of insurance coverage. Sadly, we are not currently aware of any health insurance plans which cover the monthly costs of an approach like the Gerson Therapy.

18

December Healing Crisis— CA-125 and Liver Enzymes

One month after the trip to the Gerson Clinic in Mexico we had Sun Hee's blood tested on August 20, 2008. The CA-125 came back at 24.9, which was down from 30 prior to going to the Clinic. Sun Hee was always as nervous as can be, right before each blood test was taken, worried that she might see a sudden spike in the CA-125 result. When I got the email with the blood tests result, Sun Hee was ecstatic, practically shouting for joy.

On September 24, 2008 we tested again, and the results came back at 21.7. This was the lowest CA-125 level Sun Hee had ever achieved. She was again on cloud nine saying, "Finally, I feel like I've got this thing under control." The October 22, 2008 test came back at 17.6, and again Sun Hee was elated. All seemed to be going well until the December 22, 2008 test came back at 35.2, representing a doubling. Sun Hee was stunned. In addition, the liver enzymes shot up dramatically. Sun Hee fell into a deep despondency. Her five months of joy had ended. Sun

Hee was crushed—feeling her hope and her world were ending.

I got the December blood test result late in the afternoon on the 23rd of December, but held it for a day while we scheduled a conference call with Dr. Hernandez, for the morning of the 24th of December. Then I gave Sun Hee the blood test results, exactly one hour before the conference call with Dr. Hernandez. I reasoned that, in this way, Sun Hee would only be depressed for one hour, rather than a whole day. I was counting on Dr. Hernandez to explain to Sun Hee that this was not the end of the world—that it was in fact, a major healing reaction. Sun Hee took the news of the CA-125 increase very hard. She was totally deflated, depressed and discouraged. She was thinking that all of those months of taking the juices and applying the coffee enemas had come to naught—the cancer would come back in the end as the victor. She would not be in the select group of women who beat stage III and stage IV ovarian cancer with alternative therapy. I tried to help her see the positive point of view—that it was likely the big chemo healing reaction that Charlotte had warned about.

Finally, at the scheduled hour of 11 a.m., we called Dr. Hernandez. Surprisingly, he was pumped up like a college basketball coach, whose team had just won the NCAA championship. "Did you see it?" he said, "The liver enzymes spiked up dramatically— it is the best healing reaction I have ever seen." He assured us that the CA-125 spike up was also part of the healing reaction, and that both would come down in a few months. Sun Hee was very much heartened by Dr. Hernandez's mood. I was more analytical, asking if there was any other possible explanation for the spike up in the liver enzymes and the CA-125. Dr. Hernandez stated that in some cases where the cancer spreads to the liver, a similar effect could be seen. But he was rather confident that this was not the case. Below are my notes taken after the call with Dr. Hernandez on December 24th, 2008:

> *"Dr. Hernandez thinks that the 12/22/08 blood tests result is showing a major healing reaction. The liver enzymes have doubled or tripled as is typical in a major healing reaction. Cholesterol and triglycerides are also way up, which is also typical. The only other explanation is liver disease or cancer to the liver, which he doubts. CA-125 has moved from 17.6 to 35.2 which concerns Sun Hee. After next blood result in January, we can discuss possible CT scan in February to see for sure. Wants eight daily juices and three enemas and other changes. He will send an updated program."*

Dr. Hernandez has had so much experience helping patients to fight cancer that it was always very reassuring to speak with him. He definitely has the healer's touch, much like Dr. Gerson, who was known for inspiring confidence in his patients.

The chart of the impressive liver enzyme reaction follows on the next page.

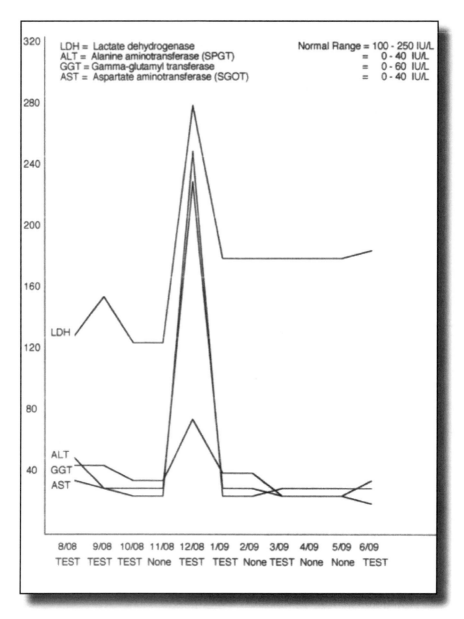

GRAPH OF LIVER ENZYMES: showing Six-Month Chemo Healing Reaction—predicted months in advance by Charlotte Gerson while we were at the Gerson Mexico Clinic in July 2008. (See Chapters 16 and 18 for further discussion.)

19

Healing Reactions
After December Crisis

Sun Hee was now a bit on edge as she had seen the CA-125 go up from 17.6 to 35.2 in the December 2008 blood test. Therefore, she looked to the January 27, 2009 blood test with nervousness. Would the CA-125 drop back down because it had been part of a healing reaction, or would it continue upward, signifying that the battle with this cancer was being lost? When we drove to the blood drawing center Sun Hee was agitated. A few days later we got the bad news. The CA-125 had risen from 35.2 to 51.5. Sun Hee went into a deep depression.

Again, we had to arrange a telephone conference call with Dr. Hernandez, with the hopes that he would be able to explain what was happening. He did not disappoint us. Here below are my notes after the call with Dr. Hernandez on January 29, 2009:

"Yesterday we got the new blood test results and here are some

highlights. WBC up to 3.5 from 2.9. Liver enzymes down from 240- 280 range to about 26 to 30 range—in other words, back to normal after a huge spike up in December. Sun Hee has been depressed that CA-125 went from 35 to 51—but Dr. Hernandez was very happy overall with the progress, and he was not concerned about the CA-125. He feels the big news is the liver reaction, which is a healing reaction wherein the liver is discharging the chemo. The CA-125 being elevated is normal also for a healing reaction. He feels CA-125 is useful for original diagnosis but not so much for follow up. This is the opposite of what the oncologist said. Dr. Hernandez says that when the body is killing cancer cells, these cells circulate in the blood, and are then discharged by the liver during and after these healing reactions. This can cause the CA-125 to spike up.

After speaking with Dr. Hernandez, Sun Hee was much relieved, and her depression over the CA-125 result lifted. Dr. Hernandez feels an x-ray and a sonogram is not a substitute for a CT scan, which he would like to see every six months or so, though he feels there is no big rush if Sun Hee wants to wait a few weeks."

On March 26, 2009 we did blood work again. This time the CA-125 dropped from 51.5 to 27.3 so that Sun Hee was finally happy again, feeling that things were normalizing and the big six-month chemo healing reaction was drawing to a close. But smaller chemo healing reactions seemed to be taking place at periodic intervals. Here below are my notes from May 19, 2009:

"Sun Hee is getting a mild healing reaction today. Tingling in the bottoms of feet, her ears get warm like when she used Zophran during chemo. Strange feeling in chest region as she has had many times before, during chemo. But all these symptoms are mild today. When chemo gets discharged by liver thru bile duct, the digestive system then reabsorbs some of the chemo. Sun Hee then re-experiences being on chemo again."

On June 11, 2009 Sun Hee had blood work done, and on June 22nd we spoke again to Dr. Hernandez. Here are the notes from that conversation:

"Call to Dr. Hernandez. He said Sun Hee needs to take yogurt 2x per day with 4 oz each time, as the 8 ph of the urine is too alkaline and having the yogurt will bring it down. Yogurt has friendly bacteria that is beneficial. 13 juices of 8 oz is best and 5 enemas which can still be 1/2 strength. Sun Hee is detoxing nicely. During healing reaction, the liver has to work very hard getting rid of toxins, and this drives up the liver enzymes.

Because Sun Hee has had an arthritis flare up it is best to cut out orange juice and lemons, in other words, no citrus fruit.

Triglycerides are high due to the body giving off fatty acids. Good to walk after meals, as this will help burn the calories and bring down the triglycerides. Triglycerides are high if resting too much. LDL is a bit high as is typical for Gerson patients. Use clay packs on the fingers to help with the arthritic fingers.

Can use (designated amount) of Novotirol 2x per day instead of synthroid and (designated amount) of lugol's per day. This may help the energy issue. Can get Novotirol from Ishi Company. Overall blood work is very good, improving in all ways. Among liver enzymes, LDH is the most important and is in fact a real tumor marker. He believes in this more than the CA-125 test, which is unreliable."

Finally on July 7, 2009 Sun Hee had a CT scan (the first one since the fall of 2007). The result was generally very favorable though some question marks remained. Sun Hee met with Dr. Ryan and discussed the report in detail.

Attached on the next three pages is this report:

Report Display   *SUH HEE LEE*   7/7/09   Page 1 of 1   ①

Patient name: LEE, SUN H Sex: F Date of birth: ▇▇▇▇▇▇

Mrn: 00725531-8 Accession number: 5103873 Primary Acn: 5103873

Scheduled date: 2009.07.07 08:30 Completed date: 2009.07.07 09:48

Report Date: 2009.07.07 09:55 Department Code: BODYCT

Referring Physician: ▇▇▇▇▇▇ MD

Exam: CTCE/ct chest enhanced Exam status: Final

Comments: PT RESCHED / BXBS / PILOT
CTCE/CTAE/CTPE

History: SPOKE W/BRENDA - SHE'LL CONFIRM PILOT

Diagnosis: MALIGNANT NEOPLASM OF OVARY

Diagnostic Report

Diagnosis:

1. Resolving right pleural effusion and minimal nodularity seen along major fissure. In the setting of known ovarian neoplasm, recommend a short-term follow-up to exclude progression secondary to pleural metastases.

Comments:

Contrast enhanced CT of the chest was performed from lung apices through lung bases following administration of 100 cc of Isovue administered at a rate of 1.5 cc per second via right antecubital approach. Comparison is to October 20, 200▇ abdominal and pelvic portions of the examination are reviewed and reported separately.

Heart size is normal. There are no enlarged axillary, hilar or mediastinal lymph nodes.

The previously seen large left pleural effusion has resolved. There is minimal nodularity seen along right major fissure on image 27. There are no pulmonary nodules or evidence of infiltrative interstitial lung disease.

There are no lytic or blastic osseous lesions to suggest metastases.

Radiologists:
Responsible providers: ▇▇▇▇▇▇
Contributing providers: ▇▇▇▇▇▇

http://oasis▇▇▇▇▇▇fm/MrnReportsDisplay/report.cgi?ris_exam_id=5103873&pid...   7/9/2009

Patient name: LEE, SUN H Sex: F Date of birth: ▓▓▓▓

Mrn: 00725531-8 Accession number: 5103874 Primary Acn: 5103874

Scheduled date: 2009.07.07 08:30 Completed date: 2009.07.07 09:48

Report Date: 2009.07.07 11:35 Department Code: BODYCT

Referring Physician: ▓▓▓▓ MD

Exam: CTAE/ct abdomen enhanced Exam status: Final

Comments: PT RESCHED / BXBS / PILOT
CTCE/CTAE/CTPE

History: SPOKE W/BRENDA - SHE LL CONFIRM PILOT

Diagnosis: MALIGNANT NEOPLASM OF OVARY

Diagnostic Report

CLINICAL STATEMENT: Ovarian cancer

TECHNIQUE: Following administration of oral and 100 ml of Isovue 370 nonionic intravenous contrast, serial helical 5 mm sections were obtained from the domes of the diaphragms to the [symphysis pubis].

FINDINGS:

A CT scan of the chest performed with this examination is interpreted separately.

Comparison is made to prior CT scan of the abdomen[and pelvis] of 9/27/07 performed at Presbyterian Hospital prior to the patient's surgical resection.

There is a small amount of ascites anterior to the liver.

A minute too small to characterize 3 mm hypodense lesion in the posterior segment of the right hepatic lobe on image 17 of series 5 is stable, and likely benign. A 1 x 1.3 cm cystic homogeneous lesion in the left hepatic lobe located superiorly on image 9 of series 5 is unchanged, and therefore may be benign. No other hepatic lesion is identified. The gallbladder, spleen, pancreas, and adrenal glands are normal in appearance. The kidneys are without mass or hydronephrosis.

New since the prior 2007 examination is the presence of heterogeneous retroperitoneal lymphadenopathy in the left paraaortic region, with conglomerate masses measuring up to 2.3 x 2.7 cm in diameter (image 36, series 5). This is in keeping with metastatic disease. There is some mild thickening and minimal nodularity of the peritoneal surfaces, for example in the left paracolic gutter on image 26, suspicious for peritoneal tumor seeding. Surgical clips are noted in the lower left paraaortic region.

Scans of the pelvis demonstrate the patient to be post hysterectomy and bilateral oophorectomy. No masses are seen at the vaginal cuff. There is a small amount of ascites in the pelvic cul-de-sac, with mild thickening of the peritoneal surface noted on image 65. There is mild diffuse thickening of the wall of the urinary bladder that is nonspecific. No pelvic lymphadenopathy is identified.

There is no bowel dilatation. Administered oral contrast does progress distally to the proximal transverse colon without evidence of obstruction. No osseous or soft tissue abnormality seen that would suggest metastatic disease to these sites.

IMPRESSION:

1. Status post hysterectomy and bilateral ophorectomy for ovarian cancer.

2. New left paraaortic heterogeneous lymphadenopathy, in keeping with metastatic disease.

3. Small amount of ascites with mild peritoneal thickening raising suspicion of peritoneal carcinomatosis.

4. Mild diffuse thickening of the urinary bladder, likely of inflammatory origin.

Results were discussed by telephone with nurse practitioner▬▬▬, on 7/7/09 at 11:35 a.m.

Radiologists:
Responsible providers: ▬▬▬
Contributing providers: ▬▬▬

http://oasi▬▬▬fm/MrnReportsDisplay/report.cgi?ris exam id=5103874&pid...   7/9/2009

This report was very hard to interpret. Dr. Ryan noted that the CA-125 at 26.8 was in the normal range and showed an apparent remission; and while the scan was generally good, there were still some question marks. He suggested Sun Hee follow up with a PET Scan, to be sure all was okay. However, due to cost and a desire not to take too many tests, Sun Hee put off the PET scan. Then we spoke to our oncologist friend from Kentucky and he said: "It is a very good report, an eight or nine on a scale of 1 to 10, so you should be very happy." Charlotte Gerson weighed in to say that Sun Hee was 85 percent healed so we should be optimistic. We then spoke to Dr. Hernandez on July 14, 2009 and I wrote the following notes on his interpretation of the CT scan results:

"Dr. Hernandez finds that the CT report is good. He considers the chest clean. Thinks the minimal nodularity is scar tissue from previous trauma or disease. A person's history leaves scar tissue. He sees that there are no lymph nodes showing in entire chest region. Thus CT of chest is clean. Liver is clean. The cyst could be due to a parasite or some other reason.

The item called new mass, may have been there before, and perhaps it was not noted on previous scan. It could be due to surgical scaring, or the building of tissue around the surgical clip, that was left in the same area, as a protective reaction.

Thought blood from two years ago would be absorbed by now. Minimal ascites is just that, minimal. Resolving pleural effusion at right is resolved in Dr. Hernandez' view. Having a very minimal abdominal ascites is not uncommon, considering patient had ovarian cancer.

Thinks the report is written to scare Sun Hee back into chemo, by raising the specter of each item being bigger than it is. He said he knows the games that the hospitals play. They want her back as a patient on chemo. As for PET Scan—can have it to be sure. But he thinks Sun Hee is OK and he has no problem, if Sun Hee wants to delay this test."

By August and September 2009 Sun Hee was looking and feeling much better. Here below are notes I took on August 3, 2009 (which is about one year after the visit to the Gerson Clinic in Mexico):

"Sun Hee has in the last week begun taking a walk in the morning at about 7:30 am to 8:00 am. This is new. She used to only walk at 6 pm if at all. She has also said that the heaviness she used to have with her legs, is now largely gone in the last three weeks. That is really good news it seems to me. Sun Hee's usual pattern is to drink six double-sized juices each day. (This is not the ideal Gerson Way to take juices, but it makes it easier.) She is taking four enemas per day. Plus food and supplements and B12/crude liver extract. We will have a blood test in this month. Hernandez is interested in the TSH, which has still been high. We are now using (designated amount) of thyroid medicine."

On September 27th, 2009 I took the following notes:

"Sun Hee skipped enema last night and woke up with headache. In the morning she was thinking of taking tylenol, but did an enema instead. As soon as the enema was done, her headache was gone. Toxins are still coming out. Detox process is ongoing. Sun Hee gets a lot of compliments on how she looks. People at Temple Music prep did not recognize her, with her elegant gray hair (no longer dyed black) and shiny healthy skin."

On September 29, 2009 I took the following historic notes:

"Today was two year anniversary of beginning Gerson Therapy for Sun Hee on Sept. 29, 2007. I note that Sun Hee has picked up the girls from school every day this year—for the first time in two years. She looks good and seems stronger than before, say one year ago. Yesterday she had some pain on left side in chest cavity. Today it is gone. She has had symptoms of chemo like this, on and off every month, for the last year since stopping chemo in June 2008. Tingling in feet, heaviness in calf muscle and chest pain are the most common chemo-like symptoms. Occasionally she gets red flushing in face and ears like when she used Zophran."

On September 30, 2009 I had a dream and made the following notes:

"Had a dream last night of a meeting with Sun Hee, Dr. Ryan and Dr. Allen. In the dream, Sun Hee was pushing for PET Scan and Dr. Ryan said best to wait, as cancer always comes back and chest cavity is seeded with cancer all over, so it will come

back. I spoke up and told Dr. Ryan he was being very bad to project failure and scare the patient.

I then said, do you not realize what Sun Hee does every day— eight hours everyday—taking green juice and carrot-apple juice and the detoxification program, plus vegetarian food and getting a foot massage each day. Then I chastised Dr. Ryan, saying the future of medicine involves combining mainstream medicine with alternative medicine just as Sun Hee has done. How many patients with pleural effusions have done as well as Sun Hee? Dr. Ryan replied that many are gone in just a few short weeks. Dr. Ryan then left the room and Dr. Allen continued to talk to us."

On October 16, 2009 I made these notes:

"Today Sun Hee had redness in ears and warmth in ears as the chemo keeps coming out. Before she used to get redness and itching on forearms, cheeks and ears—now only on ears.

On November 21, 2009 I made these notes:

"Sun Hee has had red ears after eating breakfast each morning for the last few months. She has also had red rashes and itching at the same time after eating breakfast, on her back, hips, etc. Then she takes the morning enema and after that the red ears and the red rash disappear. This appears to be a continuation of the healing reactions she has had over the last sixteen months since returning from the Gerson Clinic. It may be the chemo is in

the fatty tissue right under the skin and this is now coming out. Regarding the ears: Zofran—when she used it—had a similar reaction. It made the ears red."

On or about December 25, 2009 I made these notes which show the continuing pattern of detoxification.

"Sun Hee had discomfort in chest like when on chemotherapy in the past. Also the tops of the feet felt strange. Ears got somewhat red. These symptoms lasted 4 days."

LIVING IN THE PRESENT MOMENT

This brings us to the present—October 2011. It has now been over four years since Sun Hee was diagnosed with stage IV ovarian cancer with malignant pleural effusion in September 2007. She has made a remarkable recovery. The pleural effusion has been gone for some time. The last CT scan report on the chest cavity was excellent. The CT scan report of the abdominal cavity was excellent, with a few question marks. While Sun Hee appears to be fully healed and is living a normal life, the last scan is subject to interpretation, and she is still suffering from lingering but diminishing side-effects from chemotherapy. She is not yet five years out from diagnosis, in any case. At this point we celebrate a remarkable recovery to date—a much longer life and a much better quality of life, than is typical for such patients.

Can Sun Hee achieve a true five year cure—as a result of the authentic and deep healing work she has done—and go on to live an extra 30 years? We think it is possible, but only time will tell. In truth, we simply focus on each day, each week, as it comes along. Sun Hee is determined to thrive and prosper, so she can be there for Arianna and Julianna. This is a major motivation, which keeps Sun Hee focused every day on the relentless hourly tasks (about eight to nine hours per day) of the Gerson Therapy.

While Gerson and Macrobiotic advisors said not to do it, we have in certain ways combined aspects of both healing systems, and we got results. While today Sun Hee uses primarily the Gerson system, she also regularly uses macrobiotic vegetable miso soup as well as grain-vegetable porridge seasoned with miso. In addition she uses brown rice twice daily, not once per week as is typical for Gerson patients.

Knowing the huge benefits of carrot juice, carrot-apple juice, green juice, coffee enemas, and other Gerson elements, Sun Hee could not imagine proceeding only with strict macrobiotics for healing. At the same time, knowing the benefits of miso soup, miso porridge and regular brown rice, neither could she proceed without them. Perhaps it is her Asian upbringing, but she needs her rice! Today of course, Sun Hee eats only brown rice, which has such good fiber and minerals, and which helps to prevent constipation.

The Zen Buddhist monks—whose thousand year old traditions formed the foundation for modern macrobiotics as a humble and healthy diet based primarily on grains, vegetables, beans and miso soup—are very relevant to a world losing its physiological, psychological and spiritual bearings. And doctor Max Gerson—who used research, intuition, keen observation and clinical experimentation to create his own unique healing system based on organic foods and juices, supplements and detox—is also as relevant as ever. Truth, goodness and beauty never go out of style or lose their enduring value and relevance.

Today Sun Hee and I are simply focused—with contentment and even joy—on the next Gerson meal, the next pot of Hippocrates soup {or Miso Soup}, and on the preparation of the next glass of carrot-apple juice or green juice. As the old Zen saying goes, "Chop wood, carry water."

20

Healing Phases In Recovery Process

Sun Hee went through six healing phases, using either a Gerson or a macrobiotic approach or a combined approach, which we summarize below:

Phase I: First two weeks after diagnosis (Sept. 29 to Oct. 14, 2007)

MODIFIED GERSON THERAPY:

(1) Gerson meals including: oatmeal and fruit for breakfast with a glass of juice; for lunch and dinner we had the special Hippocrates soup, large salad, steamed vegetables, potato and yam or brown rice, and a glass of juice.

(2) Gerson eight ounce juices: eight or nine times a day. Typically three carrot-apple juices, two green juices and three carrot juices. For more detail on juices see the book, *Healing the Gerson Way,* by Charlotte Gerson and Beata Bishop.

(3) Gerson detoxification by three coffee enemas daily. It is a 15 minute retention enema. For details on how to make the coffee enema see the book: *Healing the Gerson Way,* by Charlotte Gerson and Beata Bishop.

(4) We did not use the Gerson supplements, or the injection with the Vitamin B12 and crude liver extract, during these first two weeks. We did not have these items on hand, and were not comfortable with them at that time.

Results from this approach in the first two weeks were very dramatic and are described in detail in Chapter 4 and in Appendix III.

Phase II: First two weeks after Surgery (Oct. 21 to Nov. 3, 2007)

PARTIAL GERSON THERAPY:

(1) Gerson meals as described above in Phase I.

(2) Gerson juices two times daily for the first two weeks after surgery: one being green juice and one being carrot juice.

(3) No coffee enemas during this period.

(4) No supplements or Vitamin B12 and crude liver extract injection during this period.

Phase III: Third to Sixth week after Surgery (Nov. 4 to Nov. 28, 2007)

PARTIAL GERSON THERAPY:

(1) Gerson meals as described in Phase I.

(2) Gerson juices three times daily, eight ounces each: one carrot juice, one green juice and one carrot-apple juice.

(3) One coffee enema daily.

(4) No supplements or Vitamin B12 and crude liver extract injection during this period.

Phase IV: Chemotherapy period of seven months (Nov. 29, 2007 to July 6, 2008)

MACROBIOTIC DIET: with some Gerson and Korean influence.

Due to the damaging effect of chemotherapy, Sun Hee felt she needed regular brown rice and miso soup, along with the Hippocrates special soup and occasional fish—to give her strength during the chemo period. She also used salads and cooked vegetables regularly at every lunch and dinner. She used no salt or oil in cooking. Her program in this period is described in more detail in Chapter 12 and summarized briefly below:

(1) **BREAKFAST:** Oatmeal and miso soup, or oatmeal and fruit plate. Kukicha tea and slice of toasted whole multigrain bread.

(2) **LUNCH and DINNER:** Gerson Hippocrates soup, large salad with many ingredients with olive oil and balsamic vinegar dressing, two cooked vegetables (cooked without salt and oil), potato and yam, brown rice. White meat fish or salmon, two or three times per week. Occasional bean or tofu dish, or tofu pieces added to miso soup.

Kukicha tea.

(3) **JUICES:** Sun Hee drank three juices of eight ounces each daily: one carrot, one green and one carrot-apple, taken between meals.

(4) **DETOX:** No coffee enemas daily during this period. (*Healing the Gerson Way* by Charlotte Gerson suggests one enema daily during the chemotherapy period, if one is using three juices and vegetarian meals.)

(5) **SUPPLEMENTS:** No supplements or Vitamin B12 and crude liver extract injection during this period.

NOTE TO READER: Because she had been on chemotherapy, Dr. Hernandez modified the program to ease Sun Hee into the Gerson Therapy, so she would not detoxify too quickly. In addition, as seen below, we modified the program ourselves and where we did we noted these adjustments in brackets { }.

Phase V: First six Months after Gerson Clinic in Mexico (July to Dec. 2008)

FULL GERSON THERAPY: adjusted for patient who had chemo.

(1) **BREAKFAST:** Oatmeal with fruit plate, orange or carrot juice.

(2) **LUNCH and DINNER:** Gerson Hippocrates special soup, large salad with many ingredients with flax oil dressing, two cooked vegetables with apple cider vinegar dressing, potato or yam and {regular brown rice}. Carrot Juice or tea with meal. Sun Hee used

peppermint tea {or the macrobiotic Kukicha tea}. One or two slices of 100 percent rye bread baked with no salt and oil, usually toasted— purchased from French Meadows bakery. Plain nonfat yogurt, eight ounces per day, beginning on August 28, 2008.

(3) **JUICES:** Sun Hee took nine juices of eight ounces each = 72 ounces daily: three carrot, three green and three carrot-apple, taken at regular intervals throughout the day. Beginning October 28th it was changed to eight juices of 10 ounces each = 80 ounces per day.

(4) **DETOX:** Two coffee enemas daily during this period. Beginning October 28th it was increased to three per day.

(5) **SUPPLEMENTS:** Supplements, including Vitamin B12 and crude liver extract injection during this period, per schedule provided by Dr. Hernandez. For typical schedule of supplements, see the book, *Healing the Gerson Way,* by Charlotte Gerson with Beata Bishop.

Phase VI: Next 24 months (Jan 2009 to December 2010)

FULL GERSON THERAPY: adjusted for patient who had chemotherapy.

(1) **BREAKFAST:** Oatmeal with fruit plate, slice of 100 percent rye bread. {Oatmeal and Miso soup a few times per week.}

(2) **LUNCH and DINNER:** Gerson Hippocrates special soup, large salad with many ingredients with flax oil dressing, two cooked vegetables with apple cider vinegar dressing, potato and yam or brown

rice. Twice each day four ounces of plain nonfat yogurt. Carrot juice with meal or tea after meal. Sun Hee used peppermint tea or {Kukicha tea} after meal. One or two slices of 100 percent rye bread baked with no salt and oil, usually toasted, at the end of meals or between meals as a snack. Rye bread was purchased from French Meadows bakery. {Miso soup two to four times per week instead of Hippocrates soup.}

(3) **JUICES:** Sun Hee took 10 juices of 10 ounces each = 100 ounces daily with two carrot, four green and four carrot-apple, taken at regular intervals throughout the day. Beginning in June 2009 it was changed per Dr. Hernandez to 13 juices of eight ounces daily. {Though we actually typically took six juices of 16 ounces each, starting in the summer of 2009.} We found that juicing 12 or 13 times daily was too exhausting.

(4) **DETOX:** Four coffee enemas daily during this period in 2009 and two to three per day in 2010.

(5) **SUPPLEMENTS:** Supplements and Vitamin B12 and crude liver extract injection during this period, per schedule provided by Dr. Hernandez. For typical schedule of supplements, see the book: *Healing the Gerson Way,* by Charlotte Gerson with Beata Bishop. {In 2010 we eased back on many of the supplements for financial reasons.}

21

Can Incurable Cancer Be Healed?

Whenever I look back at the June 16, 2008 chest x-ray and the June 16, 2008 x-ray report—which we received from Sun Hee's doctor on February 3, 2009—I am both hopeful and shocked. Hopeful, since the report indicates the pleural effusion is gone. Shocked, since I discover that few, if any, other patients from around the world, under the management of the conventional medical doctors, seem to be able to achieve the same results.

In fact, in the medical literature I have seen, there only seems to be discussion of the management of pleural effusions, and absolutely no discussion of curing or healing the patient of the pleural effusion. Perhaps Sun Hee is the first and only patient with a malignant pleural effusion, to have such a clean x-ray as was taken on June 16, 2008. You can see the June 16, 2008 x-ray and its report in Chapter 4.

It is interesting to note what Dr. Steven A. Sahn, M.D. wrote in an article entitled Management of Malignant Pleural Effusions:

> *"PROGNOSIS—The biochemical characteristics of a malignant pleural effusion can be useful in determining a patient's prognosis. Survival is usually only a few months when there is pleural fluid acidosis (pH less than 7.20 or 7.30 and glucose (less than 60 mg/dL {3.3 mmol/L}).*

> *"TREATMENT OPTIONS—Approaches to the management of a malignant pleural effusion are shown in the figure.....Patients who have symptoms caused by a malignant pleural effusion should initially have a large volume thoracentesis performed. The rate of reaccumulation of the pleural effusion, the patient's prognosis, and the severity of the patient's symptoms should guide the choice of therapy."*

> *Article by Dr. Steven A. Sahn, MD was found at: http//www.utdol.com/utd/content/topic.do?topicKey=pleurdis/7405&view=text#*

It is most interesting to note that there is in Dr. Sahn's writing an assumption that the pleural effusion will reaccumulate. This is because modern medicine is unable to effectively treat or heal this condition. Therefore, the baseline assumption is that it will reaccumulate. According to my oncologist friend, the cells which make up the lining of the chest cavity must constantly secrete a lubricating fluid, so that the lungs can expand and contract within the chest cavity, with a minimum of friction. These cells must also reabsorb the fluid; otherwise, this fluid will build up in the chest cavity. When cancer comes here, these cells lose the ability to reabsorb the lubricating fluid. The result is that a pleural effusion develops.

I have also found in the literature on Crohn's Disease, that conventional medical doctors only seem to be able to manage the symptoms, with drugs or surgical procedures. As Virginia Harper and Tom Monte demonstrated in their book, *Controlling Crohn's Disease—the Natural Way,* the conventional medical doctors typically seem not to have a healing plan, which outlines what to change in the patient's diet and lifestyle, so that the underlying medical condition can be healed or cured from the inside out.

However, in the alternative literature of macrobiotics and/or Gerson Therapy one can find evidence of true and authentic healing—from the inside out—of so-called incurable cancer or Crohn's Disease. I am impressed with the books written by Elaine Nussbaum, Mina Dobic and Anthony Satillaro from the macrobiotic literature, and *A Time to Heal* by Beata Bishop, from the Gerson literature.

In Appendix I, many Healing Resources are listed, from Gerson and macrobiotic approaches—the two finest natural healing systems with which I am familiar. A careful reading of this literature will reveal the answer to the question: "Can Incurable Cancer be Healed?" I think the answer is yes—if the patient does not rely only on what the medical doctors offer. I encourage each person diagnosed with cancer to reread Chapter 3, The Secret—The Trinity of Natural Healing, and to think deeply about this trinity of healing. Is an embrace of truth, goodness and beauty the missing aspect of modern medicine and even perhaps our modern lives?

22

Conclusion: A Path To Healing In Ten Steps

H
ere is summarized my condensed wisdom, in ten steps. My hope is that it inspires you, the reader, to realize a simple truth: there is hope and there may be a solution to your cancer or your friend's cancer, through an integrated approach combining conventional and alternative methods.

(1) **MAINTAIN YOUR HOPEFULNESS:** A diagnosis of cancer is not a death sentence, though it may feel that way at the time. Keep your wits about you. Focus on discovering the best and most appropriate conventional and alternative treatment for your health crisis, as both are critical.

(2) **BE PRO-ACTIVE:** Don't expect the doctor to heal you. It won't happen. You must heal yourself, by activating your own immune system. You must take responsibility. Pick up the phone and make your own future. Consult your doctor and get a second medical opinion.

Consult alternative healers and alternative doctors, such as can be found in Departments of Integrative Medicine in major hospitals, and in non-profits such as the Gerson Institute, the Kushi Institute or other healing centers.

(3) **THE DOCTOR IS NOT GOD:** You will need your medical doctors. They are experts at diagnosis, surgery, chemotherapy and radiation—but may know little about natural healing methods such as the Gerson Therapy. Be prepared to ask your questions. Don't be passive in the relationship. They will likely say that alternative approaches don't work, and may discourage you from them. This is a result of their own lack of knowledge and familiarity with natural healing methods, and the results that are possible.

(4) **TRUST YOUR OWN INTUITION:** Do not give up your own mind to be pushed around by anyone—on either the conventional or the alternative side of the equation. Find doctors and healers you trust—listen to them, respect them—but in the end the decisions must be yours.

(5) **EDUCATE YOURSELF WITH BOOKS:** Learn very quickly, not only about the conventional side but also the alternative side. We especially suggest reading: *A Cancer Therapy—Results of Fifty Cases* by Dr. Max Gerson, *Healing The Gerson Way* by Charlotte Gerson, and *Dr. Max Gerson—Healing the Hopeless* by Howard Straus.

(6) **EDUCATE YOURSELF WITH DVD MOVIES:** We especially like *The Gerson Miracle, Dying To Have Known* and *The Beautiful Truth* by Stephen Kroschel and *Healing Cancer from Inside Out* by Mike Anderson.

Get these documentary movies and watch them as a family, and get inspired.

(7) **SEEK OUT RECOVERED PATIENTS:** Call the Gerson Institute and ask for names of recovered patients you can speak with. Ask the oncologist the same. Call and ask these patients how they recovered. Ask them what were the ups and downs and what would they do differently. Take notes and follow up with them, to continue a relationship, if possible. We gained much knowledge and inspiration this way. Communicating with successful role models is really critically important to your recovery.

(8) **BEGIN DIET THERAPY ASAP:** Begin alternative diet therapy immediately or as soon as possible. Do not wait until you have been through two years of conventional-only medicine, and are on your death bed, before trying an approach such as Gerson Therapy, or macrobiotic diet. Everyone—including a cancer patient undergoing conventional treatment—has to eat and drink something. So why not adopt a diet that has a proven record of success, such as the Gerson Therapy or macrobiotic diet?

(9) **CONSIDER A HEALING SOJOURN:** After you have had treatments and interventions from the realm of conventional medicine as needed, consider going to the Gerson Clinic. While we like the Gerson approach very much, other approaches have also shown results as well. You can get information on Gerson Therapy and the Gerson Mexico Clinic from The Gerson Institute in San Diego. If you prefer a macrobiotic approach, contact the Kushi Institute which is located in Beckett, Mass.

(10) **BE CREATIVE and GATHER SUPPORT:** Many cancer patients have financial problems and are devastated emotionally. Let your family and friends know that you need help. Perhaps they will come and pray with you. They may even organize a Benefit Concert or another type of fund raiser. (One Canadian patient we met at the Gerson clinic had been the recipient of a benefit concert that was attended by 2,500 people!) Church members can be a huge help as well—with prayers, meals and encouragement.

Appendix I

Healing Resources

Gerson Web Resources:

The Gerson Institute .... www.gerson.org

Charlotte Gerson Health Restoration Center .... www.gerson.org

Cancer Research Wellness Institute .... www.cancer-research.net

Gerson Support Group in UK .... www.gersonsupportgroup.org.uk

Gerson Health Media .... www.gersonmedia.com

Gerson Books and Movies:

Healing The Gerson Way .... by Charlotte Gerson and Beata Bishop

Dr. Max Gerson—Healing the Hopeless .... by Howard Straus

A Cancer Therapy—Results of Fifty Cases .... by Max Gerson, MD

A Time to Heal .... by Beata Bishop

The Gerson Miracle (DVD movie) .... by Stephen Kroschel

Dying to Have Known (DVD movie) .... by Stephen Kroschel

The Beautiful Truth (DVD movie) .... by Stephen Kroschel

Macrobiotic Web Resources:

Kushi Institute ....www.kushiinstitute.org

Strengthening Health Institute ....www.strengthenhealth.org

Denny Waxman ....www.dennywaxman.com

Christina Cooks .... www.christinacooks.com

Christina Pirello Health Initiative ....www.christinapirello.org

Tom Monte ....www.tommonte.com

Meg Wolff ....www.megwolff.com

Eric and Sanae .... www.loveericinc.com

Virginia Harper... www.youcanhealyou.com

Mina Dobic ....www.minadobic.org

David Snieckus .... www.davidsnieckus.com

Karin Stephen .... www.yogamacro.com

Macrobiotic Books:

Recalled by Life .... by Anthony Sattilaro MD with Tom Monte

The Macrobiotic Way .... by Michio Kushi

The Changing Seasons Macrobiotic Cookbook .... by Aveline Kushi
and Wendy Esko

The Macrobiotic Path to Total Health ....by Michio Kushi and Alex Jack

The Cancer Prevention Diet ....by Michio Kushi with Alex Jack

Barefoot Shiatsu ....by Shizuko Yamamoto

The Great Life Diet ....by Denny Waxman

Cooking the Whole Foods Way ....by Christina Pirello

Becoming Whole ....by Meg Wolff

Controlling Crohn's Disease .... by Virginia Harper with Tom Monte

Recovery from Cancer ....by Elaine Nussbaum

My Beautiful Life ....by Mina Dobic

Mayumi's Kitchen .... by Mayumi Nishimura

Integrative Web Resources:

Keith Block, MD ....www.blockmd.com

Burzynski Clinic ....www.burzynskiclinic.com

Francisco Contreras, MD.....................................www.oasisofhope.com

Nicholas Gonzalez, MD ....www.dr-gonzalez.com

Issels Immunotherapy ....www.issels.com

Bill Henderson....................................www.beatling-cancer-gently.com

Jay Kordish... www.JuiceDaddy.com

(Gerson patient in 1946)

Ralph Moss ....www.cancerdecisions.com

Ruth Sackman ....www.rethinkingcancer.org

Sarto Schickel ....www.CancerHealingOdyssey.com

Mike Anderson ....www.RaveDiet.com

Terry Thompson..................................... www.newcancerstrategy.com

Natasha Campbell-McBride MD ....www.doctor-natasha.com

Integrative Books:

Life Over Cancer..by Keith I. Block, MD

Beating Cancer .... by Francisco Contreras MD, and

Daniel Kennedy, MC

One Man Alone..by Nicholas J. Gonzalez, MD

Cancer: A Second Opinion..by Josef Issels, MD

Cancer-Free ....by Bill Henderson

The Juiceman's Power of Juicing..by Jay Kordish

Cancer: Curing the Incurable ....by William Donald Kelley

Questioning Chemotherapy.. by Ralph W. Moss, PhD

Rethinking Cancer..by Ruth Sackman

Cancer Healing Odyssey ....by Sarto Schickel

A New Strategy for the War on Cancer...........................by Terry Thompson

Healing Cancer From Inside Out..by Mike Anderson

AntiCancer: A New Way of Life............by David Servan Schreiber, MD

Knockout..by Suzanne Somers

Gut and Psychology Syndrome...................by Natasha Campbell-McBride MD

Schickel Family Books and Web Resources:

Sacred Passion: The Art of William Schickel...................by Gregory Wolfe

The Illustrated History of the Schickel Motorcycle..............by Ken Anderson

Mary Frei Schickel—What a Woman!.........................by William J. Schickel

WilliamSchickelGallery.com ....Art of William Schickel
(Gerson patient in 1952)

ElizabethRobinsonFineArt.com ....Art of Elizabeth Robinson

MaryhillClayWorks.com ....Art of Jacques Schickel

SchickelDesignGroup.com ....Design of Sarto Schickel

Appendix II

My View of Dr. Max Gerson

Max Gerson, M.D. was a doctor, teacher and cancer healer—born in Germany in 1881—whose early work in curing migraine headaches by dietary changes led him to cure skin and lung tuberculosis by diet as well. When a woman with incurable cancer demanded he treat her cancer with his tuberculosis diet—Dr. Gerson was quite surprised when, in fact—the woman recovered her health rather quickly. Like many historic moments in science, it was an accidental discovery.

This one case led to a lifetime of work in treating—and in many cases healing—cancer with the Gerson Therapy. Dr. Max Gerson died in New York City in 1959, one year after publication of his classic book, *A Cancer Therapy—Results of Fifty Cases.*

Dr. Max Gerson, M.D. understood the big picture (the totality) regarding genuine healing. This allowed him to take "incurable and terminal" cancer cases, sent home with no hope by the mainstream hospitals, and to heal so many of them. In his book, Dr. Gerson outlines an amazing variety of advanced cases that were healed by the effectiveness of the Gerson Therapy—and the keen intelligence, insight, and deep compassion he personally demonstrated for his patients.

This is the book which has inspired people around the world to heal their cancers, and numerous other diseases. In it, Dr. Gerson shows that cancer can sometimes be healed, even in advanced cases—with a regimen of between eight to thirteen freshly made juices daily, including organic carrot juice, carrot-apple juice and green leaf juice, as well as three specially prepared vegetarian meals, a special soup, and certain supplements. In addition, the program includes between three to four daily coffee enemas, for detoxification. See the book, *Healing the Gerson Way*, by Charlotte Gerson and Beata Bishop, for a detailed description of the Gerson Therapy.

Reducing toxicity (via the coffee enemas, which dilate the bile ducts and thus help the liver to discharge) and providing abundant organic nutrition (via the food, juices and supplements) was Dr. Gerson's focus. Indeed, Dr. Gerson's therapy does not attack the tumors directly and specifically as do the conventional cancer therapies. Instead, it brings the entire organism into a state of optimal functioning by abundant nutrition and detoxification, which then boosts the immune system. The restored and optimally functioning liver, kidney, pancreas, and other organ systems—and the entire immune system—then heals the cancer.

In his own lifetime, Dr. Gerson was ridiculed by his contemporaries. But Nobel Laureate Dr. Albert Schweitzer, called Dr. Max Gerson, "... one of the most eminent geniuses in the history of medicine." Dr. Gerson had cured Schweitzer's wife of lung tuberculosis. Professor of Medicine, Dr. Yoshihiko Hoshino, M.D. found Gerson's book around 1990, and with its guidance, cured himself of colon cancer that had metastasized to his liver. He and others at the Loma Linda Clinic in Fukushima, Japan, have treated hundreds of patients with Gerson Therapy with stellar results. Dr. Hoshino's story, and many others are told in Stephen Kroschel's 2006 documentary movie, *Dying to Have Known.*

Toward the end of Kroschel's movie, you will find the story of my uncle Bill—whose example of embracing the Gerson Therapy in 1952 laid the foundation for Sun Hee's recovery nearly sixty years later. In fact, in the last two years of his own long life, Bill Schickel showed great interest in Sun Hee's progress on the Gerson Therapy, calling many times to check up on her. About one week before he died, he called and said, "Sarto, I'm just so happy that Sun Hee is doing well." These were the last words I heard from my dearly loved uncle. Even on his own death bed, Bill was reaching out to others with a message of love and concern. It was the way he had lived his entire life, bringing beauty and hope to others. It was a precious gift from a man almost 90, who had received the gift of healing direct from Dr. Gerson 57 years earlier, in 1952.

Appendix III

Daily Schedule Sheets

The eleven pages of sheets which follow show daily progress, starting the day after Sun Hee's definitive diagnosis on September 28, 2007. Even though these sheets are not so pretty, I feel it is important to show them here, for inspiration to others with cancer. They show how we began to implement an imperfect and modified Gerson Therapy, on an hour by hour basis, the day after Sun Hee was diagnosed.

Even from Day 1, which was September 29, 2007, you can see from the written comments that there was immediate benefit from being on the modified Gerson Therapy program. It consisted of approximately nine juices per day, three vegetarian meals (with no salt and no oil used in the cooking) and three coffee enemas each day. We did not use any of the supplements that comprise the fourth important aspect of the Gerson Therapy. Thus, while we implemented the Gerson Therapy imperfectly, it was still enough that Sun Hee's health improved dramatically—with the cough going away and with the pleural effusion reducing quite significantly in only 10 days. See the x-rays of chest cavity with the disappearing pleural effusion in Chapter 4.

Therefore, we feel that Appendix III is one of the most important parts of this book. It shows how Sun Hee—under the shock and despair of a stage IV cancer diagnosis—responded with intelligence, and began to help herself with simple, humble, organic vegetarian food and juices. Using God-made natural food and drink—stuff that grows from the ground—rather than the concoctions of the food and drug industry, she extended and very probably saved her own life. Truly a case of "God helps those who help themselves."

Working to save one's own life requires, first of all, a great will to live. This truth was greatly emphasized by macrobiotic teacher George Ohsawa. Secondly, it requires humility in which the patient acknowledeges being part of the problem and says in essence—*mea culpa*—mine the blame. Thirdly, there must be some belief or understanding involved in what George Ohsawa called the order of the universe, or the order of nature—which inspires the patient to follow closely to the way of nature, whether it is called Gerson Therapy or macrobiotics. (Can the patient understand the impact of an apple vs. a glazed donut?) When these three realities are present: will, humility and understanding, then the patient has the best chance to recover.

The humble and challenging dietary and detox work shown on the next eleven pages illustrate this principle in action, as Sun Hee worked her way back to much better health in only eleven days.

Day 1—on Modified Gerson Therapy—10 juices, 4 coffee enemas, 3 meals.

> *"Feeling somewhat better. Less coughing is positive.*
> *More positive outlook. Ruth visiting helps."*

Daily Schedule: Date: 9/29/17

Time:

#	Time	Activity
1	8:00 Am	Breakfast Oatmeal, Apple CJ.
	9:00 Am	Coffee En.
2	9:30 Am	Green Juice
	10:15 Am	Nap.
3	10:40 AM	Carrot juice
4	11:50 A.M.	Lunch & Carrot Juice
	12:30 pm	Coffee En.
	~~12:55 pm~~	~~Carrot Juice~~
5	1:15 PM	Juice (Carrot)
6	2:30 Pm	Carrot Apple Juice
	2:30 Pm	Sushi – Brown Rice, Apples
7	3:30 P.M.	Green Juice with Apple
8	4:50 pm	Carrot Juice
	6:20 pm	Coffee En.
9	6:50 pm	Carrots – Apple Juice
10	8:00 pm	Pizza with Carrot Juice
	10:30 pm	Coffee En.

Feeling somewhat better. less coughing is positive. More positive outlook. Ruth visiting helps.

2 Green
5 Carrot
1 Carrot Apple

175

Day 2—on Modified Gerson Therapy—8 juices, 3 coffee enemas, 3 meals.

"Feeling a bit weak today. Perhaps did not eat enough for meals."

Day 3—on Modified Gerson Therapy—9 juices, 3 coffee enemas, 3 meals.

> *"Feeling somewhat better today. Very little cough and lighter in tone. Healing pulse sensation in abdomen."*

Daily Schedule: Date: 10/1/07

3

Time:

	7:00 A	Coffee Enema
	7:30 A	Breakfast, oatmeal + banana, orange
1	7:45 A	Carrot Juice
2	9:45 A.M.	Green Juice
3	11:20 AM	Carrot Juice
4	12:45 pm	Carrot - Apple Juice
	12:30 pm	Coffee Enema
5	1:00 P.M	Carrot - Apple Juice
6	2:30 P.M.	Carrot Juice
7	3:30 pm	Carrot Juice
8	6:30 pm	Green Juice
	6:45 pm	Coffee Enema
9	9:00	Dinner with Carrot Juice

Feeling somewhat better today. Very little cough
And lighter in tone.
Healing pulse sensation in abdomen.

Day 4—on Modified Gerson Therapy—8 juices, 3 coffee enemas, 3 meals.

"Virtually no cough. Bloated liquid in abdomen seems to be mostly gone. Considerable coughing after visit to hospital. Dr. _____ confirmed there was no palpable fluid in abdomen."

4

Daily Schedule: Date: 10/2/07

Time:

	6:45 A.M	coffee enema
1	7:30 A.M	Breakfast, Oatmeal & Apple & orange & Carrot Juice
2	9:30 Am	Green Juice
3	10:30 Am	Carrot Apple Juice
	11:15 Am	Coffee enema
4	12:00 noon	lunch with carrot juice
5	3:30 pm	Carrot juice
6	5:10 pm	Carrot apple juice
7	7:30 pm	Dinner with Green Juice
	9:30 pm	Coffee Enema
8	10:00 pm	Carrot - Apple Juice

Virtually no cough. Bloated liquid in abdomen seems to be mostly gone. Considerable coughing after visit to hospital.

Dr. ████ confirmed there was no palpable body fluid in Abdomen.

Day 5—on Modified Gerson Therapy—8 juices, 3 coffee enemas, 3 meals.

5

Daily Schedule: Date: 10/7/07

Time:

    7:30 A.   Coffee Enema

1 8:30 Am   Breakfast, oatmeal, banana, carrot juice

2 9:30 Am   Carrot Juice

3 11:30 Am   Carrot-Apple Juice

4 1:00 pm   Lunch + Green Juice

    1:45 pm   Coffee Enema

5 3:00 pm   Carrot Juice

6 4:30 pm   Carrot apple Juice

7 5:50 pm   Green juice

8 7:30 pm   Dinner with Carrot Apple Juice

    9:30 pm   Coffee Enema

Day 6—on Modified Gerson Therapy—8 juices, 3 coffee enemas, 3 meals.

"Persistent cough is completely gone! Hurray! Sun Hee is being verbally more positive projecting success in recovery, thinking positively about the future."

Day 7—on Modified Gerson Therapy—8 juices, 3 coffee enemas, 3 meals.

```
                                              7

   Daily Schedule:              Date: 10/5/17

   Time:
 1    8:∽ A.M      Breakfast: oatmeal, orange, Carrot Juice
 2    9:45 am      Carrot - Apple Juice
 3   11:00 am      Green Juice
      9:15 AM      Coffee enema
 4   12:∽ P.M      Lunch x Carrot Juice
 5    2:∽ P.M      Carrot - Apple Juice
      3:∽ P.M.     Coffee enema
 6    5:∽ P.M      Green Juice
 7    7:30 P.M     Dinner, Carrot Juice
 8    8:30 pm      Carrot Juice
      9:30 pm      Coffee Enema
```

Day 8—on Modified Gerson Therapy—7 juices, 3 coffee enemas, 3 meals.

"Sun Hee pretty tired and weak today and yesterday. Fogginess in head of yesterday cleared this afternoon. Cough at night now gone as well as during the day."

Day 9—on Modified Gerson Therapy—8 juices, 3 coffee enemas, 3 meals.

9

Daily Schedule: Date: 11/9/17

Time:

	Time	Activity
	8:30 A—	Coffee Enema
1	9:15 A.M	Breakfast, Orange Juice
2	10:15 A—	Carrot Juice
3	12:00 Noon	Carrot Apple Juice
4	2:45 pm	Green Juice
	1:00 pm	Lunch + Supp.
5	4:30 pm	Carrot - Apple Juice
6	5:30 pm	Carrot - Apple Juice
7	7:00 pm	Green Juice
8	9:—pm	Carrot Juice
	10:00 pm	Coffee Enema

Day 10—on Modified Gerson Therapy—7 juices, 3 coffee enemas, 3 meals.

> *"Sun Hee is very energetic today. Cough gone in day and night for several days. Maintaining weight—not losing. Less shortness of breath. Less tired. Sun Hee was too active today, tried to work too much & did not rest enough."*

Day 11—on Modified Gerson Therapy—6 juices, 3 coffee enemas, 3 meals.

> *"Chest x-ray today show(s) pleural fluid is further reduced since draw down. Cough came back a few times last night—no doubt due to too much working yesterday & not enough resting. Today—no cough."*

Appendix IV

Integrative Healing Paradigm

There has been a profound divide between the worlds of conventional medicine and alternative medicine, with each side, unfortunately, down-playing the value of the other. The result is that the patients are often conflicted, confused, and in many instances, poorly served.

In some cases, sincere religious people attempt to heal with the use of a Mind & Spirit Program only. This may greatly upset the medical professionals, who feel that these patients are avoiding the beneficial use of Medical Programs, to their own detriment. In the case of children, doctors may go to court to challenge parental custody of children, and for example, ask the court to force the use of chemotherapy, in cancer cases. Passions can get very activated on both sides of this issue.

A very constructive complement to conventional medicine comes from the alternative worlds of Gerson and macrobiotic methods, which have a track record of many documented healings from degenerative diseases. These methods work strongly in the areas of Nutrition, Detoxification and Mind & Spirit—the Trinity of Natural Healing — three areas that are largely ignored by conventional medicine.

Sharlene Stump, a nurse who had tumors in two breasts, one lung, the breast bone and a lymph node, began Gerson Therapy for one month while waiting for chemotherapy to start at the Mayo Clinic. A PET scan just prior to chemotherapy showed that the tumors had cleared from both breasts, the lung and the breast bone, with the lymph node more stable. While not all cases respond this way, the Gerson method simply cannot be ignored. Positive results for over sixty years need to be studied rather than swept under the rug. Sharlene's stunning testimony in an online video is most impressive and definitely worth watching. Search for: *Gerson Therapy—A Nurses Testimonial.*

And yet, as powerful as these Gerson and macrobiotic dietary-based methods are, there are no doubt times when conventional Medical intervention is critically needed. Surgery certainly can be very helpful, especially in acute cases or where the tumor or tumors may be very large. Chemotherapy and radiation are more controversial because they leave considerable damage to the patient. And yet, there is a very serious need for more research on integrative approaches, which combine conventional and more natural alternative methods. My wife Sun Hee has had success with an integrative approach for recovery from stage IV ovarian cancer, using both conventional and alternative medicine.

The Integrative Healing Paradigm is a broad philosophical model that says if patients are only getting Medical intervention they may be very poorly served—by receiving only 1/4 of the care and support they truly need. Medicine, without a proper and broader philosophical perspective, seems to have become so focused—so specialized into the arena of medical intervention—that the totality of what the patient really needs often gets lost. A detailed and effective Nutrition Program, a Detoxification Program, and a Mind & Spirit program are three critical but often missing elements. These three comprise the Trinity of Natural Healing.

The Gerson and macrobiotic approches have a strong track record of success with thousands of improved or recovered patients, who have found relief from a broad range of illnesses, including many types of cancer as well as diabetes, heart disease and other conditions. Despite these impressive successes, often with very sick patients, these alternative methods have not been embraced by the mainstream medical establishment. There are, for example, no hospitals in the U.S.A. that provide Gerson Therapy or serve macrobiotic foods.

The great tragedy for patients is that the conventional and alternative camps communicate very little with each other. Some alternative practitioners simply condemn all conventional cancer medicine, for example, and the oncologists typically do the same in return. The patient is left poorly served, not knowing whom to trust or where to turn for advice that has integrity. The Integrative Healing Paradigm graphic which follows at the end of this Appendix, outlines the key elements in an integrative model: a Mind & Spirit Program, a Nutrition Program, a Detoxification Program and a Medical Program—thus creating a more full and balanced approach for patient recovery. This is a model that simply has never been tried on a large scale.

The diagram on the next page summarizes the numerous items that would be included in an Integrative Healing Paradigm—a marriage of modern Medicine and the Trinity of Natural Healing. If the medical system as we know it today were to embrace this integrative paradigm, I believe that results for patients would be significantly improved.

Integrative Healing Paradigm
Embracing Medicine and The Trinity of Natural Healing

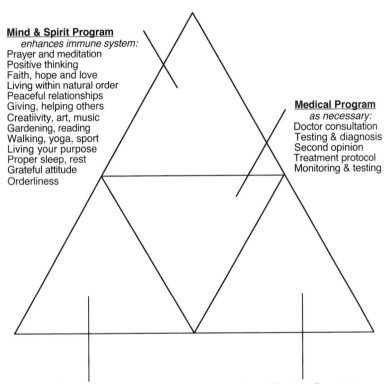

Mind & Spirit Program
enhances immune system:
Prayer and meditation
Positive thinking
Faith, hope and love
Living within natural order
Peaceful relationships
Giving, helping others
Creatiivity, art, music
Gardening, reading
Walking, yoga, sport
Living your purpose
Proper sleep, rest
Grateful attitude
Orderliness

Medical Program
as necessary:
Doctor consultation
Testing & diagnosis
Second opinion
Treatment protocol
Monitoring & testing

Nutrition Program
enhances immune system:
Natural, organic, whole foods
Selected foods only
Fresh vegetable/fruit juices
Fresh vegetarian meals
Vitamins and supplements
Sunshine and fresh air
Shiatsu, Reiki, Pilates, massage
Distilled or spring water
Family meals with laughter
Plant-based diets such as
    Gerson, Macrobiotic, Paxdieta

Detoxification Program
enhances immune system:
Clean skin - body rub & shower
Clean liver - coffee enema
Clean cells - via freshly made juices
Reduce to normal weight
Non-toxic home/work environment
Transmute stress and negativity
No drugs, smoking, alcohol
No hair dye, cosmetics, cell phone
Normal digestion and elimination
    is the best detoxification system
Sauna or warm bath - sweating

Philosophical framework—not medical advice.
Sarto Schickel, Author and Speaker

191

Appendix V

Paxdieta Healing Recipes

During her recovery Sun Hee developed her own way of cooking a unique combination of Gerson and macrobiotic food. We call it PAXDIETA (peace diet) to distinguish it from Gerson or macrobiotic recipes and patterns. I think of it as basic. It is not fancy or gourmet, in any sense; but it is definitely delicious and wholesome as it fosters good digestion, which is a key ingredient in good health and personal peace. Perhaps it could be said that it resembles humble monastic fare from olden days.

This food suits Sun Hee very well and has been instrumental in her recovery from stage IV ovarian cancer. It has also kept my daughters and me in good health, though we provide some "regular food" to my daughters as well.

For breakfast we have a large portion of oatmeal with a glass of tea, water or juice. For lunch and dinner, Sun Hee typically prepares (1) a rice dish, (2) one to two vegetable dishes, (3) a vegetable soup, (4) a large green salad, and (5) a glass of homemade juice. We call this basic pattern *BVM-SJ* which means *B*rown Rice, *V*egetables, *M*iso Soup, *S*alad and *J*uice. To consistently prepare meals with these elements looks simple, but requires about an hour for each meal. In some cases we would have tea at the end of the meal instead of juice, which we would often have between meals.

(1) PRINCIPAL FOOD—BASIC GRAIN DISHES

OATMEAL FOR BREAKFAST

Purchase organic rolled oats and prepare per instructions. We generally use the oats that require about five minutes to cook. Usually we cook the oatmeal plain with spring or distilled water and then serve with raw apples cut into 1/2 inch squares. It is crunchy and delicious. For variety we may cook the oatmeal with dried raisins, apricots or prunes, in which case we may not add the raw apple on top. In winter we may have a cup of hot kukicha tea with the oatmeal, or even a bowl of miso soup.

BROWN RICE VARIATIONS

Boiled brown rice
Boiled brown rice with 1/3 millet
Boiled brown rice with 1/3 barley

Cooked with one part grain and 1.5 parts spring or distilled water. Presoak in cooking water for two to four hours. Bring to a boil for three minutes—then turn to low keeping top on for 20 minutes, then simmer for 30 minutes. No salt in cooking. Serve with ground sesame seeds without salt. (If a person is very sick it may be necessary to prepare Soft Brown Rice using much more water and much longer cooking time.)

BROWN RICE STIR FRY

Brown rice leftovers with water-sauteed garlic, onions and scallion
Brown rice/millet leftocvers with garlic, onion, cauliflower and broccoli
Brown rice/barley leftovers with garlic, onion, bok choy and celery

This is an ideal way to use brown rice leftovers from the previous evening meal. We often have this dish as the grain for lunch. Saute the minced garlic and chopped onion for six minutes on a medium flame—then add other vegetables and saute for six minutes. Finally, add the brown rice and stir in with vegetables and cook for six to eight minutes.

BROWN RICE PORRIDGE

Brown rice porridge with onion, cabbage, bok choy and fresh corn, seasoned with miso
Brown rice/millet porridge with onion, carrot, cauliflower and celery, seasoned with miso
Brown rice/barley porridge with onion, kale, celery and scallion, seasoned with miso

Place generous portion of cooked leftover rice in a large pot and cover with water so that water level is above top of rice by about half an inch. Bring to a boil and then add vegetables beginning with chopped onion. Cook on medium flame for 10 to 15 minutes and then simmer on low for 20 to 40 minutes. Finally, add miso to taste (we use about one level teaspoon of miso per bowl of porridge) by first dissolving the miso in 1/4 cup of water, then adding this puree to the porridge. Stir gently to integrate miso with the porridge and simmer (do not boil) for five to eight minutes.

(2) QUICK STEAMED CABBAGE DISHES

Steamed cabbage

Steamed cabbage with kale and asparagus

Steamed cabbage with broccoli and cauliflower

Steamed cabbage with red radish and summer squash

Place vegetables in pot with 1/2 cup of spring or distilled water and bring to a boil. Once at a boil, turn to low and cover. Cook for five minutes and serve dribbled with apple cider vinegar.

(3) NISHIME VEGETABLES

Steamed carrot

Steamed carrot with onion and winter squash

Steamed carrot with onion and parsnip

Other variations per macrobiotic or Gerson recipes

Place vegetables in a pot with 1/4 cup of spring or distilled water. Simmer on low with top on for 60 minutes. This is the nishime method—long slow steaming on a low flame with little water. We serve these sweet vegetables plain.

(4) BOILED VEGETABLES

Potato, many varieties

Yam, Sweet Potato, many varieties

Beets

Place your choice of root vegetables in a pot 1/2 covered with spring or distilled water and bring to a boil. Turn burner to low and cook for 10 to 15 minutes. Yam or sweet potato can be cooked in same pot as potato, but beets should be cooked separately. We often serve these root vegetables dressed with plain non-fat yogurt.

(5) **GREEN SALAD WITH FRUIT**

Romaine lettuce, red leaf lettuce, carrots, celery, peppers, red cabbage, apple, grapes, pears or peaches are typical ingredients. Use Flax oil dressing dribbled on the salad. For family members not on a strict diet, use olive oil and a touch of balsamic vinegar dressing.

(6) **VEGETABLE MISO SOUP**

Place spring or distilled water in a pot and bring to a boil. Turn burner to medium high and add finely sliced onions, cooking for five minutes. Next, add carrots cut into match sticks. After a few minutes add thinly sliced white cabbage. Then, a few minutes later add cauliflower and simmer for two minutes.

Next, add miso in the following manner: remove some of the water from the soup pot into a small bowl and add one level teaspoon of miso, per estimated bowl of soup; stir and dissolve miso completely in the water; then add the pureed miso back into the soup pot and simmer on low for six minutes. Immediately after add scallions or even broccoli florets as a garnish and let them also simmer for this final six minutes.

NOTE: Once miso is added, never boil the soup, as this will kill this beneficial probiotic culture. We typically make miso soup for lunch, then reheat it on simmer for dinner. While it can be kept overnight in the refrigerator and reheated the next day, it is best to make it fresh each day.

(7) HIPPOCRATES VEGETABLE SOUP

For Hippocrates soup cut these ingredients into half inch squares and place in a pot—celery root, leek, onion, potato, tomato and a bit of garlic. Cover with spring or distilled water and bring to a boil, then turn to low and simmer for 90 minutes. Put all ingredients through a food mill to make a creamy soup. Garnish with parsely and serve. This soup can be saved in the refrigerator and reheated in small quantities for two or three days.

(8) HOMEMADE JUICE

Carrot juice

Carrot and apple juice (usually 2/3 carrot and 1/3 apple)

Green juice with romaine, red leaf, endive, escarole, chard, beet tops, watercress, green pepper, red cabbage and green apple (or other apple if green apple not available)

(9) DESSERT and SNACKS

Fresh peaches, plums, watermellon, apples, pears, grapes, cherries, persimmon, mango, kiwi or other fruit—with the exception of pineapple, strawberries, blueberries and other berries which are forbidden on a Gerson diet

Stewed fruit—apples and pears are favorites

Plain rye bread, or multigrain artisan quality bread, toasted

Saltless brown rice crakers

Corn on the cob with umeboshi plum

Oatmeal with apple leftovers

Brown rice porridge leftovers

(10) **TEA** (after meals or between as needed)

Kukicha tea

Peppermint tea

Chamomile tea

Roasted barley tea

Roasted corn tea

(11) **PROTEIN DISHES** (rarely used)

Boiled lentils with onions

Aduki beans and winter squash with kombu

Hummus spread for bread with lettuce

Tempeh

Salmon

White meat fish

(Whether these high protein foods were used by Sun Hee depended on whether she was favoring the Gerson or macrobiotic diet in each phase of her recovery. These foods are forbidden on the Gerson diet and are acceptable in moderation on the macrobiotic diet. In general Sun Hee used these types of foods rarely or very occasionally as she recovered from stage IV ovarian cancer.)

SALT and OIL

In the Gerson world salt is forbidden, and oil for cooking is also strictly forbidden. Flax oil is used as a dressing on salads. (See the book *Healing the Gerson Way* by Charlotte Gerson for further details.)

In the macrobiotic world a pinch of salt is added to many dishes and sesame oil, dark sesame oil and olive oil are commonly used for healthy people, though oil is sometimes restricted for cancer patients. (See *The Cancer Prevention Diet* by Michio Kushi with Alex Jack for further details.)

Sun Hee generally observed the Gerson dictum of no salt during her recovery from ovarian cancer, with the exception of using miso—which is not allowed on the Gerson protocol due to salt and soy content. Miso does contain some salt and is derived from soy—though it is no longer "soy" in my opinion, due to the transformative fermenting process that creates a beneficial probiotic culture.

For myself and others in the family—sometimes we used a sprinkle of gomasio as a condiment on brown rice dishes. Gomasio is a mixture of 16 to 20 parts roasted sesame seed and one part sea salt, ground together in a suribachi. Sun Hee generally refrained from use of gomasio.

LEARNING BEYOND THE BASICS

When you have mastered these Paxdieta Healing Recipes, and are looking for more variety, you may want to learn more in the realm of macrobiotic and Gerson recipes. For this purpose we suggest that you acquire these three impressive books full of healthful recipes:

Healing the Gerson Way by Charlotte Gerson and Beata Bishop
The Changing Seasons Macrobiotic Cookbook by Aveline Kushi and Wendy Esko
Mayumi's Kitchen by Mayumi Nishimura

PAXDIETA PREVENTION PLAN

The two charts which follow attempt to summarize what it means to combine wisdom from the Gerson and macrobiotic traditions to create another way, which we call PAXDIETA (peace diet). Thus the PAXDIETA PREVENTION PLAN evolved naturally and grew because Sun Hee and I had experienced the benefits of both systems, but found several critical incompatibilities. In the end we were not comfortable living within the restrictions of either the Gerson or macrobiotic traditions.

In particular we did not like the Gerson rejection of the beneficial probiotic culture called miso and the Gerson heavy use of the potato and very light use of brown rice. We preferred regular use of miso soup and regular use of brown rice, millet and barley with less use of the potato. The evidence for the benefits of miso soup and brown rice is strong in the macrobiotic literature.

At the same time, we did not like that traditional macrobiotics has not embraced a serious raw food juicing program and use of coffee enemas for detoxification for those who are suffering from serious degenerative diseases such as cancer. The benefits of these practices are very strong in the Gerson literature.

The two charts which follow show PAXDIETA, the middle way between the Gerson and macrobiotic traditions. It is this pathway that we now follow for ongoing prevention and continued good health.

Paxdieta Prevention Plan - Food Guidelines

GRAINS (3 per day)

Oatmeal (with apples or raisins)
Brown Rice
Corn on the Cob
Barley
Millet
Rye Bread (w/o salt or sugar)
Multigrain Bread (w/o salt or sugar)
Soba & Udon Noodles
Pasta and Pancakes (avoid if sick)

VEGETABLES (10 per day)

Carrots, String Beans
Broccoli, Bell Pepper
Cauliflower, Celery
Summer Squash, other types
Onion, Garlic
Watercress
Collards, Kale
Daikon, Red Radish
Tomato
Lotus Root
Lettuce, many types (esp. romaine)
Parsley, Cilantro
Chard, Bok Choy
Beets
Cabbage - Red and White
Potato, Yam, Turnip
Note: Eat two large salads each day

PROTEIN (1 or 2 per day)

Lentils or Aduki Beans (occasionally)
Other Beans (occasionally)
Chickpeas or Hummus (occasionally)
Plain non-fat Yogurt (regularly)
White Meat Fish (occasionally)
Salmon (occasionally)

SOUPS (2 per day)

Variety of grain & vegetable soups
Vegetable soup with miso
Hippocrates special soup

DRINKS (typical serving 8 FL OZ)

Carrot Juice (1x per day)
Carrot/Apple Juice (1x per day)
Freshly squeezed OJ (4x per week)
Kukicha Tea or Barley Tea (4x per day)
Peppermint Tea (2x per day)
Green Leaf Juice (1x per day)
Spring Water (4x per day)
(Adjust to season and activity level)

AVOID THESE FOODS

CANNED FOODS
PROCESSED FOODS
CHICKEN
BACON & EGGS
BEEF
HAM and PORK
SEAFOOD
HOTDOGS
BUTTER and CHEESE
MILK and SOYMILK
POTATO CHIPS, ETC
DONUTS & PASTRIES
COMMERCIAL BREADS
SUGARED CAKES
ICE CREAM
CANDY and SUGAR
COFFEE and SALT
HARD LIQUOR
SUGARED SOFT DRINKS
MSG and ADDATIVES

Many of these foods clog
arteries & cause constipation.
Therefore, they are best
avoided to reduce risk
of developing *heart/artery*
and *digestive diseases* as
well as *obesity, diabetes*
and *cancer.*

FRUITS (2 to 4 per day)

Stewed or Raw Apples
Stewed or Raw Pears, Plums
Peaches, Papaya, Kiwi
Mangoes, Oranges, Persimmons
Cherries, Grapes,
Bananas, Tangerines
Cantaloupe, Honeydew
Dried Apricots, Raisins, Prunes

COOKING STYLES

Steamed - little water, low flame
Blanched
Water saute
Saute with sesame or olive oil (rarely)
Baked
Soups: simmered
Boiled
Raw salad/ flax oil, or olive oil + vinegar

QUALITY

All food should be organically grown

Paxdieta Prevention Plan compared to the Standard American Diet—some examples:

PAXDIETA PREVENTION PLAN	STANDARD AMERICAN DIET
(natural, organic, whole food)	*(many processed food products)*

WATER
Pure well, spring or distilled water

GRAINS
Organic oatmeal with apples or raisins

Organic brown rice, millet, barley

Organic soba or udon noodles

Organic artisan quality whole grain bread
with a few essential ingredients

Organic saltless brown rice crackers

Organic wholegrain pizza with vegetables

Corn on the cob with umeboshi plum paste

VEGETABLES & FRUITS
Organic fresh salad with many
ingredients - with olive oil or flax oil

Organic fresh vegetables of many
types - raw or cooked

Vegetable soup seasoned with miso

Organic baked or boiled potato

Organic sweet potato with non-fat yogurt

Organic fruits - many types - raw or stewed

Organic fruit smoothie

Organic apple - raw or stewed

Organic fresh fruit plate

Organic baked pear with prune

JUICES & OTHER DRINKS
Organic carrot juice

Organic carrot and apple juice

Organic green juice

Kukicha tea, grain tea, other

PROTEIN FOODS
Organic hummus on artisan quality bread

Organic tempeh and sauerkraut

Organic lentils, other beans with brown rice

Salmon, white meat fish
used occasionally

WATER
Tap water (has chlorine and fluorine)

GRAINS
Commercial sugared cereal with milk

Commercially grown white rice

Spaghetti or other refined white pasta

Commercial breads with 10 to 30
ingredients - added to extend shelf life

Commercial crackers with sugar and salt

Pizza with cheese and meat (typically)

Sugared pastries or cakes

VEGETABLES & FRUITS
Salad and commercial dressing with sugar

Vegetables grown with pesticides and
chemical fertilizers, often frozen, canned

Commercial canned soup with salt and sugar

Potato chips with salt, sugar and oil

Ice cream made with dairy and sugar

Fruits grown with pesticides

Ice cream made with dairy and sugar

Glazed donut

Canned fruit cocktail

Chocolate candy bar with sugar

JUICES & OTHER DRINKS
Sugar sweetended sodas or fruit juice

Alcohol - numerous types

Commercially made beer

Coffee with milk and sugar

PROTEIN FOODS
Hot dog on commercial bun

Hamburger on commercial bun

Commercially raised chicken

Feed-lot beef raised with antibiotics
and growth hormones

Appendix VI

Reflections on Health

Health is a creative process
requiring keen insight and disciplined actions.

Keen insight means a sound set of principles
that are based on scientific reality and/or sound tradition.
It means that one is constantly learning, integrating
and adjusting based on new insights being learned.

Disciplined actions mean that one has developed
good daily habits and that through self-discipline one is
able to implement a program, which is in turn
supported by a sound set of principles.

Through daily eating we create ourselves.
The food and drink choices we make largely
determine whether we will be sick, weak and depressed
or healthy, vibrant and happy.

There is endless insight, love and creativity that can go into
cooking and meal presentation as well as all aspects
of dwelling in a home. The culinary and domestic arts
are critical for good health.

Insight allows us to appreciate and discern Truth.
Love inspires us to appreciate and generate Goodness.
Creativity allows us to appreciate and produce Beauty.
All three are essential for health.

If we are doing things right, ultimately beauty
and love will shine through—as true health is naturally
expressed as a profound and comprehensive
sense of beauty, love and peace.

A healthy person is good-humored and
well-mannered, peaceful and joyful, taking delight
in the beauty all around us—and at the same time working
to solve the many problems that confront
humanity and the planet.

". . . for when you go to sleep you come over here and you counsel, and our chore has been to help you hear yourselves, to let yourselves be energized and moved in your hearts, your souls.

"Well, you have truly danced the dance of angels over here; you have felt a new electricity, and you have declared permission to shout your truth, to sing your songs."

—The Spirit, "Dr. Peebles," to the authors

"An old soul is nothing but a very *slow* learner."
—Dr. Peebles (his favorite joke)

TO DANCE
with ANGELS

TO DANCE with ANGELS

An Amazing Journey to the Heart with the Phenomenal Thomas Jacobson and the Grand Spirit, "Dr. Peebles"

DON & LINDA PENDLETON

ZEBRA BOOKS
KENSINGTON PUBLISHING CORP.

ZEBRA BOOKS

are published by

Kensington Publishing Corp.
475 Park Avenue South
New York, NY 10016

ISBN 0-8217-3755-4

First Zebra trade paperback edition: June, 1992

Printed in the United States of America

For each of you, with loving allowance for your own personal plateau of acceptance; communicated with respect; directed to your own cognitive center of self-creation.

DON AND LINDA PENDLETON

This book is especially dedicated to the memory of Paul S. Weisberg, M.D. (1932–1989) who has gone on to a larger practice of love and healing. God keep.

Acknowledgments

A manuscript is not a book—it is little more than a hope and a promise, competing with thousands of other manuscripts at any given moment—so the authors warmly thank Walter Zacharius and Roberta Grossman, chairman and publisher respectively at Kensington/Zebra, for quickly seeing the promise of this work in its potential effect upon human affairs, and for moving boldly forward to make the work public.

And we could have asked for no kinder hand from heaven than the one that sent us Lydia Paglio and Ann La Farge, our delightful editors, who brought forward enthusiastic hearts, great talents, and fine sensitivities to the material. Their contributions to the final shaping and presentation have greatly enhanced the work and made the reading of strikingly "different" material far easier.

Of course our most profound thanks go to all of those named within the book who voluntarily stepped forward with direct contributions, putting aside their rightful veils of privacy in a purely selfless sharing of personal experiences and/or convictions. Special thanks also must be given to all the beautiful "friends of spirit" who facilitated our access to printed and recorded material and provided warm support all along the way.

Our family took part in the endless discussions of spirit and spiritual psychology with openmindedness and interest. Cindy Stephens Steele helped us transcribe miles of tape, allowing our more direct labors to move a little faster, and all gave unstintingly of moral and intellectual support. So our gratitude must here be expressed to Bob and Cindy Steele, Eric and Frances Stephens, Rose Abrams, Michael and Jennifer Dalto, Stephen and Ellen Pendleton, Derek and Erin Pendleton, and Jeff and Melinda Margulies for sharing our enthusiasm.

Thanks also to "Joseph" and "Susan" for sharing some special moments with us.

The adventure has brought into our lives an ever-expanding circle of friends, and each has touched our lives in very special ways. We'd especially like to mention the gang from the Gathering Place: Connie, Mark, Doug, Steve, Nita, Sue, Susan, Sally, Maria, Jay, Pamela, Summer, Lionel, Henrietta, Danielle, Lee, Carol,

Gary, Jefferson, Arnette, Jack, and all the others with whom we pleasurably interacted over the months.

And we send big hugs to our friends on the spirit side for their inspiration and direct communication, without which the book would not have been written.

Contents

Introduction

Do you often have the feeling that an unseen presence is guiding or influencing your thoughts or actions? Do you sometimes awaken in the night with an eerie certainty that someone or something has been there in the room with you—something not exactly human? Have you ever looked up from some private task and thought for an instant that you saw a flesh-and-blood apparition of a departed loved one, or perhaps felt a gentle touch upon your head or shoulder? Do you feel that you have guardian angels, that prayers are frequently answered, or that you often receive information that is not available to you through any of the five senses?

We are here to suggest to you that such feelings and experiences can be very real and entirely valid, and we hope to offer you understanding and encouragement that you may further a meaningful relationship with the wide universe of spirit.

Or perhaps you are merely curious about life in general, who you really are and where you really are, where you came from, where you are headed, and why. Maybe you have been feeling lately that you are going nowhere, that nothing seems to mean anything, that life has come up empty for you or that it is in total confusion.

Possibly we can help you with all of that too. First you need to know that you are not alone in any of this. And then it may be helpful to realize and understand that the earth experience is meaningful but also playful, serious but also humorous, and that you have eternity to work it all out—so maybe you can be encouraged to relax a little, lighten up, and enjoy the process.

A wise old gentleman whom you will meet in this book has told us: "It is impossible to have humor without the ability in a given situation to see beyond one single truth. If you are going to understand your own sense of humor—or lack of same—just go into multiple truths and you will discover the natural humor of the universe—which, in fact, is only wisdom—wisdom that is expressed, that embraces the multiple points of view. And then what can you do except laugh?—at yourself and at others."

But of course laughter in and of itself is not humor. A fine sense of humor can sometimes make us weep, for there is pathos, too, in all humor, and "the natural humor of the universe" touches us in all its aspects. Who wants to laugh their way through life anyway? Inappropriate laughter is more often than not the sound of appalling ignorance and/or fear. We hope to encourage you to honor your tears as well as your joy, to honor the human experience in all its ramifications, and to honor yourself first of all.

We undertake this task with a lot of help, so we are not alone—and you approach it in very good company, so you, too, are not alone. Recent Gallup studies have shown that most forms of mysticism are on the rise and growing quickly among middle-class Americans. In that same vein, the University of Chicago's National Opinion Research Council recently released the results of an eleven-year study that shows that forty-two percent of American adults say they have been in touch with the dead. That same study produced the surprising suggestion that some twenty million of us have experienced profoundly mystical experiences, including healing. But your good company is even stronger than that. The Gallup studies reveal that fully ninety-four percent of Americans believe in a supreme being and that a great majority feel that they receive supernatural guidance in response to prayer or other spiritual communion.

Perhaps your next-door neighbor never talks about such things, but that does not necessarily mean that he or she would not love to do so if given the opportunity. If you feel that way too, you are not alone, and you need to know that you are among a strong majority in your feelings and intuitions. In this book we attempt to encourage you to give free rein to those feelings and intuitions—and more, to give yourself the nobility of freedom to chart your own exhilarating course through life.

Our debt to science and its noble practitioners is so great that one hesitates to venture a word of criticism—but scientists are merely men and women like the rest of us. They err, and they have limitations, imposed by their own approaches to truth. It is not criticism but merely a statement of the obvious when we say that scientists throughout the modern age have tried to discourage and discredit the persistent and growing human fascination with mystical values. Since the scientists to whom we usually turn for answers have pointedly avoided the subject and placed themselves outside it (because they cannot investigate it under their own ground rules), there has developed throughout the world a great unexpressed yearning for some substantiating evidence that life is meaningful beyond the moment, that human existence is the result of something more than the chance combination of chemicals, and that human destiny is strongly intertwined with some worthwhile cosmic purpose.

We hope to give you comfort in the knowledge that you are among a swelling majority of twentieth-century men and women who have a strong curiosity about their place and their role in this magical marvel called *life*, who want to know where they came from and where they are going, and who want to learn how to make the most of what they've brought here with them.

We also wish to suggest that you have come to the right place to begin or extend your search.

Welcome to our magical, wonderful world of spirit. And may you never be the same again.

yearning for some approaching existence that ... is measurable,
beyond the moment, that human existence is the result of obscuring
more than the mind's compulsion to ... ... and that ...
identity is among ... ... and ... worthwhile compulsion
you ...

We hope to give you caution in the truth that you are
among a swelling majority of twentieth century men and women
who have a strong ... to know where ... ... in this
... ... where they are going and who want to know how to find the
... ... help with this.

We also wish to suggest that you have come to the right place
to begin to extend your ... ...

... ... part of a wonderful world of spirit and may
you ... be the same again.

1

The Adventure

Begins

*"There is no death; there is only change.
There is no failure; there is only growth."*

Dr. Peebles

The adventure began on a cool and misty spring evening in Southern California as six of us arrived in three cars at an exclusive seaside neighborhood and searched for parking spaces along a narrow hillside lane beneath towering eucalyptus trees. We regrouped in the drive of a fashionable home tastefully set into the flora of an urban forest and chatted nervously about mundane things while taking final inventory of a miscellany of tape recorders and their supplies.

We had been waiting two months for this appointment with spirit. We were four women and two men—ourselves the only married couple. Our interests were diverse. Helen was in her fifties, widow of a top security consultant who had traveled and lived throughout the troubled Middle East for many years, a lady of considerable sophistication who was facing the prospect of growing old alone and was now seemingly filling her days in a search for spiritual enlightenment. She was accompanied by a lifelong friend, Bea, who apparently had come out of mere curiosity.

Susan was a longtime friend and had come with Linda and me. Very pretty, late thirties, Susan was recently divorced and still a bit numb from that trauma. She, too, was a searcher and lately had been experiencing some troubling psychic phenomena; she wanted to talk to spirit about that.

Joseph was another old friend who lived in the vicinity and had elected to meet us there. He is an entertainer, musician, singer, songwriter—and very good at it—but that is just what Joseph does to pay the rent. The real business of his life is the search; and he is the quintessential searcher. He has been into every awareness gag and consciousness nook that has sprung from the California collective in recent years; Joseph has meditated atop thirty-foot poles and walked on glowing coals in the search for that truth with the capital T. We invited him along because we knew he'd love a one-on-one encounter with spirit, and also because he'd been having relationship problems of late—and if that is not the business of spirit, then what is?

Why were Linda and I there in that nervous group at Palos Verdes? Well, you see . . . we had a professional interest. We are novelists, and I had lately been writing a series of novels with mystical slants, so this kind of material qualified for the research budget. But that is not why we were *really* there. We were there because we, too, wanted to encounter spirit one on one, and we'd decided that this could be the place to do that.

We had heard Dr. Peebles twice on a KABC-Los Angeles radio show called *Open Mind,* a three-hour late-Saturday-night weekly happening hosted by Bill Jenkins and guaranteed to open the receptive mind or close it forevermore. Obviously the show was opening a lot of minds—or else there already existed legions of open minds in that broadcast area—because it was a top-rated show and Bill Jenkins was among the most popular radio personalities in a town bulging with same.

Linda was fascinated by Dr. Peebles from the first time she heard him on *Open Mind.* I was impressed, too, sure, and I even grandly condescended the judgment that it didn't matter whether he was legitimate or not because he had such beautiful thoughts— like, you know, judge the tree by its fruit, not by where it has planted its roots.

We took to arranging our social lives with Saturday nights free so we could stay home with Bill Jenkins and his *Open Mind,* where we were regularly treated to UFO contactees, crystal freaks, astrologers, psychics, and all the court jesters who have migrated to the southwestern United States in recent years. In all fairness, Bill had a lot of interesting people on the show. It was, after all, conceived as an open forum of ideas—what could be more healthy than that in a democratic society? But far and away the most interesting guest, to me, was Thomas Jacobson and his spirit sidekick, Dr. Peebles.

Thomas would go into trance, see, right there in the studio, and bring forth Dr. Peebles. Now Thomas is an engaging guy, very bright and articulate and interesting, but this guy Peebles was spectacular. He always appears with a rush of words delivered in a loud, clear, ringing voice that rises and falls in eloquently expressive patterns, almost musical in its color and richness. It is a late-nineteenth or early-twentieth-century voice, one that you would associate with the lectern or pulpit, cultivated during a time when a lot of store was placed on projection and elocution, a time before modern electronics and power amplifiers.

I love the voice, yes. I could sit and listen to that voice even if its content were drivel. But this voice does not deliver drivel. This voice delivers pure wisdom and a consistency of view that stretches across every conceivable subject; it delivers warmth, great wit, compassion, and nobility of spirit to all those listeners of *Open Mind* as well as direct personal counseling to those who are lucky enough to get their call in before the switchboard is flooded. Thomas sits there, in a trance, for two hours or more while Dr. Peebles takes the calls and waits out the commercial breaks, kids with the host and keeps the radio audience alternately awed and chuckling.

I wanted to check out the guy in person, sure. Besides, I owe it to my readers of mystic fiction to stay up-to-date on this stuff. And Linda was fascinated. That is why I was there.

Linda was there because she already knew the truth about Dr. Peebles. She knew it much earlier than I did. But I was about to get that truth, too, in probably the only way a guy like me can get it.

Thomas Jacobson met us at the door wearing a sweat suit and running shoes. He's a good-looking guy about six feet tall, weight around two hundred, with clear hazel eyes and a warm smile—maybe just a bit shy or self-conscious about the whole thing himself. I pegged him at maybe forty years old, give or take a couple—about the same age as Joseph. It turns out he was thirty-eight—close enough. We shook his hand as we filed inside (introductions by first names only) and stood in that early discomfort of invading a stranger's home until he led us through the sprawling house and tucked us into his study, made us comfortable, and helped us plug in our recorders and get it all ready. Then he sat down on a simple, hard chair, closed his eyes, and went to work.

Ten minutes later my aching chest reminded me that I was

forgetting to breathe. I'd meant to be very objective about the whole thing, to watch my companions for their reactions, to analyze Jacobson's body language and other physical actions; instead, I couldn't even remember to ventilate my own lungs. Not that there was anything spooky going on. This was not a séance. The room was well lighted, snug, comfortable. There was not even a table to tip—no crystal balls or Ouija boards or spirit trumpets. There was just this very nice-looking guy sitting there in a sweat suit with his eyes closed and hands folded on his lap, nothing moving but his jaws and lips, talking like God.

But there was a presence in that room, a presence that none of us had brought and which had not been there until Thomas Jacobson went into trance. It was dynamic and electric, and it affected us all. Joseph's mouth had fallen open at Dr. Peebles's first words and remained that way until it was his turn to ask a question; he was gawking like a schoolboy at his first circus, visibly affected and shaken, as was I. Soon, though, as the personal interactions began, there was as much chuckling and giggling in that room as awed hush. Spirit has a great sense of humor, and great wit. George Burns, I realized, was well cast as God in the movie "Oh God." Spirit kidded us, lovingly chastised us, praised us, taught us, counseled us—individually and collectively—and tried his best to make us understand ourselves.

He told Joseph, for example, to stop being a metaphysical tramp. Not in just those words (Spirit is kinder than that) but he told him that the end of all wisdom is to bring life closer together, and that he needed to lay off the search for truth and concentrate on his relationships. That scored big with me.

Spirit told Helen that there is much in astrology that has substance but that also there is much in astrology with very little substance. He told her that mental depression is a belief that one has no options, no power, a feeling of helplessness—a feeling of death—a subconscious desire for death to avoid responsibility—that deep depression is a mental form of suicide as self condemns self—that certainly it can be related to biological activity, too, chemical imbalances, but that those chemical imbalances are motivated and created by self. The therapy, he suggested, is to realize that life is endlessly full of options, that power is self-created, and that death is not the end of anything but an awakening to more responsibilities, more options, endless life. I liked that one too.

Spirit told Susan that she was picking up psychic static because she had closed off other lines of communications with life—that she is too contained, too quiet, thinking that she is playing it safe by turning away from human relationships—and that now what is happening inside her is like a nuclear activity, and that inward movement has become like an explosion, and it should be, so that the passion of her soul and her heart comes into life again as never before, so it is for her to be as lava in a volcano, to let herself come out of her body. How? Through self-expression, by expressing her feelings and interacting intimately with life. I bought that, too, because I know Susan and what she had been going through since even before her divorce. But Thomas Jacobson did not know Susan except as a stranger who appeared at his door in the night and introduced herself by first name only. Same for Joseph, for Helen, for all of us; but the guy had us nailed.

Bea declared that she had no particular question in mind. Dr. Peebles replied with a twinkle in the voice: "Well, then, my dear, we have no particular answer in mind." Spirit does not invade, you see; you have to ask.

I won't tell you what he said to Linda and me because it is too personal and there is no way we can disguise ourselves as we have disguised our friends by changing their names. I will say that he nailed us one hundred percent and forever changed the way we think about ourselves, our lives, our reality. But this book is not about us; the book is about you—so I must deliver fair warning at this point: You read further at the risk of learning the truth about yourself. Some people cannot handle that. If you are one of those, please put the book down and walk away.

But as Dr. Peebles would say, you shall inevitably face that truth someday, somewhere, so you may as well get it over with and get on with your business . . . your very, very important business of life.

It is paradoxical that all mankind yearns for world peace yet cannot get along with the neighbor next door; that all mankind prays to God and bargains with God and yearns for the touch of God—for comfort, for inspiration, for understanding—yet cannot feel that touch when they need it most; that all mankind, even those who are most isolated within themselves, reject the idea of their own mortality and dream of life eternal but scoff at anyone who offers evidence that the dream is more than a dream.

Linda's three-year-old grandson, Brian, gave us quite a lesson in humility the other day. He was looking at a photo of his great-grandfather, who died some years ago, and he asked Linda's mother, Rose, some direct and penetrating questions, as the young do best. "Where is your grandfather?" Brian asked Rose.

She smiled, understanding his confusion over relationships,

and explained to him: "He was my husband, your great-grandfather. He is not with us now."

"Where is he?" Brian persisted.

"He died," Rose replied quietly. "He is with God now, in heaven."

"How did he get there?" continued the prosecuting attorney, boring in for the whole truth. "Did he drive his car?"

Rose laughed, searching for the answer on a blank wall of her mind, then she bent her arms and flapped like a bird, gazed skyward, said nothing.

Brian lost interest immediately. "Oh," he said, in closing, "my dad does that all the time."

Mundane stuff, Brian; you bet. No big deal about flying from here to there, not anymore. Routine event. So is dying. So routine that it does not command the interest or even find a model in the three-year-old mind. Heaven could be no different than Cleveland or Disneyland to our Brians. And death has no meaning to them. They may cry if Dad flies off to Cleveland or Disneyland *or* heaven without them, but the tears are tears of separation, not of tragedy, and the mental model of Disneyland for Brian is of roughly the same quality as the mental model of heaven for Rose.

Rose does not know with any sense of certainty where her John has gone. She cannot see him, touch him, hear his laughter, feel his hand upon her cheek—she has but a vague and shadowed trust or hope that he does still exist somewhere in some form and that she will join him there one day. But she is in precisely the same boat as little Brian when his daddy flies off to St. Louis or Kansas City or other esoteric and unimaginable places.

It occurs to me that all of us are in the same boat with Brian but in a much rougher sea. We do not even know where we are, or why, or where we're going, or how, or even whence we came.

Wouldn't it be nice to know? For *sure?*

So please come along with us beyond the illusions of separation, where self meets self . . . and where self meets God. It is, as the good doctor will tell us, the only business at hand.

If you are still with us, then welcome to the adventure. Our initial meeting with Dr. Peebles, related above, occurred on April 8, 1987, in Palos Verdes Estates, California. We did not directly encounter Dr. Peebles again until June 1, at which time we had intended to state our interest in writing about him and to request his permission and active cooperation. But he already knew about it, and he had some ideas of his own to contribute. We set up a series of interviews and went to work. The result is what follows.

The adventure has begun. It is now up to you to say how far it shall travel. The future truly is in your very own hands.

2

Doorway to

Intimacy

*"The object of all knowledge is intimacy,
and intimacy is love. Ultimately, all is
God."*

—*Dr. Peebles*

Thomas Jacobson is a most engaging man—bright, articulate, open. He's a bit hard on himself, in a humorously self-effacing way and, I think, a bit troubled and undecided about the phenomenon within him. He is brilliant, make no mistake about that, and he could do well on his own as a spiritual teacher and therapist, which may partly explain the discomfort he sometimes feels in the shadow of Dr. Peebles. By and large he seems to have accepted the situation and is appropriately awed by it, but still there are moments when obviously he would like to assert his own identity and get some credit for being more than a ventriloquist's dummy.

He is much more than that, and he deserves recognition as a remarkable man in his own right. Born in Ohio and raised in the small town of Rochester, Michigan, one of three sons of a Congregationalist minister, he experienced a normal American upbringing. Don't be fooled by the "minister's son" idea. He had about the same exposure to theology as any kid who attends church regularly, perhaps not even as much. His dad left theology at the workplace, never imposing it at home, and though Thomas grew up with love and admiration for his father, he confesses that he was never really turned on by the traditional approaches to God.

He did develop a great love and feeling for music early in life, however, and began focusing on that as a career interest while a junior in high school, even though this meant turning away from an almost equally strong interest in athletics. His primary instrument was the clarinet, with emphasis on the classics, and he later earned various prestigious honors and scholarships for advanced study. Midway through his second college year, however, he realized that he was heading into a career as a music teacher and this was definitely not what he wanted to do with his life.

Trouble was, that decision was an entirely negative realization, bringing with it no motivation whatever toward another kind of work. He felt confused and "de-fused"—totally adrift with no direction and no point to his life. A counselor suggested that he try a short stint with the military—as a good place to regroup and redirect his energies, develop some self-discipline—so Thomas joined the marines and served for two years with the marine band at Parris Island, South Carolina.

He came out of that experience more confused and adrift than ever. He tried college again; tried falling in love; tried work as a policeman, as a salesman, tried a variety of unsatisfactory pursuits before coming to grips with his real problem: the realization that he was a bum and a drifter and that he always would be unless he could find some *meaning* to life.

He had moved from disinterest to agnosticism to a vague atheism. He felt utterly alone in the world, disconnected from any meaning or purpose, disconnected even from himself because he could not believe in anything.

That can be a rather jarring place to find oneself at the age of twenty-eight. So Thomas committed himself—committed his life, in the real sense—to the discovery of something that he could believe in. This quickly translated into an experience in agony. He withdrew in every possible way from the world he had known, worked at menial jobs for a pittance, barely enough to support minimal physical requirements, and became a seeker of truth. He read voraciously and gave himself tirelessly to every opportunity, every opening for personal growth and understanding.

As a result of one of those openings, he bound himself as a student to a group seeking spiritual enlightenment via meditation and direct inspiration through trance states. His teacher was a man who claimed to be a trance-channel for a discarnate entity. Thomas was not so sure about that, but this teacher "spoke wondrously" while in trance and Thomas came to the conscious decision that it did not matter where the teachings were coming from—he would not worry about that; he could suspend doubt long enough to absorb the teachings and come to a decision later as to where they were really coming from.

I believe that Thomas is still—at times anyway—suspending that decision, even though he has had spectacular success as a channel himself for the past eight years. Dr. Peebles has informed me, speaking through Thomas's own mouth, that Thomas chose his name (before birth, as do we all) as a constant reminder of his doubting nature—and Peebles also has spoken with loving understanding of the stubbornness of his channel.

Thomas's success as a channel did not come easily. During the course of an interview on June 1, 1987, he told Linda: "I had made the decision that if I was going to do this, I was going to go all the way—and all the way meant exploring mediumship on purpose, because I felt that if I could have a spirit inside me, it would not be theoretical anymore. It was an amazing time, and also the most painful time in my life. Dr. Peebles had told me [through another medium] that he would be coming through me when I was ready. I just said 'Sure' . . . I wasn't even convinced at the time that he was coming through *him*. But I was taking these classes, a series of guided meditations in which we were merely trying to open ourselves to the possibilities of mediumship.

"These were group classes with ten to fifteen people in the group and a couple of so-called mediums as guides. I think I was challenging something to happen, not really opening to it, and that's why it was so painful, because I was really torn inside, wanting it so bad but at the same time demanding evidence before I was ready to receive evidence.

"I gave it up many times—you know, just gave up and walked away—'okay, that's it, to hell with it,' and I'd walk away, but always being drawn back to try again. I really hated those classes. I felt like such a jerk. But then I began to get these experiences—physical experiences, like involuntary contractions in the solar plexus. I didn't make a big deal of that either, though, at first—it was very subtle—but I was told later that they [the spirits] were preparing me at that time, working with me on my breathing and . . . other internal adjustments.

"I was still very skeptical—there was this push-pull inside of me—love-hate, attract-repel, I was like a yo-yo going out and back, out and back. It was very painful. But I was committed to finding *meaning* to life—because if there was no meaning, then I just didn't give a damn—but I didn't really trust the experiences that were leading me to meaning.

"As for those meditation classes, there were two people who were supposed to be channeling for the class. No way, as far as I was concerned at the time, were they mediums—or was anyone a medium for that matter. Just to let you know my frame of mind at the time, I felt so embarrassed for them; I could hardly stay in the class—everything I saw was embarrassing to me personally—I just couldn't *buy* all that stuff—still there was the battle inside my head.

"But see, at this point everything was still theoretical—it was all mental, analysis. These 'spirits' kept coming through [the mediums] and saying 'bless you' and all this lovey-dovey stuff—I mean I couldn't hug anyone, not even a woman, much less a man. I was so isolated inside myself without even knowing it.

"So I was in this class and weeks would go by and nothing would happen, I'd just listen to these two crazy people, embarrassed for them and everything, and still nothing had really happened right up into the last week of the class. So I decided to give up again and I knew this was final. Either it really wasn't real, or at least it wasn't going to happen to me. I mean I came to that right there in class.

"I vividly remember what a deep feeling that was, of giving up. And at that moment—a very emotional moment—I had the strongest contraction I'd ever felt. I mean it was huge—like being hit in the solar plexus with a big hammer—a very strong contraction, almost like vomiting when there's nothing there to come up—with a force . . . as though this huge wind were coming out of me.

"I knew everything that was going on, and . . . he said his name was Ordin and started trying to talk without much success. It was just these guttural sounds. It was awful. You think I was embarrassed before, you can imagine now—I was *so* embarrassed. People told me later that I had turned beet-red. But I didn't seem to be able to stop it. In a way, it was exactly the phenomenon I had been looking for, but then experiencing it—even though it was phenomenal—it didn't really change anything for me. I still had the doubts somehow.

"So that's an example of a series of experiences where I got evidence and it really didn't prove anything, didn't make any difference for me. I was so embarrassed while it was going on. It was so crazy sounding, like my IQ had suddenly gone down to forty. I joke about it now—it's like I wanted Socrates to come through, and instead . . ."

Ordin was the first spirit personality to come forth for Thomas. There were others, as he renewed his resolve to master the technique, but none much more satisfying than that first experience with Ordin. And it did not always work.

Thomas continues his story: "I kept trying, and started with meditation groups in peoples' homes. We were all experimenting together. I would put myself in position and it would happen a little bit, then a little bit more, then I would close off and it would stop— a real tug. It went on like that for quite some time.

"Eventually it reached a point where people were coming pretty much to hear me, I guess, to see me in trance, and it seemed like just about every other time I'd sit down, get ready for it to happen, there would be nothing, not a thing.

"I was furious. I finally went to talk to Dr. Peebles [through another medium]—angrily, I got real angry with him—'What's going on? How could you do this to me? If this is real, then why isn't Spirit coming through? I'm sitting there, people are waiting to see me, and nothing's going on, you're not there. Why is it vacant all of a sudden?' "

Linda: "Okay, so at this point he was already coming through?"

"No, not Dr. Peebles. I was talking to him about these other, whatever they were, coming through. And he just smiled, inside William [the other medium], very patient and benign, as usual, and he said, 'Well that's exactly why we're doing it . . . so that you understand that it is not you doing it; it is us.'

"I guess I sort of surrendered and relaxed into it deeper after that, and the improvement was rapid from that point on. Several different ones started coming through with pretty good regularity. Ordin, and then this female . . . called Miriam . . . and that was my next humiliating experience. 'Cause she would come through . . . I couldn't even believe it, because at this time I was not only totally aware of what was going on, I remembered everything afterward. It was just as we're talking here now; there were no shades of gray. And she would come in and . . . I was used to this big powerful thing, and instead this was sweet, gentle, a soft little thing just gradually building, at first so subtle that I wasn't sure anything was really there. But it kept growing and glowing—real slow, though, it was just the opposite kind of experience . . . drove me crazy. The feeling moved into my mouth and started going into this big, huge, ridiculous ear-to-ear grin . . . not the grin of a beautiful woman, to me, but more the grin of a moron, you know, in an insane asylum —oh, God, and . . ."

Linda: "And what kind of voice did she have?"

"Oh, it's got to be the highest female voice in the history of mankind. So high; I mean you'd think—I thought to myself at the time: 'Miriam . . . I mean you'd think you'd have a little consideration for my—for me here. I mean, you know, why does it have to be all the way like that?'

"Well, those were my lines of thought. I just couldn't handle it. She was never able to come through for very long because I was so . . . so chauvinistic, and such a jerk about it. She's around me to this day, and I still can't handle it. It was the first I became aware, I guess, that I—well I guess I am a male chauvinist. I can't handle it just because she's a female, I guess.

"So . . . that happened, and then Dr. Peebles started coming through—and I was afraid of that . . . because of the comparison with William . . . he would come through and say, maybe, five words . . . barely . . . I mean not him barely but me barely letting him come out, through me, and that was even a greater battle than all the other battles. I did not want him coming through me. It would be ridiculous. I just didn't want it to happen.

"I wanted it to be some other spirit, not Dr. Peebles, because William was already channeling Dr. Peebles. I didn't want the comparison—and I thought . . . well, it would seem so obvious to some people that I was taking it on just because I'd heard it coming through William—and there would be all these comparisons.

"But over a period of about a year he kept coming on stronger and stronger, so I just quit fighting it. And I asked him—I didn't like different spirits coming through—it was as if I were being ripped up and down and it was very uncomfortable—so I asked Dr. Peebles to fix it so I could just have one spirit coming through, and that's the way it's been."

That is the way it has been, indeed. "Doubting Thomas" has apparently become a favorite channel for Dr. Peebles, although he does continue to work through many other mediums around the world. George Meek, an East Coast researcher, refers to Thomas as "one of the clearest windows [to the other side] in the world today."

We purposely set it up so that Linda would conduct the first direct interview with Thomas as Thomas. Then it was my turn, a short while later, to converse directly with Dr. Peebles. It was quite an experience, and I found myself stammering through the early part in almost total subjectivity. He was patient with me, though, and gentled me along with warmth and humor until I could settle down and ask the questions I had prepared. I still found myself often wandering from my own format, diverted by things that he had brought forward. It is such an electric experience—a truly intimidating confrontation—that sometimes the mind almost glazes over in the attempt to handle what is going on there.

Despite my nervousness and the total flight of my professional objectivity, we did get some amazing stuff in that first interview. It had been my intention to begin with very mundane subjects and work gradually into the deeper material. However, as you will see, the very first "mundane" question elicited a response that became very deep very quickly. I transcribe that for you here:

DON: Could you describe for us, as you understand it, as it is from your point of view, the process that we all now know as trance channeling, and give us an idea of how it really works?

DR. PEEBLES: The state of trance is accomplished by any personality of life on earth suspending self-interest, suspending one's self-image, suspending one's own drive and passion. Trance channeling, or the state of trance, is an automatic and natural space where different zones of time and vibration converge into a powerful explosion. The explosion is so rhythmic and so equal in its mathematical relationships that the point of contact—the human mind and heart, for example—is almost sung to sleep, is induced into a state of calmness, of sleep, of total acceptance of another being, another presence, another point of view. There is no greater love in life than the doorway through what is called trance. This is accomplished, for example, in your day-to-day lives through sleeping at night, night sleep; when you go to sleep you are going into your own deep trance, by suspending significantly your fears of the day, your self-interest of the day, your assumptions of the day. Thereby you enter in an act of love, of intimacy between yourself and the universe, yourself and the rest of the planet Earth, yourself and other points of view. You surrender into contact, into oneness, through merging yourself with the rest of life. Obviously this is activated through certain beliefs, self-created—even illusion, if you wish, of safety from the rest of the world. Ironically, what takes place is that self becomes intimate, becomes one with the rest of the world, as a result of sleep, in your astral body and in your spiritual mind. Trance is also accomplished in daydreams, precisely the same as that of sleep, but with a little bit less surrender. This is a state of invention, problem solving, innovation, reevaluation, where one's points of view are again suspended or laid aside or at least relaxed for a moment, and through the doorway of the imagination and the house of fantasy come forward new structures, structures that can become reality if the conscious, cognitive mind chooses to present them to the physical world. Because in the state of daydreams, approaching sleep, there is less and less demand by the critical mind for exactly what you were talking about, Don—less demand for the validations, for the credibility, and more for faith or simply fun in unusual points of view. And that is when true problem solving, invention, insight, become successful. As well during the state of orgasm and after the state of orgasm, in sex, physical sexuality, is a state of trance. Again the result is intimacy, contact, oneness, surrender of self—a pattern, a vibrational pattern that is so equal in its mathematical proportions that the point is lost, the self-image is lost, for a moment, and there is union of the astral body with the universe; it is—a fertile ground then is created; and immediately after the orgasmic experience, as well, is a time of great insight, great invention, and, of course, healing. Do you understand?

DON: Yes, I do. And beautifully put. Thank you. That is quite a remarkable insight into the mechanics of sleep.

DR. PEEBLES: It's a fascinating study for even greater depth, because again, Don, you see . . . people fall asleep either because of their exhaustion from resisting or fighting the world, or desire to prove self to the world—the exhaustion is so great that even fear is bypassed or overcome—or more readily, more often, it is because fear is suspended long enough to surrender sufficiently into a state of love, of bliss, but . . . because one is in the bedroom and doors are locked, they feel safe. Well, the challenge of life, the magic of life, is how can you create that same attitude out there in public as well as in your bedroom. You'll have the same results, that good feeling you have after you've had a good night's sleep. That is intimacy, you see.

DON: Yes, yes I do. It brings up another interesting question. Is this why infants will fight sleep so hard?—that will to remain conscious—does this have to do with fear or unwillingness to surrender?

DR. PEEBLES: Yes. Both. Newly upon the planet Earth, in some cases it's a drive more than a fear, to be awake, to be alive—"Let's get on with it! I want to be fifteen years old now, not fifteen months old." It's a genuine excitement, more often than with the adult. However, on other occasions it is a fear—a desire to crawl back into the womb—

and to crawl back through the womb to the spirit, upon the newly born. However—again, more often than not—the infant and the child are in a state of sleep, you see, are in a state of trance, the soul slightly projected from the body, floating around, eyes asleep, the nipple of Mother in the mouth, a feeling of security and love, an understanding that Earth is a place of contact—"for here is my mother, giving of herself to me. I feel held, I feel warm. Earth is not just a place of survival," the spirit says to itself, "but a place of love; here is my mommy." And as discipline comes into childhood—more often than not from the father—then life becomes more real in some ways but also the spirit and love become less real. And this concept is something that educators and families will concentrate on more readily, more directly as the years and decades pass. But more often than not, the child is asleep in a state of trance as a bridge from the spirit world and trying to come alive, trying to be more and more awake and in the body. You understand me?

DON: This is why in infancy the sleep periods are much longer than they are in adults?

DR. PEEBLES: Yes, exactly right. As the spirit comes forward . . . if the child was not able to have that state of trance and extended sleep, in many cases a psychological disorder would come forward and become so prevalent that there would be a psychological suicide or an actual death —suicide in the physical body—for Earth is a jarring experience for the spirit coming forward in the way that birth is taking place in some so-called civilized societies, and as birth becomes more gentle—the use of water, the use of sound and soothing environments—the bridge will become more rapid and the result will be the need for less sleep in the child. And they'll become more alert more rapidly, you see.

LINDA: What effect, if any, does difficult natural childbirthing, where there is a lot of pain, have on the baby and the mother?

DR. PEEBLES: The difficulty of natural childbirth, all right, let's see here . . . well, to address this is first to address certain implications inherent in the question, I believe, Linda, and that's the nature of pain. We see pain as a blessing, not as a curse. It's a signal to create change, and to identify resistance.

It is quite possible to bear child in a—as you call it—

a natural state with very little pain. It's all equal to degree of resistance on the part of the mother—fear of failure and so forth—and upon the part of the child coming forward —fear of life—and, according to that mixture, there is pain.

Use of anesthesia, chemicals, and so forth, to minimize and put aside the pain, is certainly an act of love, but in effect it reinforces in the child a priority of avoidance, avoidance of pain, avoidance of confrontation, avoidance of directness—very subtle influence but relevant nevertheless.

So we encourage natural childbirth with proper supervision. There would be spiritual counseling before that birth regarding the nature of life and death, relationship between child and parent, where parent is a hostess and a host more so than a mother and a father feeling responsibility to sculpture the body that is about to come forward.

There would be a clear spiritual discussion about the purpose of birth unto Earth, and so forth, all of which would equal a much greater sense of relief, and thereby a desire to release and surrender rather than to resist, so that the muscles of the abdomen and the body are used with the intention which is to facilitate the entry of the child into the world.

This muscular activity is resisted more often than not, and so it is experienced as pain and trial instead of joy and love.

LINDA: So the use of meditation or the Lamaze method with the breathing—natural childbirth methods—that just helps to—

DR. PEEBLES: Absolutely. Whatever pain might be taking place is a healthy, important communication that both the child and the mother are cultivating and aware of before the fact. I believe your original question was phrased from the point of view of the child—"Is the pain of childbirth traumatic to the child?" Well, the answer is yes, it is traumatic. But it is healthier for the child, in the long run, to allow the pain of birth, whatever be its level, to manifest, to take place.

So often the child has come forward—you know, we see some human beings walking around for years in a mild dream state, in part affected by the anesthesia given at birth. You understand me.

DON: There is another effect that is frequently noted—that is the baby who cries all the time, literally, night and day. A whole new branch of pediatric medicine is developing around this problem. Puts a tremendous stress on the household because it seems that nothing can induce these infants to stop crying. This syndrome is often given as the cause of some child abuse—apparently some parents go a little crazy with this incessant crying for about the first six months of life—so it is a serious problem. Could you comment on that?

DR. PEEBLES: Yes . . . if you were able to engage these children in verbal discussion, you would find that they are living out nightmares, nightmares within the soul before they were born. As statisticians and professionals in the health field look at numbers of children with this effect, there is, of course, a desire that it have some chemical or biological source, that is understandable.

Whatever such source might be there, however— when the child cries constantly and no physical reason is obvious—is only subservient and responsive to the spiritual psychology, a dread of life, a belief that there is nothing outside the nightmare. And then the greater experience of physical reality, a change of reality within the body, magnifies and exaggerates the very same nightmares.

A possible resolution of this problem is for the mother to be guided into her child as a translator or facilitator between the healer and the baby—to understand that the mother's mind can enter the child's mind. That entry, with proper guidance by a therapist, can bring forward clear emotions and stories as if that child were an adult, so if a therapist communicates with that level of awareness, then within a period of, oh, thirty days—sixty at the most, I believe—there can be total resolution of this condition. The child would for the most part stop crying, and within sixty days if not sooner. You understand me.

DON: Yes, thank you. I think that may be very helpful to a lot of people. The figure I have heard is one in ten children suffering this problem.

DR. PEEBLES: Yes, well, it's about . . . four in ten are souls who have lived often on Earth. Another two or three out of ten are souls who have lived on Earth before but not too often, relatively new, and the other two or three are souls incarnating for the first time. The one out of the ten who live inside these nightmares are more often than not the middle range, those who have lived less frequently on Earth but are not new nor old, experienced on Earth, and are in a state of shock, feeling that they are in the midst of some kind of unfair punishment by having to reincarnate again.

To the disbelieving mind who might read these words or hear them, this would sound as fantasy, of course, but I say if you apply the process prescribed with sincerity you will find clear results of success. Not a hundred percent, for there is free will within the human, within the soul, no matter what the age.

DON: So the mother should try to engage the baby's mind with her own mind—

DR. PEEBLES: Yes. For example the mother will hold the child to her bosom and there would be loving and firm suggestion, tones, that the mother surrender her self-image and regress herself into her own womb, during the time of labor.

When she begins to live that out, then the therapist will more likely than not achieve some real success in helping the mother project her mind into her baby, at which point the therapist can take the child backward to a moment just previous to incarnation into her womb. The child will then be encouraged to see the light of Earth through Mommy's womb, and to allow that light to pierce the nightmares brought from the spirit side.

Then the child can be brought forward into a reenactment of birth—through soothing sounds and images that reveal Mommy's great love for this being, for has she not given of herself that this soul may journey again upon the earth?—does he not suck at her breast and enjoy her total care and devotion?

These movements of the mind, through Mommy's loving heart, will clear away the fog and allow the child to wake up to the light of day on Earth. It will be successful more often than not. There will be exceptions.

Some of these children, for example, believe that they are in eternal hell. They believe they are in a region of the universe which, according to previous beliefs, is eternal damnation—and so how could they possibly believe that they are finding love and nurture? They believe that they are just going through another part of hell here, through their mother. It's a terrifying experience within themselves. That is one example. You understand me.

DON: So these babies are actually frightened.

DR. PEEBLES: Petrified, yes. It is a crying of the soul, in other words, not just of the body, as some would prefer to believe.

DON: We need to talk about this more at a later time, maybe as part of an in-depth look into the problems of early childhood. For now . . . could we talk a bit more about channeling? How do you know when Thomas is ready for you to come through him?

DR. PEEBLES: Well, if we waited for that, you know, we might never come through! So we don't wait until he's totally ready; we wait until he's approaching that . . . oh, as long as three minutes, while he is trying to fully dislocate . . . uh, disassociate from his experience, his physical experience, then we come forward. Ask Thomas about this —he has a pattern, a series of inner movements he makes that would be interesting to you, that are very specific. When he's completed that last particular movement, we have an agreement—we're very aware of it—then we come forward, but he's not totally gone yet. We have to . . . we assist him out of the body by the force of our presence. That's accomplished through union, not disregard for Thomas, it's a very deep love affair. He is held— he is, uh, as a child in the bosom of mother—he is taken and held in great love, he is nurtured and invited to another vibration.

DON: So it's not a matter of him just being nudged aside.

DR. PEEBLES: No, it's not force. No, it—it's a—I'm not the only one here. There is myself, Dr. Peebles, but there are other beings and teachers here, and some of them work solely with the channel. Others work with the people in the room, such as the two of you, to help you go into a state of trance so you hear a larger depth of truth . . . about self, you see, and the world. Otherwise it might be difficult; so, everyone's lullabied a little bit—you, and my channel, and even ourselves; we all just relax and come together.

DON: Sounds wonderful. That partly explains, then, the almost total subjectivity I'm experiencing here; I'm being lullabied. Well, it's a nice experience. Thank you.

I have been asked to clarify something with you. Some of us have difficulty understanding how it is that you and other spirits seem almost at the beck and call of the channels—that is, the instant availability that allows a channel the confidence to schedule an appointment and assure someone that the spirit will be there for them. I have been asked about this. People wonder if this doesn't somehow interfere with Dr. Peebles's life or process or whatever is happening in the spirit world, or are you always instantly available for this sort of thing?

DR. PEEBLES: Well, first of all, for the vast majority of spirits it would be an interference. Correct. Most are not involved with the planet Earth but are involved with their own lives, and it is best that they not have anything to do with the planet Earth; quite correct.

Whoever said this, they are—there is accuracy, there is truth in their belief, their statement and question; however, there are a few spirits, such as myself and others, whose life *is* communicating with earth. That *is* my joy; that *is* my day and my night; that *is* my greatest joy. It is both my greatest recreation, greatest pleasure, and most extraordinary growth, to continue to communicate with the planet Earth, and so it is not a detour or an inconvenience, it is a blessing, it is an act of love.

It is a total love, and to come forward at what some humans would call the beck and call is in fact merely an act of love on our part.

We *want* to be there. Why would we want to hurt or disappoint anyone and not be present when they call upon us? We want only to be loving and to respond and to be available and it does fit, in our case, to *our* life which is communion with the planet Earth.

It is further of value, for any soul who asks this question, and a reasonable question, why would they think— why would they ask a question in those words where there would be a suspicion for a spirit to always show up, to always be available in love?

So when someone asks that question, they must look into their own life. Do they have a fear of always being available to someone?—at their beck and call? Do they call it beck and call and feel it as demand?—and when they become more loving enlightened, instead of feeling they are being called and "becked," will they instead realize that it is the greatest experience of life to respond . . . to respond to life, not to remain separate? Do you understand?

Yes, I understood that I was conversing with a being who could not be offended by impertinence or disbelief. This was almost like a conversation with God, and he was being so patient with me, so lovingly patient, allowing the dumb questions and treating them with respect the same as a sensitive father sitting down with his little boy to straighten out a misunderstanding.

I have found this to be characteristic of Dr. Peebles. He is not defensive, nor is he offensive. He communicates with respect, and he is always as direct as is possible when discussing difficult concepts. Another characteristic is the consistency of his message and the character of his thought, no matter what the subject. There are no direct contradictions anywhere, though the conversation may range from theology to quantum physics to classical metaphysics, and he often synthesizes spontaneously from several different disciplines in making his points.

My biggest problem throughout has been to remain objective and to question realistically from a human intellectual point of view instead of continually nodding my head and saying, "I see." What he has to say is always so totally sensible, so thoroughly packaged, that you're always being challenged to ask for more than he is giving. I always feel totally relaxed and at ease in his presence, but I also feel totally awed much of the time. It is, yes, somewhat like a dialogue with God, but Dr. Peebles would reprimand me gently for saying so.

3

Illusions of

Separation

"The greatest illusion is that you are alone; never are you alone. The second greatest is that you are unloved; you cannot escape love, for it is the invisible essence of all things."

—*Dr. Peebles*

Faith has been defined as a willingness to believe without proofs or evidence. Skepticism is the opposite case. A true skeptic will insist that any inquiry into truth must be a process of doubting, and he will demand overwhelming proofs and evidence to support even an obvious conclusion.

"The sun is shining today," I declare.

"I doubt it," replies the skeptic.

"Look out the window," I suggest.

This is where we sometimes get into trouble. A reasonable skeptic will look out the window, note the sunshine, and become a believer. But not all skeptics are reasonable. Suppose the skeptic demands that I bring the window to him before he will consider changing his point of view. Or suppose he involves me in a pedantic discussion of the meaning of the words *sun* and *shine* and *today*. Or, as the worst case, what if he goes to the window to check the truth of my proposition just as a heavy cloud moves in front of the sun? He may never believe me again about anything. "Don lied to me, told me the sun was shining; it wasn't. Don't believe anything that guy tells you."

Everyone reading this book knows a skeptic and probably has operated from the skeptical point of view from time to time. We all do it. Often we are not only skeptical but also downright cynical, especially in the areas of politics and commerce. It becomes a learned point of view. Aren't we usually somewhat skeptical of product claims in television commercials, cynical about campaign promises? We learn to be discriminating, don't we, because we grow accustomed to being misled—and it is simply common sense not to accept everything we hear on faith alone.

We even begin to equate skepticism with intelligence, and sometimes our skeptical reactions are primarily to guard against being thought a fool. The Smothers Brothers have raised this type of reaction to high art, the one brother being cast as something of a half-wit but still smart enough to think that the other is trying to make a fool of him and so he is constantly on guard, skeptical of statements which would be perfectly acceptable to any intelligent person. With the Smothers Brothers it is hilarious comedy. In real life this brand of skepticism is anything but funny.

The true scientist is also something of a natural skeptic, necessarily so because of the dictates of his profession. This form of skepticism can also be exaggerated, however, with similar results. If the scientist demands that I bring the window to him, then refuses to look through it except with a device that blocks sunlight, how am I to demonstrate to him that the sun is shining? If you took a camera into the deepest jungle and wished to demonstrate the miracle of photography to a witch doctor, how could you convince him that you had actually captured his image inside the camera if he demanded that you develop the film in broad daylight with the whole tribe looking on?

Skepticism is a natural and healthy exercise of human consciousness, but it can also mislead and defeat us when not exercised intelligently. Just as skepticism is not synonymous with intelligence, science is not synonymous with truth. The entire history of science has been revolution, not evolution, with today's "truths" becoming tomorrow's lunacies and vice versa. What many scientists do not bother to tell us is that "faith" is the true engine of science, skepticism merely the brakes. The "scientific method" does not produce scientific breakthroughs, it merely verifies them after trying its best to discredit them.

Even in its purest form—as a means to evaluate knowledge—

skepticism is mere negativity. That's okay if it is exercised intelligently and with a desire to learn the truth. It is not okay if the skeptical attitude is merely a mask worn by a closed mind trying to hide from truth. This closed-mind form is what we had in mind when we raised the question with our friendly Spirit. It bears directly on any discussion of the "illusions of separation," so we wanted to discuss that aspect first.

DON: You've always been most patient and thorough when responding to skeptical or merely curious questions, uh . . .

DR. PEEBLES: Certainly; because the skeptic truly is the lover who wants to understand. The skepticism is worthy of attention but not as *the* priority.

DON: He's just working through his blocks, in his skepticism?

DR. PEEBLES: His fear of being in love. Uh, his or her. It is more often *he*—those *males* of the planet Earth—hear us, hear us! It's time to experience more of the female inside you! Go ahead and shake and quiver at the concept, but open to the female inside of you, my friends. There is a magic place, as yet not taken advantage of, understood, and expanded to its greatest power. The experience of skepticism is a—really!—a soul who's afraid to fall in love, afraid to let passion overcome him and who almost desperately wants to stay in control of everything within him and around him—and skepticism becomes a brilliant, perhaps subtle technique to maintain that state of control. So it's really not intellectual, it's really not an exercise of the intellect, it's really not even a state of disbelief; it's a desire, a plea, in times of desperation, to maintain control; and the fear of falling in love is one of losing control and then finding oneself alone again through rejection. You understand.

DON: Yes, I do. I would like to make note of the fact that there has recently been established in this country a professional organization of skeptics who have taken it upon themselves to shoot down the various phenomenal ideas and interests in the public mind. Could we interpret this as being a mass defensive mechanism . . .

DR. PEEBLES: Yes, it is. And really the numbers are very small. The organizations around the world, religious and otherwise, who wish to understand and who do believe, are a thousandfold more numerous, and that's because the truth lies therein. The skeptic—again, however—is the lover—

we love this organization. Indeed, it has been somewhat through the inspiration of the spirit that they have organized themselves, and we support them in their work; for this will prove to themselves their own passion. They will realize that they are not objective, but instead they have passionate points of view that they wish to maintain, and through their collective reinforcement they will become increasingly clear and honest about their own bias rather than demanding to isolate the bias of another. Furthermore, it's their way of coming to God, and it will lead them to God, because the truth is contained within the spirit, within God, the magic of life—so they are accelerating their quest and they will find the truth, one by one by one.

DON: So you see it as a positive movement.

DR. PEEBLES: Yes, yes we do. That doesn't mean we're going to address them in their terms all the time. Sometimes, yes; not all the time.

DON: I would think that probably many people who think of a spirit teacher would have an expectation that a grand Spirit such as yourself, or a spirit teacher, would be almost totally concerned with theological issues. I'm sure you know what I mean. Would you care to comment on that?

DR. PEEBLES: Yes, uh . . . the spirit that wishes to teach and to learn is concerned with truth . . . truth as translated through the human mind, and the philosophies of the universe—or as some might see it, the physics of the universe. What are the relationships?—one particle to another particle? What is their give and what is their take? What is their response to each other? The relationship between the smallest of particles is relevant and reflective of the relationship from one human soul to another, for example. And so it is impossible to avoid the philosophy of life, or the physics of life, when one quests—one wishes to understand God. There is no other search. All activities of life, be they the business or commercial world, be they the educational world, be they the world of the child, or of the elderly, the ill, the handicapped or the healthy, be they criminal—each and every one of them is a search for God. There is no other subject. All subjects are contained therein. So the higher perspective, if you wish, is a little more direct about that. You understand.

DON: Yes, thank you.

DR. PEEBLES: Theology is the search for God, to know the

purpose and meaning of life. Translated, it is the belief of God translated by mankind. It is worthy of greatest respect and reverence; however, mankind all too often finds not only permission but comfort in delineating and isolating and intensifying illusions of separation rather than diminishing the same through the search for God. It is a great paradox, similar to the great paradox that all humanity craves intimacy, in one form or another, and yet for all humanity that is the greatest fear—intimacy. It is the paradoxes of life that can be studied to understand higher truth.

We would like to add the observation that the issues of skepticism and faith often have that contradictory context as well, most notably when one has been exchanged for the other and from one extreme to the other. Saul of Tarsus, for example, persecutor and bitterest enemy of the early Christians, was "converted" by a remarkable personal experience on the road to Damascus and, as Paul, became the virtual founder of the Christian Church and staunchest defender of the faith. As the opposite case, consider anyone you know who has been betrayed by love and now is cynical about romance.

Both skepticism and faith are dependent upon one's perceptions of meaning and purpose in the world about, and are the reactions to those perceptions. The mainstream of modern psychological thought tells us that the way we perceive the world, as well as the way we react to those perceptions, is produced from childhood models of reality which often are greatly distorted and can produce inappropriate behavior in the adult.

When Dr. Peebles speaks of the illusions of separation, he is referring to a basic, all-encompassing and all-pervading state of consciousness that perceives, identifies, and defines the world in which we experience being at this moment. This world we inhabit is very real—no illusion—but our perceptions of it create the illusion that our world is composed of material aggregates that exist separate and distinct from one another when actually there is no such separation, no real distinction, except in consciousness.

Our particular form of consciousness operates at a frequency of being that resonates with certain aspects of the total universe but not with all aspects. What we perceive, then, is limited to a narrow band of effects and we never glimpse the true cause of anything. Imagine the effect if you were seated in a darkened drive-in movie with no screen. You would see only a beam of light passing overhead and disappearing into the distance. If you turned and looked behind you, perhaps you could note the source of the beam as it flows from the lens of the projector, but you would be hard put to explain the beam as anything but light if you had never seen or heard of a movie projector. You would be even harder put to infer a forty-million-dollar collection of Hollywood talent and expertise that infuses that light with purposeful activity.

That beam of light is actually just that and nothing more, a beam of light, but a beam with certain programmed interruptions and discontinuities that will appear as reflected patterns of light and shadows that seem to be constantly changing pictures of people and objects if someone erects a screen to intercept the beam. The genius of Hollywood is realized upon that screen, diffused into nothingness without it.

It seems that our brains function somewhat as a movie screen making sense of a flow of energies in which we are totally immersed. What results is called consciousness, but it is a limited consciousness because our "screens" do not react to the total energy available. We therefore experience distortions of the total reality, and the particular limits within which our consciousness operates cause us to draw certain incorrect conclusions as to both the nature and the source of the experience.

Some of these conclusions are what Dr. Peebles has in mind as the illusions of separation. It is a difficult subject, hard to grasp, maybe even harder to believe. But let us try.

DON: When you are present, Dr. Peebles, expressing through Thomas, are you actually here with us?

DR. PEEBLES: Oh very much, yes.

DON: You are sensibly aware of the environment?

DR. PEEBLES: Well . . . some difficulty there, Don. I—it's—I'm really locked into this body, and so I don't visually see you. When I'm out of this body I don't visually see you as you see each other. I see energy patterns and waves, like heat off hot tar, but with color and change and movement —panorama, panoramic. In my channel I see blackness. However, I work with other spirits, and I am able to sense you through *some* of my channels . . . oh, you might call them psychic, sensory ah . . . ah . . . doorways of his brain, of his mind. This is where the channel can be very valuable, very important, very significant.

DON: We have noticed in the past when you have been counseling an individual that often they will be across the room from you, while Thomas's eyes are closed—and they are perched on the edge of their chair and almost wringing their hands as you speak to them, pursing their lips and preparing to break in, to speak while you are speaking, and we have seen you pause, evidently aware of their desire, and give them permission to speak. Is this . . . is that an example of the psychic sensitivity?

DR. PEEBLES: Yes. It is not because of any physical vision. It's because between all life there is connection, there is synchronicity, there is a field of energy that is disturbed or affected by every movement and every thought—and the thoughts, the emotions behind the physical wringing of hands or pursing of lips is much stronger and . . . the thoughts and emotions have a much more dramatic effect on the field of energy than physical movements. And so in turn, it's like I'm on the end of the rope over here, and the rope is being shaken—and I can feel it, you see.

DON: Yes. Thank you. Uh . . . we know you here as Dr. Peebles. And apparently that is how you were known in your last previous incarnation on earth. Is that how you are known by your contemporaries in Spirit?

DR. PEEBLES: Oh, hah! I didn't think you'd ask that so quickly, Don! Yah, you're way ahead of the game here, aren't you? All right. Let's see here. . . . We're going to wait a little while on that one.

DON: Okay.

DR. PEEBLES: I'm not sure we want to talk about that *too much* in your book. It might become a distraction. So . . . please . . . keep the question and please ask it again . . . some other time. I want to talk with some others about that.

DON: Okay, we'll skip that for now.

DR. PEEBLES: You might want to keep it simple right now. Dr. Peebles period. But we'll see.

DON: Okay. We have noted—

DR. PEEBLES: But you're right in what you are feeling. There's lots of other stuff going on. I am Dr. Peebles and I am many other things.

DON: Oh, very well, thank you . . . uh, Linda and I have both remarked on your amazing ability to show intimate knowledge of a person just from a first-name identification. Could you discuss how that works?

DR. PEEBLES: Well, there are several patterns here. First, when people give their first names, they . . . uh . . . in subtle ways . . . are unlocking their own selves. When you say your name, Don—in fact right now, Don and Linda, in a moment—not . . . just a moment, I'll ask you to say your names and *feel* the energy change inside you and around you as you say it, as if you are introducing yourself . . . you are opening yourself, you are opening your . . . ah . . . your vibratory channels and always revealing yourselves in energy as you say your name. Now I perceive and wish only to perceive and receive that information your soul will give. We have no desire or need to enter into the center of a soul without self-revelation from that soul, so even though it be unconscious, nevertheless the soul of the questioner begins to reveal itself, saying in effect to the spirit: "All right, Spirit, now's the time, here's the part we want the conscious mind, the personality, to hear . . . to look at . . . to think about . . . to be confronted by, even, albeit in pain . . . here's the free association, the free memory . . . and do with it what you will." So it is that which is offered by the soul of the questioner more so than what we offer that unearths from beneath the soil a hidden stone. Now, without question it takes . . . some skill, and particularly love for an entity —whether it be a discarnate spirit or incarnate spirit—to respond and translate and apply and, ah . . . to suggest proper relativity between all the diverse information, to be sure. But it's all really an act of love. Do you understand?

DON: Yes. Thank you.

DR. PEEBLES: The question is an act of love from the questioner, who loves himself and the world enough to invoke that information.

DON: It has almost the same connotation as . . . surrender, as your channel going into trance.

DR. PEEBLES: Ah, yes. So right now why don't you—as if you're introducing yourself—just say your first name, Linda.

LINDA: Linda. [Very quietly.]

DR. PEEBLES: Oh, no, no, do it again. Little more—little slower, [kiddingly] a little more sincerity there, Linda! I am Linda!

LINDA: I am Linda.

DR. PEEBLES: Now, did you feel any change?

LINDA: Yes.

DR. PEEBLES: Don't lie! [Spirit is having fun, here. It is blowing our minds.]

LINDA: No, I . . . felt a change from the first time.

DR. PEEBLES: So did we! Good work! [Spirit seems to have a

special feeling for Linda. The voice is always warmer and more "twinkly" when he is speaking to her.]

DR. PEEBLES: Don?

DON: I am Don. See what you mean, yes. [I am suddenly feeling stark naked, so I keep right on talking.] You know, that—that really makes me think—how difficult it is for some people to speak their names to others.

DR. PEEBLES: Exactly. [Spirit is twinkling at me now.]

DON: How some people seem to be shrinking from—from identifying. . . .

DR. PEEBLES: Exactly. Just think of the terms of normal relationships—person to person—and how others and how you say your names or don't say your names—when you say your name it's always with different notes, you might say. It's relative—if you were to record one person saying his name to twenty different strangers, twenty different occasions, twenty different days, you would not find any significant similarity between the twenty occasions. The name would be said differently each time. You would find similarities relative to the degree of vulnerability of the soul, but it's a sign that is very indicative of whatever communication is about to take place. You can anticipate it by how you say or another says the first name.

DON: Very interesting, yes. Names have fascinated me for a long time. I did a little expositional sketch in a recent novel on the significance of names and naming. When a being has had multiple lives on earth, and therefore presumably has lived under many different names, what is the significance of a name in the spirit plane? Is there another name, a spirit name, that identifies an entity for all time?

DR. PEEBLES: Sometimes. But your name in your current lifetime is the culmination of your soul. And that's in part how you chose a name for a current time. Now, when I say culmination, that does not mean inclusive of all attitudes you've ever had. It means inclusive of the deductions you've drawn, to this point, that are most relevant for you. So you are asking the world to call you—whether it's the world of the spirit or the world of earth—you are asking the world to identify you by a certain tone, series of tones, that in effect unlock the door of those toys that you want to play with most, so as grow and to learn. So, for example, my channel Thomas wanted to be called Thomas so he'd really keep looking at the doubt inside his soul— doubt about God, about himself, about the spirit, about life, about his intelligence. You hear him talk about that all the time, don't you—and, uh, and also the great compassion of Thomas, so that he will discover and feel the great compassion within the Thomas of himself, for he has been Thomas before. There are very different specific reasons for choosing a name, but it's all to unlock the door, and that continues on the spirit side as well as the Earth.

DON: As though each new incarnation represents a new plateau of development and that is now *who* the person is, who the being is.

DR. PEEBLES: Yes. It does include the past.

DON: Well, now—is the separation between the Earth plane and the spirit plane a real separation?—or is it an imagined separation?

DR. PEEBLES: Ah, very good, no, it's not real. It's an imagined separation, right. In the physics of your perception and experience you can note great ranges of diversity in sensory perceptions. Nevertheless there is a greater value in understanding similarities rather than differences, as you have inferred. So, in reality you see there is no such thing as the spirit side. There is not a spirit side. There—it's all one universe and one world with different localities inside it, and right here among physical life as you know it is interspersed spirit life, and it is according to the faculties of perception and reception of each individual as to how much they feel moved or affected by other parts of this reality called life, which includes spirit side and Earth side. There have been times, mostly in unwritten history of Earth, and in the so-called future, where that will be bridged dramatically. It will be common to communicate with Spirit as you're walking around. There are some societies in your history who have done this, who bridged that, but they were just called . . . uncivilized! That's all, you see, then everyone gets to ignore it.

DON: Uh-huh. So . . . we tend to think of life on Earth as biological life . . . but you're saying life is life whatever the . . .

DR. PEEBLES: Absolutely. Right. If anything, if one is more dead than the other, it's biological life. But that would be an unfair statement. If one must judge and compare, it would be that way.

DON: So if we insisted on thinking of separation between Earth and spirit, it would be improper to think of separation in spatial terms such as light-years, miles, hours—but it should be expressed more as a difference in vibration or frequencies?

DR. PEEBLES: Exactly—frequency, vibration. And there are a variety of localities of vibration according to the mindset of different spirits. The frequency can be very much slower than your visual color spectrum, and often it is much higher frequency, beyond your color spectrum. Uh, X rays and . . . so forth.

DON: I see. Well, on a scale of zero to ten, with man at zero and God at ten, where on that scale is the spiritual realm?

DR. PEEBLES: Well, the spiritual realm of teachers—what humans perhaps too often would call *master*—is the nine, the realm of nine. Ultimately, from the absolute highest perspective, we would have to take exception to your scale and remind you that everyone is always part of ten, everyone *is* ten, right now, no matter what their self-image, you see. But from the place you're looking, the way you ask the question, the locality of the teachers that we are, and others, it is of nine. But nine is the number of change, and the great wisdom of the true masters is not only the allowance of change, it's the ecstasy of change. For change is perceived not as separation, in a linear way, but as a voyage that is circular or spiral in nature, so that you are always participating in different realms of the divine, of ten, of God. So nine accepts change. Eight and below, to lesser and in greater factors, resist change . . . or abuse change.

DON: So the idea that man is zero and the angels are something else and the spirit masters—

DR. PEEBLES: That's the whole problem right there. That's why you're all still on Earth, because you believe that.

DON: That is still part of the illusion of separation.

DR. PEEBLES: Exactly! Right . . . and so I got to crawl along to eventually obtain ten. Well, it is to understand how you *are* ten now and you're afraid to see that because one is afraid of too much responsibility—for the misunderstanding of the true nature of love. Love does not demand—and love includes error—what you must call error. Love includes emotions and feelings that are less than smiles and joy and happiness. Love and God contain all things, you see. And so . . . forgiveness—the teachings of forgiveness, and then allowance, uh . . . have been techniques to help people quit trying to see themselves as one and two, and to see that God is ever present in self as well as in life elsewhere, even in the midst of rage. One cannot have rage unless one believes in meaning and purpose. One cannot believe in meaning and purpose unless one believes— whether they know it or not—in God, in a divine force, you see.

DON: Yes, yes. In . . . the most widely . . . taught metaphysical systems that are present on Earth, including the Neoplatonic schemes of man and God . . . they speak of hierarchies, of different realms of being . . . is this also caught up in this illusion of separation?

DR. PEEBLES: Yes, it is. But there is some truth in it nevertheless. There are realms of the spirit—or different dimensions of reality—that do operate on that basis, where spirits perceive themselves and others around them as part of that hierarchy. And so there are spirits who are loving, and who are wise . . . who operate in the realm of that hierarchy. And so these repeated insights are harbored and fostered in certain typically secret societies of mysticism, which is relevant. There is truth there, but overall that again is part of the separation, and it's only part of the truth, it's not the total truth. You see, there is a point in self where you don't need a hierarchy.

DON: We are living hierarchies.

DR. PEEBLES: Right, correct.

DON: Very interesting. We've heard of—

DR. PEEBLES: You see how he did that? *We* are living hierarchies ourselves. Very good. He just said it as if it were nothing. Brilliant, Don, brilliant.

DON: Thank you. Linda and I have been looking into the various forms of channeling since we've become aware of you —enlightened by you, I should say, and—

DR. PEEBLES: That word *should,* you know, we're not gonna use it too much anymore, Don.

DON: (*chuckling*) Okay. We have come across these various forms of channeling that are usually called something else, such as table tapping, materializations, Ouija boards, the more commonplace dreams and automatic writing and the like, but the audio channeling that we are experiencing now, with the spirit personality being so present, so dynamic, seems to me to be a really high state of the art.

DR. PEEBLES: It is. And the reason is only related to levels of fear. So you see with table tapping and Ouija boards, these forms are somewhat limited by the human's understandable need and supported desire to be in control.

DON: So you sort of have to play the game that's at hand. Right?

DR. PEEBLES: Right. It's your turf, as they say in the current lingo.

DON: So most of our restrictions in receiving spirit guidance, then, are really our own obstructions.

DR. PEEBLES: Self-imposed, right. Science can create and is going to create technology to bridge that and make communication possible, but they haven't wanted to yet. It's not because the difference is *that* extraordinary, as you suggested earlier, and it is not because we aren't there, it's because those aspects of mankind that operate in scientific ways haven't wanted to concentrate on that technology. Part of the reason for that is that science has its own pride. On the one hand, scientists want to discover, but on the other, they don't want to discover anything they don't know about. So . . . of course that varies with individuals—and on the surface it's a paradox, although beneath the surface it is not, that your less civilized cultures, historically and present day, have a closer proximity to some issues of truth, yet they are ignored, they are seen as less intelligent, you see.

DON: The so-called aborigines of Australia, for example?

DR. PEEBLES: Right. Doesn't mean they don't have things to learn. They do, but they are close to the spirit—certainly not all the realms of the spirit—but to some realms that are of great value nevertheless.

DON: It's difficult to visualize—to make a model in the mind of this . . . this reality of . . . superimposed planes of . . . I—I have to feel that you exist in some continuum that I cannot experience directly—and I have to think in terms of structure. Is the spirit world structured on lines that are similar to ours here on earth?—that is, with social institutions, governments, defined communities, families, this sort of thing?

DR. PEEBLES: Yes, it is. And as it is throughout the universe. You will never find another planet, for example, of your dimension or another, that is that extraordinarily different, as a few science fiction writers have suggested. What is going to be shocking are the similarities. Certainly—just as there are different species, different personalities, different races, so you will find elsewhere, but the similarities will be greater. So it is. The truth of the universe is that all things are one. All things want to learn and thereby they expand. As does the universe. Yet all things are one with each other, and the learning through expansion becomes a spiralic activity—albeit inadvertently at times, from the conscious mind—that returns to the center. And so, cause and effect and gravity, for example. The universe is expanding and yet there is gravity, to be closer together. And so there is always—everything is one with each other, but oneness is not everything—oneness is a state of rapture in the differences rather than a demand for the differences to change into self. Instead, self becomes in rapture by merging with the diversity that surrounds you. And so communities, villages, gatherings of people, whether in the world of Earth as you know it or in the spirit as you see it, that's the nature of things—to be together with each other, to do cooperative projects and products, to have opinions, to express those opinions, to experience the response of those opinions—that's the joy of living, that's life everywhere. That's part of exploring the constant metamorphosis of God and of the divine, through communication. Silence, of course, is hearing the communication of others, but that is as naught if there is not the ability to bring it back, forward out of self into your local environment, whether that local environment is Earth or the spirit worlds. So eventually one surrenders to that and it becomes the dance of life rather than a life of survival and competition. You see?

DON: I see, yes. One of the things that bothered me even as a child in stories about heaven is that it seemed that no one was doing anything, they were just—

DR. PEEBLES: Oh, it's very active. There are businesses, there are communities, there are projects. Some of the differences are, for example, depending on what vibratory plane you are responding to, things become things from thoughts more rapidly. So it might take two days in your experience to build a chair, where here if we want to sit we sit, with or without the chair, or there's a chair instantaneously. Or there's no need to sit. But there's a much more rapid response to thought, and the slower vibration of Earth, where there's a delay in thoughts becoming things, is by intention so that you can study the process of that. So, over here we don't need to study the process of that—it's other issues—collective work typically—over here also there is much more emphasis and gladness about collective work, where typically on earth the more people you have working together, the more problems, the more difficulty, even though there are times of celebration and joy—and that's because again people seem to believe, want to believe, that oneness or peace is accomplished by less noise, by having not any sound, by having agreement instead of disagreement. Where over here we love disagreement. Please disagree with me!—ah, we love disagreement because we want to hear different points of view.

DON: I understand. How would the spiritual communities compare with what we have as human beings here on Earth?

DR. PEEBLES: Well, for example, you would have on Earth a university which in and of itself is its own culture, its own village. You would have a village or town in a state called Montana, and another one in a country named Austria, and they would all have very distinct differences and characteristics and priorities. Well, so it is on the spirit side as throughout the universe. Like mind gathers with like mind for the purposes of loving reinforcement, encouragement, and for the purposes of loving reflection and magnification for purposes of growth.

As you fulfill yourself within one locality, you move to another. As you feel contented—or completed, rather —in one village in the world, you feel an urge to move elsewhere, to change your proximity and thereby your priorities, and so forth. So it is in the spirit world. There are many, many towns and villages, states and countries—not by your definition of same, but by collective expectation, collective desire and want, over here.

So there is great diversity. There are communities, little communities here of spirit, people who gather together to reinforce their Buddhist belief. There are others who gather together to reinforce a particular portion of their Christian belief. There are others who gather together to reinforce and explore their atheistic belief—yes, atheistic even on the spirit side—and so forth and so on.

Now, there is a movement of consciousness that humans call enlightenment. This so-called enlightenment creates an ability to penetrate some levels of consciousness and of reality, and I am blessed to be part of that environment, and we who are gathered together in this community, having lifted ourselves through and beyond the karma of life, have another experience that is more unified, more objectified, more consistent and cooperative with each other. It's one large community of light, and in that light there is a sense of freedom beyond even what words can describe, and that sense of freedom is the result of love, love of self in the light of the divine and all life everywhere, a love of learning, a love of differences, a love of intimacy. All these items tend to be the source of fear for those who have not yet achieved this state.

We are able then to move through these various villages, towns, and localities on the spirit side, as a traveler on Earth who has much means—for example, money—or other means to freely move around the world of Earth and through one culture and community and another, and so it is for us over here who you call teachers and counselors.

Now, within those villages on the spirit side, where like mind gathers with like mind, to reflect and review and magnify, there is a physical community. Unto each other within that community, they feel physical, as you feel physical to each other, because your frequency matches, and their frequency matches. When you have frequencies that match, the sensory system of self perceives it as solid, for sake of convenience. So it is over here as it is on Earth. However, it is true the frequency is of a higher resonance than that of Earth.

Let's see here . . . in these localities there are those things that you can call crime, trespass. There are those activities of sex and love and so forth. There is an overwhelming awareness of a force, or a light, an authority, or a structure within and around all these environments over here. And it is a sight to see how many souls, even with that awareness, remain stubborn, remain separate, remain disbelieving, remain hurtful to self and to others. Guilt is the greatest burden in the realms of spirit, whereas some religious and health authorities of Earth tend to think of it as healthy, for purification. This guilt drives people to be deaf, dumb, and blind . . . to their own drives, hopes and fears and wants, bias and prejudice therein.

That is where there is cultivated a need for a more striking experience of life, a school where there is a rather amplified study of separation, illusions of separation. Basically, you have what you think you want. So that is where you are encouraged, and you find yourself moving toward reincarnation, onto the school Earth.

Does this clarify, or do you wish to pursue?

DON: Yes, I think that clarifies quite a bit. What you have just been describing sounds more like just another place like Earth. This is quite contrary to the common expectation of most people in this country, who are of various religious faiths and seem to think that when they die, they suddenly become all-knowing, like God, and know everything about everything and about themselves, so now they are pure and—you're saying that this isn't quite the way it works.

DR. PEEBLES: No, not at all. When you die, my friends—when you die from the human body—you do have the encouragement and direct inspiration of friends and loved ones, teachers of the spirit world, to use as a resource. However [forcefully], you remain in control. Your free will remains dominant. And so you are able to perceive and respond to that inspiration in the way you want to. That's the stubbornness we're talking about. The desire to disbelieve the right to be loved, or the reality of this or that, can be so strong—and supported through logic—that any manifestation and experience is secondary to the drive to remain safe.

The drive to remain safe within the human consciousness on Earth is so powerful that all possible inspiration more often than not is secondary to the feeling, the desire for safety. It is no paradox, it is no irony at all, that on Earth some aspects of many religions reinforce and support that drive for safety, which again is rather contrary to your higher spiritual nature that you're trying to break into. The degree of experience at the point of death and afterward is relative to the degree of the intensity of belief or disbelief. So, for example, if you believe in hell, and that you deserve to go there—and you believe it so firmly that you are not willing to even blink your eye, then you will experience a place called hell. For a while. For the power of the divine within is so strong that you will be gathered with others of like mind, who insist on believing it as well, so you create that reality.

But if there is even a flicker of an eyelash of receptivity to an alternative, you begin to experience more light of a more objectified and consistent universe. Even when such is the case—which is the rule rather than the exception—nevertheless you find yourself moving in time and space according to your beliefs much more clearly than on the earthly realm. You find awareness much more swiftly, with much more immediacy, and you begin to become honest about your own motivations.

You choose to return to Earth again, for it's an opportunity to slow it all down and look at it piecemeal—piece by piece by piece—for you have a sense of separation between thought and the manifestation of thing, called time. So, yes, you continue to believe, for the most part, what you believed after you died. This is altered in greater or lesser degrees by real and direct proximity of inspiration, according to your own karma and dharma. You understand me.

DON: So our access to that inspiration and that learning is somewhat enhanced when we're in spirit.

DR. PEEBLES: Yes, it is. It is somewhat enhanced, but the point again is that the will of self is so large, it is so profound and so massive—and properly so—that it's a consistent experience to see human beings inspired and yet habitual in their beliefs and feelings. To study that, merely look at yourselves on Earth.

DON: So the power of our will really does create our own reality, even our own sense of heaven.

DR. PEEBLES: Yes, and when I say by intent the will is so profound and so strong, it is because your movement as a soul is to discover God within you. Not God within you as opposed to God where you believe there is lack of God in others, just God within you as well as God within all life. To do that, you must experience the results of your own choices over a period of time, and see how always there is a new morning, a new sun, a new opportunity—no matter how great your vengeance upon another, or their vengeance upon you. You understand.

DON: I see, yes. Is the astral body the body that is spirit?—or is this—is it a substance uh—

DR. PEEBLES: Not quite.

DON: What I'm trying to get at—are you able to identify one another by the way you look?

DR. PEEBLES: Oh, yah!—well . . . yes. But you would have to redefine "look." The astral body is also a subcontainer, it's also a vehicle, the physical body is a vehicle for Earth, the astral body is a vehicle for the . . . vast aspect of the spirit world, and there is a point in the evolution of the soul where that vehicle is shed as well, and there is communication in all directions, all the time, for any reason, with no demand, no expectation except the song of life. So to "look" we experience all colors of another party, and that is because we are not threatened by any one band in that color wave. And we experience colors that you don't see there on Earth. Typically we can—it's as if you were looking through your instruments of optics—we are able to see a person, another being, a fellow being, another vibration, from a distance and up close at the same time without asking them to move forward or without us moving forward. For we transpose—and I use that word advisedly—we transpose time. Uh . . . yah!—so we'll talk more about that another time. That's the physics of the spirit side. Let's leave that for another occasion.

DON: Very good. But, if I may, in that line of thought, one more . . . do you have formal entertainments such as music and the arts, or is this peculiarly a human—

DR. PEEBLES: No no no. The only difference is, over here it's all the time, and on Earth it's only once in a while and then most people don't go—we don't know why—over here it's all the time, it's one big party but it's not a party of withdrawal and suppression of the senses, it's a party of heightening the senses—how are our senses heightened?—through contact, through intimacy, through party, through different points of view, a rapture of the differences rather than a fear of them. And the sense of being God, the sense of being divine, or alive, is heightened accordingly, through collective activities or parties or celebrations.

DON: Is there anything there that corresponds to physical sex?

DR. PEEBLES: Yes. Now, again, there are different worlds here, worlds that are more fluid in their activity. It is walking into the center of another being. So, Don, if you and I were here at the same time—has nothing to do with male or female—we would walk into each other. You would just walk over here and uh, "Hi, Dr. Peebles" and you'd just step right into me. And I would not feel invaded, I'd feel expanded. Indeed, in this particular vibration no permission is requested, it's a constant activity like breathing, people are walking in and out of each other all the time. When you become part of another being, inside them, your vibration feels different. Again, enjoying the differences rather than fearing them, and it's what you translate through the illusions of separation, and parts of the brain, into physical orgasm. It's that moment of difference. When you come to sexuality, you love the difference more than ever. Over here we love the differences all the time. So there's no orgasm, it doesn't become delayed to a moment of time, you see. It's a constant bliss.

DON: Wow, you just read my mind. [Laughter.] Okay. We hear about guardian angels and spirit teachers and guides and so forth for every person that's on Earth. At least, this would be the impression that is given—that every living human being has these people—not attending, but—

DR. PEEBLES: Good, yes.

DON: So if that is true—and considering the fact that there are some four to five billion people alive on the earth today . . . uh . . .

DR. PEEBLES: I follow you.

DON: Is the atmosphere up there getting a bit crowded?

DR. PEEBLES: Well, yes—every soul, and that includes many animals, is guided by Spirit. However—what does *guide* mean and what is Spirit, and when and why? Well, guided is to be touched with love so as to be . . . resurrected . . . to experience, for example, when you wake up in the morning, a new permission, indeed a desire to be alive, where a mere eight hours earlier you may have wanted to die. You could have the most tragic of events in a given day, wake up ready to live. But it's not because your body lay inert. It was because you went into another realm, and you experienced guidance, healing, if you will, from the Spirit, that made sense of your activity and gave permission and invoked desire to come alive again. That is the purpose of guidance. We want to inspire you, through your dreams, through your subjective mind, as opposed to your brain, to say, "Oh, now, that's all right, it's all right, you've bruised your knee; now get up, come alive again— and this is how you're going to learn. What're you going to learn?—you're going to learn love, you're going to learn that you're loved, how to love others—there is no greater joy than loving others, if it includes self-respect—uh, self-love—and that's *all* it is, and earth is a school for that. So, the Spirits who are working with you are already inside that vibration. We don't really need that help. We enjoy the communication and touch but we do not need the guidance. You on Earth need it, knowing it or not. If you cannot feel the guidance, then you do not sleep. If you do not sleep, you die. Physically. You go to a state of less and less sanity, less and less presence in mind and the body. Now, however, as you talked about earlier, Don, all of us over here are not staring at you all the time, though, watching your every move, when you go to the potty, and how you make love.

DON: You are going ahead of me here, Dr. Peebles. I hadn't asked that yet, but it's on my list.

DR. PEEBLES: Well, we helped you write some of that, you know. We have our celebrations we talked about earlier, we have our collective events, and although I am in communication with earth all the time—by choice and as an honor—nevertheless I work with millions of spirits, of beings who are on Earth—and so you're pretty much left alone to your own activity, but there's always one of your council or your family on the spirit side who is going about his or her own business, who—like that rope I was talking about?—who feels a tug of the rope, typically through great pain, or request, who responds; says, "Oh, what's going on over there with Linda; let's take a peek" —and then we respond in concert, according to the nature of the problem—different spirits have their different preferences of work, respond to you during your daydreams or most often your night dreams, your meditations or your prayers. Now . . . every soul . . . is guided likewise, no matter what their belief or their energy, every single soul. The spirit community can be a little distance away from you, pretty much leave you alone, or it can be pretty close, again according to your request, your need, and your permission level. Now, Don—in the question is a common assumption that mankind and planet Earth is it, and thereby mathematically how can there be billions of souls here now, all of whom are guided by spirits—not to mention historically, and so on. But actually, you see, if you would take quintillions and cube it several times—a few hundred times—you would begin to approach the number of souls in the universe. Life on Earth, all of your history—if you took all your history and repeated it a hundred times, it still would only be a particle, represent a slight drop in the bucket, of souls and life throughout the universe. Many, many souls have come to the planet Earth and have left it, finished, done, enlightened, and are in other spheres of growth and living. New souls come— new to the planet Earth—all the time. You see, you understand. So Earth is not isolated. I know of no soul who does not have at least three guides or teachers who are in contact and aware and concerned with its activity. Well, it's just like parents. You send your kids to school, they go through different classrooms, different teachers, different experiences, and you know you have to keep your hands off—don't you?—so they can learn. You can't do it for them, can you? Then they come home and are nurtured, and go back out there and learn. And you can't do it for them. They'll come home and say, "Come on, you say you love me, Mommy, how about doing my homework for me? Then I'll know you love me because that will take away my pain." But it doesn't work, because if you do their homework for them, they're just going to go out and create the pain, that problem again, because they didn't create the solution.

DON: Individuals who have gone into a deep depression—they are really suffering a very special form of separation, aren't they?

DR. PEEBLES: They sure are; they have illusions of separation, and their fear is responsibility; they don't like and don't want the responsible world, and they have a massive separation.

DON: They are even separating themselves, probably—would you say?—from the guidance that would be normally available to them?

DR. PEEBLES: Yes, right, they have created a shell, and the therapy and breakthrough is to break that shell, to encourage them to break that shell—can't do it for them. The first step is to understand—well, it goes both directions here. One, their attention is on everyone else victimizing them, so they have to take responsibility, but in taking responsibility they in turn must understand eventually the joy of communion that only there is their life, communion with others, and if they are operating only on themselves and their own hopes and fears, they are alone, they are dead. So, again, it's both sides, it's the whole that they must experience, and pierce the veil. Healers and patients of the future will understand, will be on the one hand much more forceful, direct, and honest about it, quit pitter-pattering around—and that part of each of you that is depressed is a, uh, a chicken—uh, you see, afraid, little chicky-chatch—and, on the other hand, each deserves every ounce of gentleness and comfort, so it's both. The compassion will come forward only with sincerity only when the practitioners recognize that they, too, are depressed, that every human on this planet Earth has at least a tiny eency bit of depression, because every human being on the planet Earth has at least a tiny bit of separation, illusions of separation.

DON: This would probably apply also to destructive addictions such as alcoholism, etcetera.

DR. PEEBLES: Oh, very much so. It all fits, it all makes sense, it's the ongoing struggle to—the belief that one has to be present but doesn't want to, the desire to be alone, believing that to be safety. Which in turn, eventually, whether it is or isn't becomes a moot point when eventually one understands that there is no greater disease, no greater pain, than loneliness.

DON: If we took a hypothetical John Doe, say that he's seventy-five years of age, he's getting ready to vacate the flesh . . . does somebody in spirit world already know that his time is coming? Is there any sort of a preparation that is made for this? Or is it something that doesn't even require preparation?

DR. PEEBLES: Very good, you know, those little last comments you make—listen to yourself do those, Don, that's a doorway for you. All right, uh . . . well, it is not—it is usually not planned to the minute, although that does happen. Usually it's simply that one knows that they are probably going to want to leave—oh, in their thirties, in the middle of their life, or maybe they want to live to an exceptionally elderly age between eighty and a hundred and twenty, but that's forty years difference there, isn't it? So the free will, according to your growth patterns—presence, withdrawal—withdrawal, presence—choices that are made, relevant to that growth, dictate as to what year and what month one is either finished—what you want to learn and need to learn in this life—or you don't care if you're finished, you want to quit, and want to really withdraw, and so you invoke your own experience. So it is predestined, and yet that predestination is hand in hand with a free will.

DON: We sort of set our own predestination.

DR. PEEBLES: Right. And you can reset it when you go to sleep every night, or at least once a month.

DON: So that you're not really committed if you came in planning to exit at the age of twenty-three . . . you can change the clock.

DR. PEEBLES: Yes, because, you see, you must remember— again, capture the assumptions about time and space, where an assumption—your understandable assumption —that the human life is a long time, even at a hundred years, well, it isn't, from our vantage point it's all just the flash of an eye. And so your day-to-day activity . . . each day is the same as a hundred years. Each day can be a lifetime in and of itself. It is not a great tragedy when one leaves before they have lived, because they are still living, first of all, and they were living before it, and because in that two years they lived, sometimes they've lived more than someone who's lived sixty years; they were more present.

DON: So the process of transition that we call death, moving from the earth plane to the spirit plane, is this a lonely process?

DR. PEEBLES: That's an important question and, Don, we're going to leave right now and I'd like to ask you to ask that question first when we start again. We'd like to spend some time on that. We are going—please understand that there will be times that we will leave quickly from the channel, from your vantage point, because we want to speak only—for you, in this project—when we are fully present, to capture the depth, so as to honor your wonderful, insightful, important questions, Don and Linda, that you have assimilated. So we must leave right now. My friends, go your ways in peace, love, and harmony; life is a joy. You are the creators always, never the victims, we love you very dearly; everything's right on schedule; relax and enjoy the process, enjoy the process. God bless you.

Thomas, who places nothing in his stomach for several hours before a trance, had developed hunger pangs. Apparently Spirit knew that, was aware of his physical discomfort, so withdrew gracefully.

But he'd left us with an awful lot to ponder.

4

Transformations

"The perfect circle is an infinite line defining a finite space. Around and around you go but always in the same place. Transform your circle into a spiral, my friends, and you touch the fabric of eternity."

—Dr. Peebles

It is okay to change one's mind. It could even be wise to do so. Less than a year before our first encounter with Thomas Jacobson I had made this statement in a novel I was writing, through the major character:

Let me get something into the record here. I have never been one of that variety of psychics who dabbles in so-called spiritualism—communication with the dead—mediumship. I have attended a few séances, out of simple curiosity, and I have known people who claim a close relationship with spirit guides who are ever ready to counsel and instruct them. However, since I have also never known anyone whose life situation seemed significantly enhanced through such "contacts," I just really never had a lot of interest in any of it. I mean, I'd never met a medium with a Nobel prize or any such measurable recognition for superior knowledge. Most of them I've met, in fact, seem to be singularly unimpressive in any area of knowledge, an observation which has not been deterred by the usual self-serving double-talk and smug mystery with which they would cloak themselves. I figure, hey, you'll know them by their fruits, not by their postures, and I've never seen much of a harvest from those trees. But then, what do I know? All of life may be no more than a posture of one kind or another— and whoever said, in this modern age, that being "fruitful" is what it's all about?

By that little tightrope act, you see, I was trying to prepare my reader for some rather bizarre developments in the story while preserving the narrator's credibility. And my own. Not just for the reader's sake but for my own sake as well. I will tell all manner of lies and enact filthy deceits through various characters in my novels —because a novel is supposed to be a somewhat valid reflection of life and the novelist is forever striving toward that end—but the *voice* of the novel, that moving statement on life and its realities, must issue from the writer's own heart and mind and it must be true to his own vision. The danger to the novelist if he is not true to that vision is not only the failure of the novel but ultimately the failure of the novelist himself—and, even worse, the loss of the novelist to himself; that is, we are what we say we are (all of us who live) so the danger of saying what we do not really believe is that we thereby tend to fulfill the lie in our own image of self.

Any novelist who truly understands that game is therefore brutally honest with his vision.

I give you this so that you may understand my tightrope act with Ashton Ford, the fictional psychic detective quoted above. Ford had to be leery of mediums because his creator was leery of mediums; it is as simple as that; the "vision" of the novelist in 1986 was very uncomfortable with an area of human activity into which he was plunging his hero—*and he did not wish to be tainted by the association.*

But when a reasonable person is confronted with convincing evidence that he has been wrong, it can be a powerfully liberating and transformational act to simply say, "I was wrong."

Okay. I was wrong. I have been convinced of that. I now have no qualms whatever about being associated with spirits and mediums, and in fact I revel in that association.

I have told you something of the transformation as it was experienced in my personal interactions with Spirit, but it occurs to me now that I need to give you the inside story of that transformation if you are to believe it.

First, then, the background. Linda and I were married late in 1985, the second time around for both of us, neither of us kids—and I am fifteen years older than she. I have to give this to you straight, with no embroidery. We had both had "good" marriages, were both still fully married when first we met—but we did meet, and we did fall in love, each to our horror, and we both went through two years of sheer hell as we tried to reconcile the absolute pain of trying to deny that love with the absolute chaos and pain to others if we did not. She was married to a very nice man; I liked and respected him. I was married to a very nice lady; Linda liked and respected her. Linda had two grown children; I had six. The two families shared a community of mutual friends; our spouses knew each other; our kids knew each other. It was a mess. Worse, it was a disaster.

Nevertheless, it was beautiful. We were two starry-eyed kids when together—which was damn seldom—and two neurotic messes when apart, which was practically all the time. And we weren't kidding anyone. Everyone knew, our spouses and children included. Everyone was hurting. We were crazy. Linda began seeing a therapist and marriage counselor. I simply retreated deeper within myself, tried to get interested in my work, could not even *find* my work.

Finally the pressures resolved themselves, dramatically so. My wife requested a divorce; Linda's husband did likewise; our kids went crazy (but have survived it very well, after all); Linda and I were married at the earliest legal date. Linda's ex-husband almost beat us to the altar with a new marriage of his own and now seems very happy; my ex-wife has found an exhilarating new creative life and says she couldn't be happier.

See how well things can work out . . . if you just let it happen? Letting it happen, of course, can be an agonizing course—and though things certainly now seem to be "nice" enough on the surface, it came at a terrible price. For Linda and me, of course, it was worth the price; we cannot speak for others. Nor did we wish to speak for the others at any time during the painful processes of change. It is one thing to assume pain for yourself, to determine that you will work through it for a positive goal. It is quite another thing, however, to work through the pain of others who can see nothing positive in the outcome.

There are scars, to be sure, upon all of us. We can only hope that they will fade quickly and that the final outcome for all will be seen in a positive and expansive light.

Speaking entirely for ourselves, we feel that we both "came

alive again" (as the Doc would say) in our new reality. I created Ashton Ford and signed contracts for six novels during that first year with Linda. She resumed work on a novel she'd begun some years earlier, completed it, and wrote another. We began a collaborative novel (still in work). I created another character, Joe Copp (private eye), and contracted three novels of his adventures. At this writing, I still owe one publisher an Ashton Ford novel; another, two Joe Copp novels. I am also a consultant to a third publisher who bought the franchise for one of my earlier heroes, Mack Bolan, and is now producing twenty-four to thirty titles per year based on my characters. Linda has another novel in work in addition to the one we are writing together.

So why did either of us need Dr. Peebles? Our lives are already booked for the next couple of years. We frankly do not know how we are going to fit it all in. So why Dr. Peebles?

The answer, we think, is that Dr. Peebles needed us. We have discovered the truth that one does not argue with the angels. To show you how far we have traveled in this direction, we have even considered the possibility that somehow all of this was foreshadowed in our first meeting, that we have been nudged and tugged through all the pain and joy and confusion and ecstasy of these past few years to our recent confrontation with Thomas Jacobson and his spirit sidekick. Certainly our lives have not been the same since that moment, just as certainly they had not been the same since that electric moment four years earlier when our eyes first met as strangers across a crowded room.

In that first meeting with Spirit, back in April, Dr. Peebles told us in explicit and precise terms of the moving forces in each of our lives that had brought us to that moment, describing in uncanny detail the pain, confusion, and chaos that had marked our transition from "comfortable" lives to blissful ones. He spoke of my "second life" and of my "resurrection" as a joyful movement into tasks and challenges that could have awaited my next lifetime. (I had a near-death experience during open-heart surgery three years before I met Linda; in a subsequent session, Spirit assured me that it was not "near-death" but death itself, that I had accepted spirit counsel to return to Earth for important new work.) He told Linda that her challenge now was to "become visible" and thereby complete the important work awaiting her. (Linda is very shy, to the extent that it sometimes interferes with her revelation of self through her writing.)

Spirit told us many other things, of course, which I will not go into here, but there was no hint during that initial session that any of our "tasks and challenges" were in any way to be involved further in a personal sense with Dr. Peebles or Thomas Jacobson. But we could not leave it alone. No one, spirit or otherwise, approached us in any discernible way to involve us further—but we found ourselves chasing Thomas around from that moment, rearranging our lives so as to attend his public appearances at every opportunity and listening to his weekly radio shows. Always at arm's length during that period, we did not speak personally to Thomas until several weeks later, when we introduced ourselves following a public session in West Los Angeles. He did not immediately remember us from the private meeting in April, but he did recall a thank-you note we'd sent him immediately after that session—a note which, he said, had touched him deeply.

We saw him again a week later, on May 18, following another public session, and this time we spoke of our books and our interest in metaphysical thought. As of this moment, as Dr. Peebles is my witness, the thought had not occurred to us that we should write about this. Thirty minutes later, however, as we were hurtling along the freeway en route to our home forty miles away, I glanced over at Linda and muttered, "I think we have to write a book about this guy."

I can still see the look on her face as I said that. Linda and I have always had some sort of mental connection; call it what you will, but we frequently vocalize each other's thoughts. I recognized the tingle in her eyes as she gave me that knowing look and replied, "I know. I was just wondering if you knew."

I think what we both "knew" at that moment was that we were already embarked on a new direction in our lives. It is okay to change the mind, yes. And sometimes that can have a powerfully liberating effect.

Paul S. Weisberg was an eminent and widely respected psychiatrist with a highly successful private practice in Washington, D.C. He was a president of the American Society of Adolescent Psychiatry and one of the pioneers in group therapy. He was also a remarkably fearless and outspoken thinker in matters of mental health, as you shall see.

We telephoned Dr. Weisberg at his Washington office on June 5 for a very surprising interview, armed only with the knowledge that Dr. Weisberg had been in touch with Thomas Jacobson at some time in the past. We did not know at the outset whether his interest was personal or professional, and hoped only that he would be willing to discuss the matter with us off the record.

He was naturally cautious at first, but he was also friendly and courteous and seemed interested in what I had to say. I went to considerable lengths in explaining the reason for the call—and I talked a bit about dissociated personalities, how I had initially considered that as a possible explanation of the phenomenal Thomas Jacobson, and asked his opinion about that.

Dr. Weisberg replied that he would comment by telling me a story. He also gave me permission to activate my telephone recorder and to quote him in the book—which instantly produced fears in my mind that he was about to blow this whole thing apart with his professional opinion. Remember, I still knew nothing at this point about the nature of the psychiatrist's interest in Thomas Jacobson.

My fears were groundless. Dr. Weisberg had virtually the same story (in essence) that I had heard already from so many others. What makes his story so compelling—beyond the obvious charm and exquisite imagery—is the context from which it is produced. Keep in mind that this is coming from a noted medical practitioner, man of letters, a past president of a national psychiatric association. Here is Dr. Weisberg's statement:

My first introduction to Dr. Peebles was via my cousin, who is some years my elder, and who is a lady in her early sixties, who's just taken a Ph.D. in some branch of psychology out there in California. We've been close life-long, although we don't see each other much. She came out to Washington on another errand in December—and she called me up and we had dinner.

[During dinner] she told me, "You know, I've had therapy and counseling and various experiences in my life, but I've never had anything like this happen to me, and I find Thomas Jacobson and Dr. Peebles, who he channels, to be really so useful to me."

As I looked at her I was astonished, because she looked ten years younger, although the last time I saw her was ten years ago.

She said, "I want to give you a present. I want you to write down some questions about yourself. I want you to go into a lot of depth. Much of the stuff you will ask, I don't know about. I'll serve as your conduit, and I'll ask your questions to Thomas when I have my next interview with him."

Well, she did that, and she sent me the tape. It was astounding. I mean, it's very clean, you see, because he didn't know who I am, nothing about me, and she very carefully kept me anonymous—but when Peebles started, he started with material that had come out of my very early childhood that I remembered clearly, and remembered kind of hiding or distancing from people around me—even from my parents, who I felt would find me rather odd if I told them. I had a birth injury, and he described it in great detail, and . . .

DON: Phenomenal, isn't it?

DR. WEISBERG: Well, it certainly rivets the attention. At that time I was feeling in kind of a slump, and the voice over the tape was aware of that, and said in all kinds of ways that I should kind of get off my duff and go into the world and take the leadership role that was waiting for me, that people were waiting for my leadership in various ways that he specified. That had—it had an effect of reaching me in a way that nothing else had.

After that interview—actually even before I had heard that tape—my cousin had called me and told me the substance of it. I was already in kind of a state of expansive anticipation. When I got the tape, I sent it to my two eldest children, who are adults and living in New York now, and they listened to it. I said, "Is this me that he's talking about?"—and they both said: "He got you just right, Dad."

They were so impressed that they both called Thomas Jacobson and made appointments for themselves, and I did too.

I talked to Dr. Peebles through Jacobson. Now in the second interview, he said, "You know, I think we've already been of service to you"—and he was absolutely right. I mean my attitude had evolved and improved, to the point where he said, "You know, I feel like your older brother." He said, "You're about at the end of your cycle of lives."

And I said, "Well, what do I do when it's done?"

He said, "You'll probably come up and be like me; you have this love of Earth and love of humanity, and you'll come up and help people. Even now you are a guide when you're between lives."

The effect of his words on me was activating, like an electric charge.

DON: Everyone uses that word: electric.

DR. WEISBERG: Yes; well, I've listened to a lot of tapes since that time. I have not talked to him again but I find that now I would like to talk to him again. I've been talking about him to some of my patients, and several of them have called him and each has had marvelous experiences with him.

The point of it to me is that it brings back another reality that is as true as the realities that we perceive around us. It helps us to redimensionalize our lives in holistic ways, sidestepping egotism and reductionism, that we have tended to forget or have been distracted from.

I'm very attracted by the position on evil, that it is a distraction rather than a positive force, because to me that is absolutely right.

You see, in my life I have had two or three encounter experiences. Each one has been very much on target with the Peebles tapes. Let me just mention one: about ten years ago, after a severe thunderstorm here, I had an experience—somewhere between a fantasy and a dream—in which I was walking down the corridor of the old Senate Office Building, which is beautiful inside. It is gorgeous, with high ceilings and fine plasterwork, and down at the end of this very long corridor was a room, and in the room was an electric-blue light, and there were fifteen to twenty people who I knew and who knew me and were very familiar.

They embraced me and they seemed to be saying, "Welcome"—and then there were kind of instructions coming out of the blue haze that meant, "You have to go back. Don't worry; it's just for a little while. You'll be with us again soon enough."

That, like other encounter experiences I've had, has given me a kind of a belief system that I haven't shared, until now, with many people—and I think that millions of people are in that category . . . of knowing, of being a little ashamed and diffident about coming forward and putting that level of cognition, that level of realization and understanding, on the line—because we tend to be reductionistic, both in terms of our language and in terms of our customs.

So on a personal level, I don't believe that everything Dr. Peebles tells us is complete, but I believe that everything he tells us is true. For instance, I wrote a paper recently on neurobiological aspects of growth and development in humans, and how certain psychological factors can negatively impact on the actual neurobiology in this kind of resonating parallelism that we set up. I call it synergy and point out that human development is not defined by nature or by nurture but from a combination of the two. I believe that to be true, and I think it ties right in to the spiritual focus. I mean, Dr. Peebles does not suggest that we have to give up our intellects, but merely that we must deemphasize the reductionistic aspects of intellect, and use our minds to expand and integrate our experience in a more holistic way.

DON: Yes; I have felt for a long time that there is a wide, a very broad and deep public interest in that very thing, mainly because we have evolved into a period where we no longer find that much comfort from a pastoral concept of God, and we aren't really equipped to deal with the complexities of modern social structures.

DR. WEISBERG: Well, you know, that comes very close to something I've felt, which is that a period of major change, in terms of cognitive forms and style, comes when there's an inability of the social structure to give meaningful gratification of people's basic needs. The falling apart of the family, the escalation of divorce, the sense of anomie that has gotten so usual and regular in our society, lets us know that our margins have shrunk to the point that unless you are really quite an unusual person you don't get it, you don't get to the point of having a satisfactory and gratifying existence—and that's the point at which, you see, an enterprise devoted to major change can successfully transform our lives. It's just a matter of which one it's going to be.

Paul Weisberg appeared unconcerned about heralding a "new age" of spiritual enlightenment. He dealt with everyday realities in his work, and he told us that there is a *practical* aspect to all this present-day emphasis on spiritual awareness. We need it in the same sense that we need food, love, and shelter. It is a basic human requirement, in other words, and it is one that has been overlooked or shelved in our race toward technological modernization and complex world politics.

Political revolutions are transformational. So is anarchy. So is social malaise. Let's not wait for that kind of transformational experience. Let's go for the good. Let's try to find out who we truly are, and what life is truly all about. We think that's worth a try. What do you think?

We spoke to many interesting and interested health care professionals who have experienced personal interactions with Thomas Jacobson, all of whom responded to our queries in terms similar to the views expressed above by Dr. Weisberg. Not once did we encounter a negative reaction or anything even approaching condemnation, dismissal, or disbelief. Some told us that they used insights gained via Dr. Peebles in their professional practice, and some have also referred patients for spirit counsel. Only a few, however, were willing to state their views for this public record, and that is understandable.

One professional in particular, an internationally educated Jungian psychotherapist and parapsychologist with an impressive background in both Europe and America, spoke to us passionately and enthusiastically and at great length of her repeated experiences with Dr. Peebles, of Thomas Jacobson's "very high class" psychic abilities and his "very outstanding" sensitivity in comparing him with other psychics whom she had investigated, though she would not commit to any judgment as to the source of Thomas's information and she later asked that she not be identified in our book.

Of course we have no wish to embarrass anyone, so we killed the interview with this "Dr. X." There is hardly any value to an anonymous testimonial. We mention the incident only to emphasize the fact that this "free society" of ours still can intimidate and suppress the free flow of ideas and information. Dr. X was worried that she would be barred from access to various professional and academic forums—not in Russia, but in the United States and Western Europe. Doesn't it seem a shame that all these great minds with such brilliant insights into the problems confronting us all are afraid to speak their truths, to shout their discoveries to the world? Who, in this atmosphere of fear, is the ultimate loser? Isn't it you and me?

Ironically, perhaps, our Dr. X is a devotee of a most fearless and innovative pioneer, the great Carl Jung, who was a contemporary and one-time colleague of Sigmund Freud. In the lay mind, Jung is usually associated with his studies into what he called "the collective unconscious." He coined the term "complex" to describe emotionally charged clusters of associations withheld from consciousness but manifesting in the conscious life as mental disorders. And he instituted radical new therapies that have become the basis for various modern approaches to human psychology and psychiatry. It was Jung who delineated the two basic personality types, introvert and extrovert, and the four functions of the mind: thinking, feeling, sensation, and intuition.

Jung's colossal breakthrough came, however, in his brilliantly insighted studies of mental symbology and specifically archetypes which he felt to be instinctive patterns of a universal character that are expressed in behavior and images. Jung was one of those rare scientists (like Einstein) who saw beautiful meaning and great intelligence locked into the mysteries of being, and he was concerned throughout his illustrious career with the relationship between man and man's concepts of God. He was much involved in the psychology of religion, regarding the Christian religion as part of a historic process necessary for the development of consciousness.

These ideas are fully elaborated in four large volumes of his *Collected Works,* including an ingenious study of alchemical symbols and their influence in modern dreams and fantasies. He concluded that alchemists (building from the ancient Gnostics) had actually constructed a sort of textbook of the collective unconscious.

I personally find it both illuminating and satisfying that there are also great parallels between the phenomenon that we now call "trance channeling" and the phenomena that parapsychologists such as Dr. X characterize as psychic abilities. Certainly it must occur to them, as it has to me, that in all phenomena involving the human mind we are dealing with very imprecise terms anytime we attempt to define what is happening there.

What is "clairvoyance," for example? No one living (or dead) has ever isolated the vehicle (or natural law) that accounts for the transfer of information from one mind to another via purely mental means. What is the route? Where is it? Of what is it composed? Not even Carl Jung could offer more than a *theory* to account for it.

But where did Jung get the theory? And exactly what is the *mind* that he used to get it with? What exactly is *thought,* and what is feeling? What is *intuition,* for God's sake, and where is the connection between this insubstantial *intuition* and the even more insubstantial "collective unconscious"?

We deal with very imprecise terms. So when I am in the presence of Dr. Peebles, what does it buy me to dismiss this phenomenon as intuition, or clairvoyance, or any other *purely mental* faculty when we do not even know what mental is, or what clairvoyance or intuition are?

I respect and admire the great thinkers and innovators such as Carl Jung—but their great disservice to humanity at large, if you choose to look at it that way, is that they have given us dumber folk an excuse to freeze around a mere idea and elevate it to the status of *a priori* truth which can then be used to explain unexplainable things.

It was the vogue before science became so powerfully influential in human ideas to ascribe all the unexplainable things to God, or to some idea of God, when God Itself was unknown and unknowable—a very imprecise term in the ultimate sense.

Now that we have science to fall back on, even the scientists invoke imprecise terms to describe indescribable events, and often with all the dogmatic conviction of the religionists.

So let's put it on the table, faceup, bare, and trembling: None of us really knows exactly what is going on here in this place called life. We don't know precisely where the place is, what its dimensions are, where it has been, where it is taking us. So let's not freeze around any imprecise idea of what it is all about. With all due respect for science, its establishment, and its practitioners, let us insist that these ladies and gentlemen speak to us not from their bias and prejudice, not from the defensive mechanisms for self-preservation, not from mere speculations clothed in sanctimonious certainty —but let us insist that they speak to us with the clarity, and the humility, and the great common-sense honesty of people like Paul Weisberg—or, as the very least, stand back and let the Dr. Weisbergs have their say without fear of retaliation. Anything less disserves us greatly and runs the danger of seriously misleading the entire human movement into dead ends of deadening convention and stultifying conformity with wrong ideas.

For the only difference between saying that Thomas Jacobson is a psychic who is tapping the collective unconscious, on the one hand, and saying that he is a physical channel for a nonphysical spirit entity who wishes to teach us how to make more effective use of our lives, on the other hand—the only difference is in the *idea* itself—because we do not *know* what "psychic" is, we do not *know* what "collective unconscious" is, and we do not *know* what "spirit" is.

For all we know, we could be talking about God Itself—because we also do not *know* what God is.

Or we could be talking about *life* itself, for the same reason.

All I know for sure is that Dr. Peebles through Thomas Jacobson knows me better than I know myself, that he touches and moves me very deeply, that he has given me new faith that the universe is beautiful and that something tremendously lovely and loving is moving it all.

I say, with Paul Weisberg, that this is a highly useful and necessary new vision for modern humanity.

But the book is about you.

So what do you say?

Before you say anything at all, let us try to give you a handle on the human reality as given to us by Dr. Peebles through Thomas Jacobson. This is merely an extract, paraphrased to present the more salient ideas gleaned from numerous in-depth interviews with

Spirit. The actual interviews, presented elsewhere in this book, go much more deeply into the specifics of this general overview:

- You are not alone in this life; have never been; shall never be—awake or asleep—whatever your situation.
- You selected your own parents, your own body, your own name, your own time and place to be born and all the conditions thereof.
- You are here on a mission—not a mission for the world at large (except in the ultimate sense) but a mission for yourself, your own growth, your own image of self.
- You are experiencing life at all times as part of a multidimensional reality that encompasses all that ever was and shall be, and you are continually in an intimate relationship with that reality, consciously or otherwise.
- You are a living hierarchy of selves all experienced simultaneously in all dimensions of being, the least of which is the physical-Earth self that now expresses the personality.
- There is no sin or evil anywhere in the universe, there is only growth; there is no death or ending, there is only change.
- Birth and death are interchangeable terms that define the same phenomenon; what is birth here is a sort of death in another dimension; what is death here is a rebirth in another dimension. Between the two, birth in the physical plane is a far more jarring experience.
- Death of the physical and rebirth of the spiritual is in fact a continuous experience that can be likened to stepping through a doorway, from the storm outside to a pleasingly comfortable environment inside, where old friends and family have gathered to greet you.
- Death of the spiritual and rebirth of the physical is precisely the opposite experience, in which one leaves the comfortable community of Spirit and steps outside to the chaotic world, through "the valley of forgetfulness" and into the hands of strangers, where the adventure begins anew.
- There is no "judgment" of the Earth experience except in the sense of one's own reflections upon lessons learned and values gained; there is no condemnation, no punishment, no "hell"—but there may be the necessity to incarnate again in the Earth environment to work out continuing problems before a permanent change of state (into the spiritual) can be attained.
- The lessons of life on Earth all resolve ultimately into the quest for intimacy with all life everywhere—not for obliteration of the self but to exalt the sensing of self in relation to the whole:

the profound realization that you are uniquely God while also all are God and God is the all.

- Your soul is bound to Earth only while you are fully conscious. In sleep, in daydreams, in meditative states, your soul withdraws to the spirit dimension for nurturing, guidance, and reenergizing.

- Consciousness cannot remain bound to Earth if the soul is deprived of these "rests"; total deprivation of sleep causes the soul to detach and release the body permanently, as do other "blocks" within the physical environment.

- In your present life you are a "deduction" of all you have ever experienced; this deduction is your personality as it reflects the progress of your soul, in all dimensions of being.

- You shall live forever, in one dimension of being or another, and you shall always know yourself as yourself except in the sense that your "self" is always changing into higher deductions of experience. (You experience this same relativity of self in the present life as you "grow" from infancy into maturity and beyond; the thirty-year-old is not the exact same self as self was experienced at six months or six years or even at twenty-nine years—but the deduction of experience continues to modify the perception of self into an ever-unfolding identification with self.)

  If this information strikes you so as to present some inner response or correspondence—even a vague attractive tug—then you have probably lived many lives upon this Earth and are nearing the completion of Earth-deductive experience; possibly, then, your next life shall be experienced within your own spirit community in another dimension of being.

- You are not a native son or daughter of planet Earth; you are here only for educational experiences that prepare you for greater unfoldment elsewhere. Earth is the College of Relationships, and you cannot graduate from this college until you have fully mastered the subject.

  Not even your physical form is expressly native to Earth; the naturally evolved animal form has been deliberately modified by "off-Earth" influences to accommodate human expression. Thus, we are the aliens. Various other life forms upon the planet also are "transplants."

- You are tied, then, by certain "karmic bonds" to these beings who regard themselves as our "big brothers and sisters" and who involve themselves in the affairs of Earth but at arm's length. They, too, though, are still in school and not that much further advanced than we except in a technological sense. Because of the karmic bond, there is sometimes an interchange at spirit level (between lives) in which souls from that "school" and souls from this school of Earth exchange places during one or more incarnations.

- There is physical life very similar to human life spread throughout the physical universe, upon planets much like Earth—and there is much more to the physical universe than as yet has been detected from Earth because there exist other physical dimensions that are not perceived by present detection devices—but all of what we commonly term "physical life" exists within the same vibrational density of the matter universe, and therefore occupies zones of reality that seem separate from the spirit dimensions.

  But this is merely an "illusion of separation" since all harmonics of the one universe coexist in the one reality and are interlaced one within the other—even within your own physical body—so that the entire universe in every dimension is ever present within the same space at the same time. Being, in other words, is a multidimensional expression of the one reality, with so-called "matter" expressing at the lower end of the spectrum in linear time, since linear time is the vehicle of expression at such frequencies. But linear time is also an illusion of separation since it is not absolute throughout the multidimensional universe but serves only to mark events for consciousness in the denser dimensions.

- The word *spirit* itself is an example of the illusion of separation, serving only to delineate the physical and nonphysical dimensions of reality whereas the delineation is "real" only from the viewpoint of the matter universe.

- Your physical body is but the base of a living hierarchy of multidimensional expression. You are thus both spirit and matter occupying both space and nonspace, time and nontime, finitude and infinity.

The larger illusion is the physical body itself and the way it interacts with space and time as a temporary structure in the chaotic dimension of material separation. All structures in this dimension are temporary and therefore illusions created by consciousness interacting with matter to produce linear time.

The interactions of consciousness as linear time produce a history of experience that is a prerequisite to the larger experiences available in nontime, or in what we term the spirit realms. Thus all of space-time experience in the physical universe is an educational process in which *self*, as a conscious entity, begins to apprehend reality through its denser vibrations and is given *time* to study processes that underlie the multidimensional reality. Thus the human form is a biological schoolhouse in which and through which "spirit" interacts with the basics of reality to produce understanding at an elemental level.

As that understanding grows, through repeated excursions in human form, "self" grows accordingly and rises to higher states of learning—much as in any educational system devised by mind—until a point is reached where continued interaction with the denser reality is no longer needed or desired, whereupon the higher dimensions of self release all attachment to temporary physical bodies to continue the educational process at finer environmental levels.

So that is the package as we understand it. There is nothing grim in it that we have seen, nothing really difficult to swallow, nothing to dread. It is a package with beauty, meaning, and purpose, and the mere acceptance of it into consciousness can transform a drab life into an electric one.

There is no urgency in the package either. We all have eternity to play with and work through, so we can take heaven now or leave it for another time . . . and that time will come when we are ready. Dr. Peebles repeatedly assures us that everything is "on schedule"—that we all should "lighten up a little" and "enjoy the process."

Maybe that is the best advice of all. It would be transformation enough for most of us to simply forget our worries, to brighten up, and to live a little.

Why not?

5

The

Process

---

*"There's nothing theoretical about
thought. It's the realest [sic] thing in the
universe. Thought moves and thought
does. It moves against and into. It is a
force, a thing, a reality."*

—*Source uncertain, but see page [64].*

We believe that it is both proper and pertinent that we tell you that
this writing is going along spontaneously as the material is being
developed. In certain respects it would be best, for a work of this
nature, to collect all the facts and information first, then scrutinize
and analyze and diagramize before committing anything to manuscript—but there is also much to be lost by that method. We prefer
the spontaneity and excitement of recording the experience directly
as it occurs, or as closely as possible—of wondering what we're
going to encounter next and how it will fit in with what we already
have—and of being able to work directly with the energy generated
by all the excitement.

As of the very moment of this writing, this page, the date is
June 19. We had our first session with Dr. Peebles on June 1, so you
can see how close we are to the initial point. Meanwhile we have
been conducting deep interviews with Dr. Peebles on a twice-weekly

basis, gathering old tapes from radio and public appearances and copying them, transcribing these miles of tape, reviewing the material, talking daily to Thomas by telephone (usually several times each day), conducting interviews both personally and by telephone with dozens of interested individuals—and somehow we are still getting enough time each day to observe the animal necessities, sleep four to six hours, and keep the writing going. We have dined with Thomas several times since June 1 and attended (and taped) three of his public appearances.

Frankly, we are both amazed by all this. We think we're getting help. We have good reason to think that, and I even got the first direct evidence of it at three o'clock this morning when I staggered out of bed with something trembling on the tendrils of the barely conscious mind, went to the study, and with eyes hardly open scribbled in a strange handwriting the epigraph to this section of the book (on page 63).

Now, maybe this is not exactly earthshaking thought, or even original. But it is original with me, and a trifle earthshaking for me since my hand was holding the pen and moving across the paper—I remember writing it—but when I awakened again a few hours later and found the note lying beside the word processor, I knew that this was not my handwriting. It resembled mine but was also very different from mine. Whereas I write with an elongated vertical lift, straight up and down on the paper with occasional flourishes in upper loops, this three-A.M. note is written in flowing script with the words leaning heavily to the right. It is wide open and carefree, with the bar of the crossed T's extending above the entire word and even flowing into adjacent words. And, hey, I would never say "the *realest* thing."

I would stop short of calling it automatic writing because I know the idea woke me from sound sleep and sent me to the notepad, and I do remember thinking that I had to write it down because I would not remember the thought later. But I also know that I was only marginally awake; and, besides, there was a little postscript at the bottom of the page, more in my own style, which reads simply "q.-p. psychic beehives," heavily underlined, which I can only take to mean that I should query Dr. Peebles about psychic beehives, whatever the hell that is.

I have to feel that the good doctor and/or his crew of spirits were behind it. Because, you see, he'd told us a couple of weeks back to expect this sort of interaction. He even assured Linda and me that we are "mutually channeling" with Thomas and he repeatedly urges us to exercise our own objectivity and literary talent in developing the book—as though he is inviting us to rewrite him.

Sometimes I get the feeling that our work with Thomas is almost a tandem linkup, with Dr. Peebles working through Thomas at Thomas's level of reception (as a clear channel in total surrender without bias) then through Linda and me as literary specialists who know how to organize the material and shape it for publication.

You see, the channel is vital to this whole process. I gather that speech and therefore language is peculiarly a development for communication of consciousness in the dense-matter regions. Spirits don't use it, don't need it, therefore don't have even the capability for expression through speech. I mean, ordinary speech and language to them must be something like primary readers to us: "See Dick. See Jane run."

We have been led to believe (or at least I have) that language more than anything else has produced and shaped the human cognitive centers in the cerebral cortex of the brain (which is man's great gift that sets him apart from the rest of the animal population). Now I have to wonder about that. Could it be that the natural and spontaneous and instantaneous flashes of thought (where thought is real, and moves and does), which would seem to characterize the mode of communication in the spirit world, was made to slow down and become mere *potential* communication in the dense realm and more or less dependent upon the development of higher brain mechanisms for their expression? If so, could this be what has given rise to language centers in the cortex, rather than vice versa? And could this be tied somehow to Jung's ideas about universal symbology in the minds of mankind? Does Spirit think in *symbols?*—wouldn't that be more efficient than linear packaging, when a single symbol can be used to convey an entire encyclopedia of thought? (Witness the Christian symbol of the cross, the Star of David, or simply the American flag.)

Does the brain produce thought from mere nerve tissue?—or, conversely, does thought arise in different form from somewhere beyond the brain and then stimulate certain neurons of expression in the brain? Is it possible that our medical researchers have put the cart before the horse?—and is that why none can locate the mind in any physical space of the brain?

I have a theory about how channeling works.

The voice I hear issuing from Thomas Jacobson *is* Thomas Jacobson, I believe, modified to some extent by Thomas himself as he surrenders his articulation centers to an expression of thought *that is not of his own origin*. The *expression* of thought is *not* Dr. Peebles—*but the thought is.*

I believe that to be the meaning of my three-A.M. revelation,

"There's nothing theoretical about thought . . ." (And that comes in at several levels of meaning.)

The thought of Dr. Peebles "is the realest thing in the universe" but it must be slowed down for resonance within the dense realm—*and it is slowed down by Thomas's brain.*

Now, Dr. Peebles had told us that mind and soul are one and the same. It is our *souls* that produce the thoughts that trickle through the dense matter of our brains to find expression in the matter universe.

He has told us also that Thomas *is taken out of the body* and held and nurtured while Dr. Peebles is present in that body. But Thomas is just outside, close enough to maintain some cognition of the event. It is then Dr. Peebles's soul (or mind, however you prefer) that interacts with the dense matter of Thomas's brain to channel the thoughts through, interacting with Thomas's own articulation centers to produce the stream of consciousness *in human terms* that we all can understand.

If this sounds complicated to you, what do you think it must be for Spirit? He is *moving against and through* a vehicle designed specifically for another soul. The firing of neurons and the unutterably complex matrix of electrochemical transfers taking place within that alien brain *must be orchestrated by the guest spirit*— which must continually contend with the automatic reflexes and conditioned responses—habit patterns, if you will—of the host brain which also contains memory, therefore bias and prejudice.

Is it any wonder, then, that researchers mourn the dearth of "high-class" phenomena and become so ecstatic when they encounter some? This kind of communication is obviously the result of a team effort, with the channel struggling to give over and surrender control, to keep the memory cleansed of conflicting dicta and to calm the animal survival mechanisms, to remain pure and loving— the perfect host—and give that guest soul a clear shot at converting thought from the spirit realm to *thing* in the dense universe; the visiting soul, on the other hand, working through some unimaginable kind of discipline to contract its universal presence into the tiny avenue thus opened *and slow down its spirit vibration* to a point where it can interact with the facilities provided by the channel. Language is one of those facilities, and it is a language absolutely peculiar to the brain that has fashioned it from the pure thought of another entity. *Thoughts become things in the dense universe along specific and well-conditioned avenues of expression.*

That is why some channels are "high class" and some not quite so. The visiting soul must use the equipment that is there. If that equipment is flawed, then so is the expression.

But perhaps that is not being entirely fair. "As above, so below" probably applies to this situation. Even in heaven, I would think, there are degrees of high and not so high. Sometimes maybe the "low-class" channel is actually providing a high-class facility to a not-so-high class entity. (Right. I simply could not use "low class" in this connection.)

That Thomas Jacobson is so distinctively high class is indicative, I would think, that the whole team is high class.

And I happen to believe that "Dr. Peebles" is somewhat more than he has led us to believe he is. I'm going to say it, Doc, and you can chide me later. I believe that Dr. Peebles could be what has been referred to in Judeo-Christian literature as an archangel. That is defined as a "chief angel." The archangel Gabriel, for example, was thought to be sort of like God's chief of staff for earthly affairs. And our Dr. Peebles may even be "higher class" than that, by whatever definition or description in Spirit. I specifically asked him; he specifically declined to respond. It is the only time I have ever known him to evade a question.

This particular section is a postscript added to the manuscript during final editing with the publisher, long after the initial writing had been completed. Our editor was curious about the "automatic writing" experience described at the beginning of this chapter. She was justifiably perplexed that we had not questioned Dr. Peebles about the incident, even though we have been in frequent contact with him ever since, and she believed that many of our readers would be interested in his response to the event.

There is a very simple explanation for the omission. I had accepted the experience unquestioningly because I did not wish to know anything more about it. It is my usual routine to produce three to four books each year, it is how I make my living, and I suppose I just did not wish to question the process. But we are speaking of "process" in this chapter, so I agreed to grit my teeth and ask "the fatal question" for the benefit of our readers—and we leave it to you to come to your own conclusions regarding the influence of spirit and the meaning of "inspiration."

In an interview with Dr. Peebles in February 1989, I said to him: "While Linda and I were writing *To Dance with Angels,* I had a rather unusual experience in which I awoke in the middle of the night and felt compelled to get up and write down something that was in my mind. The next morning I saw instantly that this note was in a handwriting different from my own, yet I clearly remembered writing it. I deduced that this was a bit of automatic writing, which I had never experienced before in my life—but then there was a postscript to it, in my own hand, which said, in a sort of a shorthand, 'Ask Dr. Peebles about psychic beehives.' Does this strike anything in you?"

The good doctor boomed right back: "It sure does! It strikes my chords—my song, my litany of life! Just a moment here. . . . All right, let's see here . . . well, you should talk to my friend, Henry. Henry is quite aware of you, he's quite a bit of a humorist. He likes to engage people in—tease them a bit, particularly if they're in the body, on Earth. He's very adept at human communication. He works with you, Don—he has a similar mode of thought to yours, and he's able to engage your intentions. He has remained with you ever since. The psychic beehives he talked about are his own symbols for my investigations when I was on Earth. I was very fascinated by the possibilities of the psychic world and the psychic mind, and much of my work and research was dedicated to trying to formulate and categorize, organize, methodize the psychic possibilities so as to help people discover their own spiritual world.

"Well, when I talked with my friend Henry, so often he would make jokes about my buzzing on and on like bees in a hive, making so much noise and excitement and flying around—it was always disconcerting to him. He always wanted me to be calm and sedate, for that's Henry. That's how he sees a man of respect. We'd be in a parlor—I'd be speaking away and he'd blush—and I'd know that he'd blush and so I'd start talking all the faster. It tickled his funny bone. So he wanted to stimulate you, to become aware of your dreams, Don—not only for personal guidance but for your creativity. You'll find yourself waking up in the midst of your dream state and writing out a paragraph and a page that will give you your direction of writing for the entire week to come, sometimes for a month. Henry, with your permission, is going to be a conduit for that, for he speaks the language of your mind. He enjoys metaphors, he enjoys the art of suggestion, and he enjoys humor, and he's very sedate. He says he respects you very much and you respect him very much. He's very—he's a noble man. You understand me."

I replied, "Yes, I do, and thank you. Please thank Henry and tell him that I will try to be more open to his influence."

But Dr. Peebles was not finished with me and my "ghost writer."

"Yes, and the writing—let's see, here . . . just a moment— Henry, come talk here . . . [Long pause]. Henry was helping you to remember an ancient life in Tibet, where you were a priest of that culture, and this was in an ancient language, a mystical language— it wasn't fully brought through you, but it was related to a symbol of leaves falling from a tree to the ground, and in the falling to the ground there was rebirth, there was fertilization and rebirth and a cleansing . . . for new abundance to come forward . . . your *processes,* Don—it's a little poem, a little parable, of that culture that, I believe, was your own writing a long, long time ago, as a high priest. You understand."

So much for that. Satisfied my mind completely, and then some. But not Linda's. She has been busily researching the terrestrial Dr. Peebles and documenting his life on Earth. She has books both by him and about him, newspaper articles, tons of biographical data.

Linda, to her satisfaction, has found "Henry"—Colonel Henry Steel Olcott—author, attorney, philosopher—who, with Helena Blavatsky and William Q. Judge, founded the Theosophical Society in 1875 and served as its first president. Olcott and Peebles were longtime friends and associates. Together they visited India and established numerous schools for the poor. Olcott settled in India and established the permanent headquarters of the Theosophical Society in Madras in 1883. He edited the *Theosophist* from 1888 until his death in 1907 at the age of seventy-five, and his *Buddhist Catechism* was published in 1881 and translated into many languages.

In one of the very rare books Linda has unearthed, Dr. Peebles speaks glowingly of his warm friendship with Olcott, who was a special commissioner for the U.S. War and Navy departments during the American Civil War and served on the special commission investigating the assassination of President Lincoln.

So, okay . . . speak to me, Henry. I guess it's all just part of the process.

We have encountered a couple of people who seem disappointed that Dr. Peebles is not omniscient—knowing everything about everything to the smallest detail—and several others who seem a bit confused about the nature of specific rather than general information. Both attitudes are understandable, and we sympathize with them while not sharing them; there is something very comfortable about absolutes, for we who are continually submerged in a reality that is forever in process.

The *process* is what we are talking about in this chapter.

And Dr. Peebles has told us repeatedly that there are no absolutes except at the very upper end of the process. One of the cardinal points of his spirit psychology—the healing message that he wishes to share with all mankind—is bound into the idea that all of us, each of us in our own way, are continually *creating* our own process. "You are forever the eternal creator, never the victim."

Some of us are understandably uncomfortable with that idea because it puts the responsibility right back into our own hands. We have gone to a psychic or a fortune teller or a channel for comfort, for a *release* from responsibility, only to be told that no release is possible. We are creating ourselves, our own heavens and hells, our own reality. That is a sobering idea because there is no escape from it if it is true. There is no escape, even, through disbelief, *because it is true whether we choose to believe or not, act upon it or not*—and the essential intelligence that resides within each of us *knows* that it is true. That is the reason for the discomfort in confrontation. We are trying to hide from the truth; we turn to another to help us hide, only to be turned back into the light again.

Sure, if you are tired and bruised and hurting from some pain of your own creation, comfort can be found in the illusion that you have been victimized; there's even more comfort in the thought that another force or power or person is going to magically turn everything back right for you again by snapping the fingers.

If you have searched for love and found none, so turn with that pain to Dr. Peebles only to have him lovingly reproach you for having created within yourself conditions that numb you to the possibility of recognizing and responding to the love that is all around you, then you may go away complaining about the "generalizations" he handed you as a gift of love even though he has instructed you quite specifically as to the techniques for coming alive that put the creation of love and happiness back into your own hands.

You wanted him to send you a lover.

He is telling you that he would gladly do so—indeed that all of life everywhere in the universe is devoted to that search—but to send you a lover while you are numb to love would be an exercise in futility. He is telling you that all of life is sending lovers into your life every day in every way, yet you are not responding. "Open your eyes and receive, my dear; we cannot open them for you, nor can we remove the numbness with which you have so carefully insulated yourself from the experience of love."

I have heard him say it fifty times in the past two weeks, in words to that effect, to a variety of people both male and female, in response to a variety of questions. *You must create your own reality.*

You are doing so even when you shrug away wisdom in the further search for comfort. You don't want to have to create anything, dammit; you want someone else to create it and hand it to you tied in ribbon. So you will seek out a "better" psychic who can put you on the road to your lover. And even if you should magically find one who can create your own future for you, the final responsibility is always in your own hands.

So you find a magical prophet and he tells you: "Next Wednesday morning at ten thirty-two you must go to the corner of Fifth and Main and there you will see a 1987 Cadillac parked at the southwest corner, license plates XYZ123, and your soulmate will be sitting behind the wheel waiting for you to come along. He is brilliant and loving and handsome and very sexy and everything you have ever wanted in a man and he will immediately recognize you as his soulmate and he will ask you to marry him."

Wow! Now, *that* is *specific*.

So you go along with the gag (though probably still doubting) and it all works out the way it was promised. So you and your "soulmate" get married and you live in ecstasy forevermore.

Really?

What if this beautiful, sensitive, loving man can never remember to take out the garbage, he cannot or will not keep a job, he sleeps around a lot, drinks too much, hates kids, sulks when he does not get his way?

And what about you, kiddo? Are you critical, nagging, insecure, anxious, bitchy, hostile, competitive, resentful, lazy?

So who the hell played matchmaker for *you* two? Has all that "specific" information from the prophet served or disserved you? And now that you are in this mess, *who created it?* Better, maybe, you should have gone along with the general guidelines and left the specifics to be worked out in your new understanding of self.

Dr. Peebles does not attempt to create process in your life. He will reveal to you, if you ask, the processes that have brought you to your present moment—and he will even start at the start—"In the Beginning"—when you first emerged as a potential from the mind of God—and he will give you a general outline of all that you have ever been. He can even tell you where you will eventually end up; but from now until then is entirely up to you; you will create your own route and itinerary, your own joys and tears, and not even God Itself can reveal those details to you *because they remain within the uncreated.*

There are those who go to Dr. Peebles with test questions. That is very understandable, even laudable. We should always try to get at the truth. We should want to know whether Thomas Jacobson is a con artist, or suffering self-delusion, or if he is a true channel for divine truth. Yet the truth about all that lies within the revelations themselves. Anyone exposed who does recognize that truth will not get much comfort from test questions because a "direct hit" on some specific date or hour or circumstance that could not possibly be known by Thomas Jacobson is "proof" of nothing whatever. It could be a lucky guess—and how will you ever be sure that it was not? It could be a genuine display of momentary clairvoyance; but what is that?—and, whatever it is, how can you ever be sure that other disclosures from that same mind are also issuing from the selfsame "momentary clairvoyance"? Surely this "psychic" is not omniscient; if so, wouldn't he be ruling the world?

Dr. Peebles does not work at that level of process. I have no reason even for believing that he could if he wanted to. Nor can I find any reason within myself for wanting to believe that he could. To the cosmic mind, details must be something like the alphabet in the mind of a gifted orator. What would the orator be revealing to you or to himself by reciting to you the alphabet? He wishes to discuss powerful *ideas* and profound understandings. Don't ask him if he can recite the alphabet. Possibly he could not. And why should it matter whether he could or not *if his ideas stir you?*

I happen to believe that Roy Clark is one of the finest guitarists in the world today, yet I learned recently that Roy Clark does not and cannot read music. Does that disturb me when I hear his magic accompanied by a full symphony orchestra?

"Roy Clark? One of the finest guitarists in the world? Why, the guy can't even read music. Turn him off."

You turn him off. This guy *creates* music! So why do I care . . . ?

Another "illiterate" genius: Lionel Richie, who creates music in his shower, then *hums* it into a tape recorder because he cannot write it down, yet has given the world so much beauty. Shall we turn Lionel off?

Relax, Doc, I'm not calling you illiterate. I am just trying to remind the people that the greatest truths and the most profound insights and the most moving music and all the most beautiful wonders of life are revealed to us not as details but as grand assumptions held in the fabric of mind, and that we react to those assumptions, not to the underlying microscopic bits of detail that make them possible.

If you are one of those who must hear the musical scales instead of the concert, then you could be disappointed with Dr. Peebles. He simply does not work at that level of process.

Tell me why, please, a grand master should concern himself with where you were and what you were doing and who you were doing it with last Tuesday night at six o'clock in a tiny crease of the planet called Earth when he has come to you from the very breast of God to discuss with you your immortal soul and its pathway to the very same breast?

The wonder is not that he does not answer your test question; the wonder is that his voice twinkles in loving allowance for your own frailty as he goes on to explain to you that you are God—even last Tuesday night at six o'clock on planet Earth—and that the realization of that truth will totally erase last Tuesday night from your consideration forevermore.

Do I have that right, Doc?

Oh . . . okay. Now *he* is rewriting *me*. Make that read "apparent frailty"—and nothing is erased; it is merely subducted, whatever that means.

The little essay just above was prompted partly by a recent experience that we set up ourselves. We had felt that we should have a record of Dr. Peebles interacting directly in an intimate environment with individuals who were experiencing him for the first time. We have miles of tape covering individual interactions in a large group environment, but we knew that Dr. Peebles goes into much greater depth in private sessions and we wanted a direct record of such.

We also knew that we could not invade the intimate sessions of others unless we set it up ourselves—and we really did not want to work with total strangers (though the scientists would prefer it that way) because we wished to see directly how our own intimate knowledge of the subjects would mesh with the revelations from Spirit. So we invited my younger daughter, Jennifer, and her husband of one year, Michael, to a consultation with Spirit. Both were interested; both leapt at the opportunity.

Jennifer and Michael are entertainers—a musical duo somewhat on the lines of Steve Lawrence and Eydie Gorme, though much younger and not nearly so well entrenched in career (but of course, from this father's viewpoint, well deserving of fame and fortune). They have worked together for the past six years and enjoy a large and loyal following in the local area; they have also worked in Las Vegas and other cities, but their dream is a big recording contract, concert tours, etc., and they shall realize the dream one day, I am sure. Meanwhile they are making a very nice living. We see each other often, so Linda and I are aware of the various forces operating in their lives; we thought they would make excellent study subjects, and we were not disappointed.

Several days prior to the appointed session we were discussing the project with a recent acquaintance, a woman in her late forties and recently remarried, who expressed a strong interest in the proceedings. We will refer to her here as Jean, but that is not her real name. We know Jean only very slightly, but we invited her to the session with the understanding that we could have full use of the material developed in her interactions with Dr. Peebles. She was delighted and accepted the invitation without hesitation.

So there we were on a Saturday afternoon, gathered in the rec room of our home, Thomas Jacobson seated in close confrontation with our three subjects, Linda and I off to the side with our recorders and notepads when Dr. Peebles entered with his usual bang and in superb form.

He began with a broad outline of the individuals' past lives, taking each in turn along the backtrack of their many lives and revealing each to self in the most intimate details of "relevant" experiences—relative, that is, to the current life. It was immediately obvious to both Linda and me that he was reading Jennifer and Michael like a book. We could only presume that he was on an equal track with Jean, though her reactions revealed nothing whatever. If anything, she seemed a bit embarrassed and perhaps detached from the process even though she had come into it with great interest.

Perhaps Jean was just not prepared to gaze into that mirror—or, to be totally fair, maybe she did not believe and was just wondering what in the world she was doing there.

At any rate, Jean became a distraction. Dr. Peebles held forth for thirty minutes with the individual broad outlines, then he asked for questions or comments. Jennifer and Michael were totally enthralled and caught up in the experience, reacting with animated appreciation of Spirit's wit and wisdom, and altogether it was obviously a valuable and delightful experience for both of them. They have not yet stopped talking about it and have expressed the desire to do it again soon.

Jean sat through the entire seventy-five-minute session with hardly a smile or other visible effect. She asked murky and misleading questions and continually challenged Spirit to read her mind. Every question was a test. Dr. Peebles surely knew that. We knew it, and later Jennifer also commented on it. Nevertheless, Spirit treated her with great patience and gentleness, and he revealed her to us if not to herself.

She wanted to know how her father had died (many years ago) but did not offer the year or any clues whatever. Spirit told her that he had been "assisted out of the body, as we say over here . . . and we do not mean helped by Spirit."

She wanted the exact cause of death, though Spirit had just told her, and later, while still probing Spirit for the precise finding, she confided that there was some discrepancy between the coroner's findings and the private conviction of the family. Spirit wondered if there was pain in her heart over it, and whether she wished to "solve the mystery." She replied that there was no particular pain, just curiosity, and declined to pursue the matter further.

Jean then wondered about her son and his present situation. Spirit painted for her the portrait of a strongly dependent personality that could not function in this world, could not face this world without constantly borrowing from the strength of others.

That was not enough. Jean wanted to know in precise terms what was happening to her son.

Spirit told *us* more about the son than perhaps Jean will ever understand—and he told her, as well, of the total relationship between mother and son that was relevant to the son's condition.

That was not enough. Jean unbent enough to speak murkily of her son's "past problems" with "external stimuli," and wanted to know "if he is still doing that."

Spirit told her what she already knew, but even that apparently was not enough, so she turned to her own recent marriage and spoke of various difficulties in adjusting to it. Spirit took her back again into past lives and pointed out the conditions there that were casting shadows onto the present marriage.

She apparently did not like that either, so she rang down the curtain in a predictable way. She set up her own rejection of the whole experience by asking Spirit the first pointed question of her day with Spirit: "Will I have any more children?"

Well, now, this lady is about to have her fiftieth birthday. She had a total hysterectomy seven years ago.

Spirit regarded her question through a moment of silence, then he put it back to her in very gentle tones: "Well, it's still optional. I would say possibly not. I believe that part is fulfilled . . . but it's up to you, what would you like? How do you feel? I'm not sure you want a whole lot—do you want more children?"

"Not particularly, but I was wondering if I—"

"I don't see it as likely. Well, you're still fertile. It still could happen, literally speaking, but I don't believe it will. [Long silence.] If it does, it's all right—you just get on your knees and praise God and say, 'All right, Spirit, I'm ready, let's go dance, come on through me.' "

I don't know exactly what was going on there. I am sure Dr. Peebles knew. And, as Paul Weisberg pointed out: "Dr. Peebles does not always divulge the whole truth but what he does divulge *is* true."

Literally speaking, maybe it could still happen for Jean. If Sarah could give birth to Isaac at the age of ninety . . . well, maybe we do not know as much as we think we know, "literally speaking."

When Spirit told Jean that she is "still fertile," how do we know what he had in mind? Perhaps he spoke of mental fertility and he was trying to get at some repressed regret that she had not completed her motherhood mission on Earth. But perhaps that is stretching too far to get a "hit" instead of a "miss."

All I know for sure is that Jean baited a trap for Spirit and invited him to betray himself.

As he has said to me, he does not always address the skeptics in their own terms, but sometimes he does.

Maybe he just decided to give her what she needed at the moment: a step backward from the truth about herself. Perhaps that mirror was just too clear for comfort, so he gave her an out. He stepped lovingly into the trap, smiled at Jean, and said to her from her own mirror: "Silly, silly; you don't have to believe a word of it."

Spirit, I am sure, is big enough to do that.

If you were given a thirty-minute audience with God, what would you want to talk about?

Think about it, please. Soberly and seriously. Here you are in the presence of the Creator of the heavens and Earth, the seat of all power and all knowledge. You have been told to prepare a list of ten questions, and that the answers will be fully revealed to you. So. What do you want to know?

It has been suggested to me recently by two different friends at different moments, men whom I respect for their intelligence and common sense, that Dr. Peebles has told me nothing that any brilliant man could not have told me. Now, these two have not yet heard everything that Dr. Peebles has told me (but only fragments) —but even if they had, possibly their reaction would have been the same, considering the mindset at work there. Nor does it serve any useful purpose to point out the difference between "could have said" and "is saying."

Now, think about this, please, because it is going to be a common reaction among sensible people, so it may be your reaction as well.

What would you have Dr. Peebles say to you that would convince you that no one on Earth could have said it?

And please remember that Dr. Peebles does not claim to be God, or omniscient, or even infallible.

So let's put the question to God Itself. If God Itself fails the test, then how can we hold a mere angel accountable to an even higher standard?

What can you tell us, God, that we cannot tell ourselves?

That would be my first question if I wanted to challenge Deity. Let's try a little scenario, just for fun.

God replies, "You live forever."

US: That's not exactly an original idea, Your Worship. Many men have told us that. Tell us something that we've never heard before.

GOD: The Earth is part of a system that is part of a system that is part of a system, etcetera.

US: Our astrophysicists have already told us that.

GOD: You are part of that same system.

US: Our microbiologists and nuclear physicists have already told us that.

GOD: You are the personification of the divine on Earth.

US: Jesus and all the other mystics told us that! Come on, now. Give us something *hot!*

GOD: You already contain all truth within yourselves.

US: We know that! Tell us something new!

GOD: Hummmmmmmmmmmmmmmm . . .

US: What? Say that again, please. We don't understand.

GOD: Hummmmmmmmmmmmmmmm . . .

US: We still don't understand!

GOD: Then I cannot tell you, can I, what you will not understand. Do you understand when I speak to you through the wind, and through the flowers, and through the beautiful animals of Earth? Do you understand when I speak to you through your own dreams, your own appreciation of beauty, your own sensing of self? What can I tell you that you will understand, unless I speak to you in your own terms?

US: But then we don't know if it's true or false!

GOD: Oh, but you do, you do, you do, hummmmmm . . .

Get my drift?

So what do we want mere Spirit to tell us? Something that we cannot possibly encompass with the mind? Let's be reasonable about this. *Spirit cannot possibly tell you something that you could not tell yourself.* The difference—the principal difference—is that he *is* telling you, and he is trying to frame the thought in forms that can be taken in and digested by the human mind. It is up to you then to decide if it makes sense, if it is useful, and if you wish to be affected by it.

It was frequently said of Jesus by his contemporaries: "Never hath a man so spake."

But in fact much of what Jesus had to say to the world had been said before in one form or another. For example, the Golden Rule was given by Confucius five hundred years before Jesus was born, and it is now felt by modern scholars that many of Jesus' teachings are from the Essenic tradition. Jesus revealed man to himself, certainly, but because he "spake," not because he invented a new speech, and because of his presence in those truths. Dr. Peebles salutes Jesus as a "divine grand master" and speaks warmly of man's religious quest, assuring those with ears to hear that every man's quest for God is deserving of reverence and respect.

But please do not dismiss truth in hand simply because *anyone* could have said it. That is not the point; the point is that someone *is now* saying it—so will you listen? Will the world *ever* listen to the truth about itself? That, my friends, is for you to say.

Linda and I both have known Michael for many years; we know him to be warm and gregarious, a devout Roman Catholic, a fantastic showman with a nice easy personality that charms on and off the stage. His Italian good looks are not overlooked by the ladies; there is always an adoring flock of them who sit at their tables gazing lovingly at him through every performance. This has been Jennifer's cross to bear—but then she gets plenty of the same admiration from the gentlemen.

Michael formed his first band shortly after he graduated from high school. He was also a sports enthusiast (still is) and made a stab at college, but music and performing commanded his life early. He is now in his mid-thirties and has spent his entire adult life before audiences—directly with Jennifer since their first meeting in 1981 when she was only twenty years old (and had to fib about her age to work in the clubs). They had an on-off romance during those early years of working together, the "off" times primarily due to Michael's reluctance to commit himself—but true love had its way and they were married last year in a lavish Roman Catholic ceremony; I think they are still honeymooning.

If Michael has a character problem, the only thing I could point to (and very faintly) is his tendency to cover deep feelings (or to distance himself from them) with a devil-may-care attitude. Anything is okay with Michael. He has a great sense of humor, laughs a lot and jokes a lot, seems to take life and its bumps in stride without getting overly involved in that stride. But I do know him to be a man of deep feelings and a reverence for life; it shows in his music, shows in his eyes, shows in his relationships. He is a very easy touch, and is forever volunteering to do something for somebody when he knows damn well there's no time to do it.

I know him to be a devoted son to his own parents, a warm and respectful son-in-law. We have a great relationship, and I could not feel more strongly for him if he were my own blood.

So much for Michael. You will meet him again in just a moment.

Jennifer, God bless her, has been a warm light in my life since the day she was born. She was a delightful child, easy to live with, a pleasure to grow up with, a total satisfaction as an adult from my fatherly point of view. But Jennifer was always essentially a very private person. She kept diaries, and I never knew it; wrote moving poetry, but I saw none until recently; was gifted with a beautiful singing voice, but I did not know it until it was almost fully developed, and I discovered it almost by accident at a high school recital.

She is now torn between career and motherhood—wanting babies so much she aches every time she sees one—but also hesitant to leave the stage just when things are beginning to look so bright.

I do not know of anyone anywhere who does not adore Jennifer. She is, in a word, adorable. You will see why in a moment.

Thomas met Jennifer and Michael for the first time just minutes before going into trance. He knew only that they were my daughter and son-in-law.

But listen to what Dr. Peebles "spake" about them:

Jennifer, you are a beautiful spirit; you came to the planet Earth as a search for the great creativity of God, the beauty of the divine. Similarly, you came into this life through the doorway of beauty. The planet Earth appeared to you to be a great rainbow of experience and of color. You came forward from other places in the universe in a great love affair; there was no hesitation whatsoever; you said, "Look at that beautiful blue place. I want to be part of that." And so you came into Earth, you immersed yourself into the physical experience, and immediately had second thoughts.

You said, "Goodness gracious, this feels like quicksand. I'm used to thoughts becoming things, *now;* how come my thought isn't yet a thing and hours have gone by?" You felt a little disconcerted; you felt—well, you were dumbfounded, frankly, and you felt as if you had lost total control.

It is perhaps wise to consider that, for that became the foundation of all of your lifetimes, dedicated to the expression of beauty from within you as the calling of God—uh, to experience God within you—with great courage on your part; and yet feeling upon a foreign land, as if you were in quicksand unable to move.

Well . . . as you went from one life to another, your challenge was—your feeling was that you wanted to overcome that loss of control. You wanted to regain control, and over a long period of time this often became a contrast or a conflict— or a challenge—to your expressed desire to communicate through your subjective nature, through your artistry, through that golden loving heart inside you.

So on the one hand you had love; on the other you had great fear, frustration, which became anger and hate. So Earth was a love-hate affair. You dedicated yourself to regaining that control and you did so, increasingly through the male experience, living as the male.

In your male lifetimes, however, you felt that you lost your sensitivity, and you did tend to blame it on the male. And so you separated from the male, quite strongly; you dedicated yourself to the study of the female and of your sensitivity, but then you had a sense of losing control again.

Here is where you became fascinated by the sexuality of the female, Jennifer. You had a series of lifetimes where your sexuality was of primary interest to you in order to experience sensitivity, and the beauty of life, and to be in control all at the same time.

It was a grand experiment. You were something to behold, my dear, with your sexuality. Busy, busy girl. You had many affairs and—with and without marriage, mostly the latter—and you lived the experiment over and over—uh, yes— uh, several lives in a row; you did it once and you said, "Well, that was pretty good, I think I'll try it again; here I am in full control—silly, silly men"—and you enjoyed it thoroughly. You were also able, of course, to maintain your sensitivity, but you began to experience that it was more of a scenario, or more of an act, Jennifer, than an actual experience—that the sexuality *and* the creativity—of your sensitivity—both increasingly were more of a performance, and this became clear to you through a series of shattering experiences in family and in community where, for the most part, you felt rejected and you felt artificial; you felt that you were accused of being cold— none of which was really true; however, you saw that there was you, Jennifer, inside yourself, and there was your outer face, and often, my dear, there was a wide gap between the two.

So your brave, courageous insight was that you must

meld the two, bridge the two—and you bring that even into this present lifetime, with notable success, bringing your inner personality, your inner self-image with your outer face, into one solid form of communication.

Well, from that series of lives you began to feel suspect, and you blamed it not only on the male, you also blamed it on the sexuality, so you did the opposite; you abstained from sexuality totally; you entered into some mystical and religious environments that justified that for you—however, now you also felt increasingly separate from your expression, your art; for your concept of thinking, Jennifer, was almost exclusively from the mind, very theoretical in nature. And that was comforting for you; it felt like a quiet place; you enjoyed it for several lives but eventually it just got plain boring, that's all, and you said, "Well, goodness gracious, this is—this is a—am I a *book* or am I a living thing?" And you—with a little bit of force—you thrust yourself into creative endeavors: how can I be sensitive?—how can I be alive?—and how can I experience the beauty inside me?—and you did do that, right from life number one, successfully experienced the beauty within yourself—and how can I balance the male-female within?—how can I know a great presence in life?

Well, there is where you dedicated yourself even more to the artistic being that you are, determined to express yourself, but with a great fear of your performance being artificial and thin; a bridge—building a bridge between your personality in life and the performer onstage—in Greece, in Rome, in Turkey, and around the world.

Well, it was difficult; it was very hard for you; there were certain demands and expectations by the public, and this created more demand upon you, and you had a choice again and again—a choice, a pivotal choice—whether to be vulnerable, and very direct and honest with that public, or whether to try to fit their expectations so as not to be booed by them.

It was the latter you chose, my dear, almost inadvertently creating a very strong state of invulnerability; for you felt that was the only way you could survive—maintain and continue your creative expression and still be alive—without going crazy.

So . . . but you come into this lifetime with counsel from the spirit that you *can* bridge the two, you *must* bridge the two, and the vulnerability of yourself, where you don't have to fit the audience; you certainly respect their requirements but you just express yourself fully, deep inside yourself, inner to the outer, outer to the inner, and that is what you are doing in this lifetime, *nicely*—discovering the beauty of all life in you and around you and the divine of all experience, a personal God within your being.

Jennifer, you are also recognizing that truth, the search for truth within you, is actually secondary to the experience of contact, of oneness, of intimacy with all life. Part of your journey in this life is intimacy and closeness with the many rather than the few. Part of you would rather have it be with the few, outside of your creativity, only with the few, but your greater soul wants that with the many. And that is the drive of your creative being, to touch other people. Now your challenge, Jennifer, is to let other people truly touch you, and move you, and you're doing a very good job of it.

God bless you, my dear. Keep up the good work.

Michael . . . you are a beautiful spirit, and we don't have a word to say to you. Next, please.

[Laughter.]

No, we tease you, my friend. All right, let's see here . . .

Michael, you came into the planet Earth as a pioneer, as an adventurer, you came to the planet Earth from other regions of space and time merely out of curiosity—no passion, no real desire, just kind of off to the left of your shoulder: "Well, what's that over there? Let's go take a look." Because that was just your drive, just curiosity, to explore the unknown —which we send you accolades for—your ability to seek the unknown, where so many fear it.

Well, that was your fundamental drive in original lifetimes, seeking the unknown. You couldn't wait to go somewhere you hadn't been, as a pilot, and you went from one country to another, one village to another, one tribe to another, one *woman* to another—uh, one man to another—one life to . . . as quickly as you could, you spent *no* time in the spirit; you'd die, you'd leave the body; with your next breath you'd be in some woman's womb again as a child, being born unto your self. And, uh, just busy, busy—you lived, oh, goodness, about a hundred lifetimes right away!—quickly!—on the planet Earth; you lived many lives in ancient community, then. I believe you're aware—perhaps you're not—of a fascination and interest with ancient history, although I do not see that you explored it. It is fundamental to your being. The reason you haven't fully explored it is because of a slight hesitation to truly embrace your past lives, for reasons that we are coming to.

Now . . . your fundamental drive, then, to explore the unknown . . . and so you were charismatic, Michael, and you attracted respect from people; often you were called upon to be a leader, for they saw this courageous being. Your lifetimes were dedicated to a sociological experience—what is the relationship between all people?—and what is this experience of leadership and demand and expectation by others and by myself? I don't *want* to be a leader; I just want to explore, I want to be left alone, thank you very much!

You found that it was very difficult to do that—and again you wanted to keep exploring, and yet you wanted to be left alone. Well, with the passing of time and lives, you realized—or rather you were told; it was suggested to you—a few thousand times—that maybe the drive of adventuring, of exploring, was also a shield as well as an honest curiosity; it was also a camouflage that allowed you to avoid staying in one place too long, before someone "gotcha" . . . actually you were hurt by that, you were offended, became a little angry about it, because you knew the truth of it unconsciously.

So eventually you understood the truth here, you saw the possibilities, and—like you are: Once you make up your mind, Michael, watch out! So immediately you put your feet on the ground—almost into the core of the Earth, figuratively, and stood fast; said, "All right, fine, you want me to be present? Here I am; present; now what?"

The effect was totally the opposite; you felt like a tree in the wind that couldn't bend, losing all your limbs as well as your leaves, and not having faith that you could grow them again, that there would be a new cycle. So it was a stormy period; it was a period of defensiveness, of defensive fighting and battles—feeling put upon and misunderstood—of severe psychological withdrawal—eventually finding that the more you withdrew, the more life came at you; and you just decided, "Well, goodness, I don't know what else to do; I think I'll just go a little insane."

So, you just lost your mind, actually, you won't have to think about it all the time—but, what happened as a result of that, Michael, was that you were taken care of. People who cared reached out to you, and took care of you despite your anger and frustration. You suspected their motives for a while, but eventually it moved you very, very deeply. You didn't really resolve the issue of being present or not—and what does that really mean?—but you did create an experience, you did feel—you made a major growth, where all this time previously you didn't really care deeply about anything; you were curious, and you were sincere, you were kind, but there wasn't that deep caring.

Well, now you were provoked and then inspired to become very caring. You dedicated yourself to service, service to others; you felt, "Goodness, that felt *so* good, when others cared about me when I wasn't very nice; so now I am going to care about others."

And you spent a series of lifetimes—most of the time, not always, but most of the time through religious dedication, to serving people, to helping them—as a doctor, as a healer, as a facilitator, a person of the mind—helping them understand, helping them love themselves and forgive themselves. Part of trying to help others, over and over again, to forgive themselves was your own roundabout way of trying to get yourself to forgive yourself. For you felt guilty that you had—oh, that you had offended humanity on occasions, and denied yourself and so forth—all of which you exaggerated greatly; no one judged you at all.

Well, in your kindness to humanity you felt a new desire to be really present, for the first time, to root yourself on Earth not as a demonstration of courage or stubbornness, but as a desire to be close.

You come into this lifetime, Michael, with multifaceted aspects of your personality. You are the gentle, gentle lover and healer who wants to help life around you. You are the power that is able to stand present and let the wind come at you; and your challenge still is to let yourself bend—let the branches bend; you are doing that now—much, much more often, and there's just a wee bit more; now let the trunk bend, as well as the branches, in the winds of life—and to have total faith that the leaves will grow once again.

You come into this life with an understanding of religion, and you have a drive to know God once again; you come into this life determined to root yourself to the Earth, where originally it was a great curiosity, because you learned to care. You bravely understood, Michael, that you must embrace Earth as a *personal* experience. And so you are also dedicated to the physical, material world—for which we applaud you—so as to bridge heaven with Earth and discover God *here* and within yourself. You are dedicated to success. And with less and less guilt. To understand that is a manifestation of your own divine spark rather than in opposition to the same.

You are here as well to balance the male-female within you; to love the female more within yourself, Michael, because you did live about eight out of every ten lives as the male, and so within your male self now you are seeking to love, to discover the female of your own being; and, again, you are making wonderful strides.

As the original traveler and pioneer and explorer, Michael, you nevertheless—despite all that's said—you still tend to allow yourself to remain a little detached, a little away from almost everything in life. And you mentally, and with your personality, are capable of showing presence and care, but in your soul it's as if you're reaching from across a fence a little bit, and remaining a little detached, so our primary invitation to you, Michael, is total intimacy with life, to let yourself be overcome by the wind, to let it tear your roots even out of the ground, to let yourself be fully moved; and, to let the *world* explore *you* . . . as much as *you* have explored the world . . . and there is where you will know joy beyond your wildest dreams and imaginations.

God bless you, my friends. And would you have questions . . . or comments?

Questions indeed, Doc, and comments aplenty. Hath ever a man spake so penetratingly and so relevantly to total strangers?

Or is it something that any of us could have said?

Ask Jennifer. Ask Michael. Each was nailed to the wall, and knew it. And they are still talking about it to everyone they know.

I spoke with Jennifer during the week following her encounter with Dr. Peebles. This is what my daughter had to say about her experience:

I think we both felt like someone else was there. I mean other than Thomas; it was someone different. Dr. Peebles was there and I really felt as if he were talking to me, that I could really trust what he was saying—as if he were right inside me —and I really believed what he was saying to me.

I'm not someone who has really ever thought about reincarnation—or if I thought about it at all, I didn't much like the idea. But I just knew that what he was saying pertains to my life now. I can't remember when I didn't feel—well, I think I was beginning to be artistic at an early age—it has always been something very important to me.

And when I met Michael—you know I didn't date in high school that much—and I just immediately committed myself only to Michael. When Dr. Peebles referred to some of my previous lives with all that exploration of sexuality—you know all that about the female sexual being, to see what that was all about, but that in this life I really wanted to concentrate on intimacy—well, that's just the way it is, that's all. I felt as though Dr. Peebles were commenting on that, on my sense of commitment to Michael—and the fact that there's never been anybody else, and I don't expect there ever to be anybody else. I really thought that he was expressing that.

Everything that he told me was just right on the mark. Everything he said about my previous lives was kind of like a lead-up to this life and where I am now. And it really made sense, everything that he said, it made a lot of sense.

And it was electrical. I mean, you could be as skeptical as you want, but when you sit in a room with this guy and he starts talking to you, you really believe what he's saying. It's really incredible. No matter what—you know, it's like—Michael has been raised Catholic, under very strict guidelines, and I really studied the Catholic faith and converted to it—and I'm still striving toward it, trying to get close to God and feel that reverence, to feel that special time for prayer and meditation. But at the same time, everything that he told us just kind of applied to that. You know, that it all fits in together in a way that we don't feel a betrayal of faith by talking to Dr. Peebles.

Everything he said made a lot of sense—and not because I wanted to believe it. In a way, I was really wanting *not* to believe some of it but—in listening to the tape over again . . . he's such a vibrant personality. And he *is* different from Thomas. Thomas is a very nice man but you know, you do get the separation; they are separate people. I felt like any question I would have put to Dr. Peebles, he would have answered to the best of his ability, no matter what we asked him.

He was very patient and very loving, kind, and humane and sympathetic, all the great qualities that you would expect someone on the other side to have. Nothing at all seemed out of place or jarring, it was just all very beautiful and just like you would expect it to be. Such a soothing—and the feeling of total love, I mean *total* love, and he makes you laugh. He *enjoys* it. You just get the feeling that he is *loving* the experience himself, enjoys talking to you and trying to get you to talk back.

I was—Dad, honestly, I don't know where he comes from, I don't know what it is, but everything that he said made a lot of sense to me, and I felt that if I had asked him anything more personal, he would have answered—if I had really gotten down to deep problems or personality things or explanations of things that I didn't know, he would have answered anything. And it only whet my appetite. I would love to talk to him more.

I *really* would. You talk to him once and you think, "Oh, God, I should've asked about—I want to hear him talk on *this* subject and *that* subject."

As far as Michael—the thing about him being an adventurer and explorer and wondering about life and everything—that *is* Michael. What Dr. Peebles said about him being a beautiful spirit, it's so true about him.

You know, when I first met Michael, I saw more a side of him of . . . new things to see and not wanting to be tied down—footloose and fancy-free, I guess you'd call it. But I also felt that he wanted to be committed but was afraid to be. So when Dr. Peebles talks about his past lives and all the things that he's done, it really does fit.

I really saw a lot of Michael in all of that. It all fit together. I saw how—when he was talking about Michael's purpose in this lifetime and his need for commitment and how he would *root* himself and just let the wind blow all it wanted—well, that's my Michael, and I've seen him growing more and more into that just since I've known him. His life is pretty set now. There's a lot to happen yet but he does have his feet planted beautifully, he really does.

He goes with the flow, he doesn't get upset, he's the most giving and *bending* person I've ever known, and the most relaxed and secure. And strong. And I can see the leadership qualities Dr. Peebles was talking about. It really fits him. I mean, Dr. Peebles knew who he was talking to.

And I feel that he described *me* very well. You know, I think that he knew me when he was talking to me. I really felt that he knew me. All the sexuality stuff—the only thing I mind about that is what people would make of it. I understood what he was telling me about that, but I wouldn't want it to become the brunt of jokes. You know what I mean. But you know he really did—I could believe everything that he said about me, I really could.

I feel very warm within myself about all that, very secure with it.

It was totally fascinating. Absolutely great.

We deeply appreciate Jennifer and Michael's willingness to share the experience with our readers; for us, it is but another testament to their beautiful fascination with life.

If you should ever be so fortunate as to find yourself the subject of one of these phenomenal broad outlines of individual history, you will find contained therein an actual personality description that cannot be easily evaded or shrugged away—not the general sort of thing encountered in horoscopes but a multilevel revelation of self in terms at once so penetrating and so profound as to strike your understanding with a force you have never before encountered. And it resonates for days, like a corkscrew turning slowly within the mind and unearthing all manner of buried fears, frailties, and foibles in a process somewhat similar to catharsis. It is a ventilation of the soul, so to speak, that explains us to ourselves. Viewed from the side, we get only a quaint story that perhaps could be interpreted in various ways; from head-on, though, we know that this is us and that we have not been condemned by our adventures in life, that we are more and better than we have ever realized, and we begin to see our deep-felt goals in different perspectives.

The general effect for most is similar to the expansive, electric activation mentioned by Paul Weisberg. A few experience a brief carryover effect similar to a mild depression; and, indeed, a lot of things are stirred up there, but in each case I have followed, the mild depression is soon replaced by the other effect as certain strong preconceptions begin to yield to the ventilation.

I have encountered only two individuals, out of more than a hundred questioned, who report very little personal correlation to the material. These could represent genuine "misses," certainly, but I would also suggest to both of these people that they submit their material to an intimate who is exposed to them daily and get a second opinion, because both of these profiles suggest personalities who are defensively rigid of thought and in strong need of help.

In that connection, it is pertinent to mention at this point that we have found several medical practitioners in the local area who now use insights gained from Dr. Peebles in their treatment of psychological problems—and we have so far been exposed to only the tiny tip of that iceberg.

We have discovered also a local psychiatrist, Dr. Richard Ferman, who for several years now has been approaching various types of so-called mental illness with the view that, instead, these patients may be beginning to experience certain psychic events which they do not understand and therefore cannot deal with. Included in this category are some who appear to be suffering various delusional phenomena usually associated with schizophrenia. This could be a whole new area developing in psychiatry, and it promises to grow rapidly as our "new age" advances and more and more of us begin to experience remarkably new direct perceptions of reality. That is a subreason for this book, and it could involve you directly because one of the most common reactions by individuals in early awareness of the spirit world is: "I was afraid I was going crazy."

Indeed, it has been a common experience throughout history that our saints and geniuses have been but a single step removed from an insane asylum—and God only knows how many "crazy people" we have in our institutions today who are there only because their perceptions of reality are a bit fuller than yours and mine.

Right now let's go have an encounter with that reality in a way not quite so disturbing.

6

The Canvas

of Life

"You are the paintbrush. Life is the canvas. Learn this, and you will never feel the victim again."

—*Dr. Peebles*

As all great teachers of the past and present, Dr. Peebles relies heavily on metaphor, simile, analogy, and allegory in dealing with ideas that may be difficult to express in a more direct manner. We get the feeling that he is forever trying to "get in tune" at our level of understanding—and, at times, with Thomas's own linguistic thresholds. Language has forever been the great barrier in trying to elucidate esoteric ideas, so it should be no wonder that symbolical representation is often used by mystic and poet alike. Dr. Peebles is both, so his expression is often very colorful.

Some may wish to view this as vagueness on his part, but surely that is never the intent. This beautiful soul is working with all his skill (and all of Thomas's pliability) to impart important understandings to any who will listen. He is never intentionally vague but always as direct as language (and the process) allows.

During the session that follows, the Spirit was trying to elaborate one of his favorite themes. We recommend it to your close attention, for he is touching the fundamentals of the life experience both in and out of the body.

DR. PEEBLES: It is a joy and blessing when man and spirit join together in search of the greater truths and awareness. Might I offer encouragement, my dear friends, as you strive to understand consciousness in the affairs of the public, to understand the nature of spirituality in the forum of your own country, to understand the nature of searching—searching within and outside of traditional religion, for parallels are alive throughout all mysteries of mankind, the clues always apparent to the seeker who works with faith and follow-through.

All right. We want to start with the issue of creatorhood and victimhood. For there begins the greatest challenge in the human mind. Do I accept responsibility as the creator of my experience in the world?—or am I in fact the victim?—and all fundamental thoughts and decisions radiate from that pivotal, critical choice.

It is in the choice of accepting responsibility that one maintains and builds the right to create change. It is in the desire to be the victim that one, instead, is the follower of change, the passenger of change. It is the latter category from which true pain radiates, and the greater conflicts in life. It is in the former that one is able not only to assert self, but as well to have the mobility, the locomotion to change one's mind and thereby work with the world rather than against the world.

In the latter case as the victim, since you are not able to create locomotion, when there are differences of view between yourself and another—well, then, it is simply a fort, or a lack of a fort, there is protection, the need to protect, rather than the ability to change.

And so the issue of creatorhood and victimhood is fundamental to the intellectual mind as well as to the spiritual journey. The ability to accept authority as the creator, also, is necessary before true creativity, artistic creativity, can take place. The "victim" cannot find a paintbrush to compose upon the canvas of life, whereas one who accepts authority, self as the creator, has the concept to *be* the paintbrush, to take the paintbrush to create your life, to draw it upon the canvas of life.

And so masterhood, enlightenment, is predicated on

that authority to be the creator. It is relevant to understand that as the creator it is not in opposition to life, again, but instead the ability through free will to move with life—different points of view, to be sure, as part of the oneness, but moving with life.

To be the greater creator is not to be necessarily the warrior but the lover, the more compassionate being. The experience of life on the planet Earth is a journey, a journey to the heart where all things are true for a moment, a journey that is a greater celebration of the diversity of life, formerly feared.

It is in the nature of life a desire to be loved, to be appreciated, to be understood. This is not possible when one is the victim, but only when one in fact is the creator. God bless you, my friends, and would you have questions or comment.

DON: Thank you, Dr. Peebles. Again you just wiped out half of my very carefully structured format for this discussion by anticipating my questions in your opening statement. How do you do that?

DR. PEEBLES: *You* do that, Don. With a little help, maybe.

DON: Oh. Really? Uh . . . so where do I start? We had the feeling during our first session that you are more interested in communicating your spirit psychology than in convincing people that they are being visited by Spirit.

DR. PEEBLES: Correct. The latter is really not relevant, very simply because each and every soul on the planet Earth is going to leave the body through death. You see, in our concept of time, your life—every human's life, animal life —is but the flash of an eye, and so everyone has life after death proven to them rather quickly, when they die and leave the body. And, indeed, those who wish to look ahead and believe in the meantime already do so. Those who don't, or don't need to, won't. The issue, you see, is not to live or not live after death. That's already settled. The issue is to use the time you are here for the growth you came here to experience. More important than one might think, Don. What is this?—a game, here on Earth? Or is it an important opportunity to move along your pathway?

DON: Yes, I understand that. But—

DR. PEEBLES: But no—we can see—it is understandable, one must be anchored. It is not my—our calling to prove the existence of life after death or to reveal the physics of the universe—that is not our specialty. There are others who feel that calling and . . . but . . . of course, Don, we are here to help in any way that is open to us. We are not impatient with your questions. We applaud them.

DON: Thank you. Very good.

DR. PEEBLES: It is just that our time, our limited time, through this channel, could be taken up with the issue of proof, which would then greatly dominate the important work of the philosophy—spiritual psychology, if you will. But we understand what you are doing and we support that, applaud that; God bless you.

DON: I understand and appreciate your priorities, so let's proceed in that vein. You've spoken of the various domains or plateaus in the spirit world, collectives and the like, and I presume that those were actually set up from Earth. In a sense, we create our own heavens. So could we say that certain rigid religious disciplines set up something like a karmic pattern that will find correspondence on the spirit side? Are there actually dimensions of truth, in spirit, where a devout Moslem would go to something approximating a Moslem reality, a Christian to a Christian reality?

DR. PEEBLES: Oh, absolutely; consistently. When one leaves the body in death, there are certain factors that predicate your locality in the spirit side. The most important and most forceful of which is your own will and belief. If a soul believes with such intensity, *anything*, with no flexibility—no flexibility whatsoever—then upon arrival in the spirit side, you will find yourself sucked into a certain locality of the spirit side, with others who have that same determined belief, with no flexibility, so that you can have mirrored and magnified to you your own self. What typically happens in these localities is some reinforcement, to be sure, but eventually rebellion. For you see yourself so clearly, so crystallized, that you are able to identify the lack of flexibility; and all of a sudden there is a movement inside where you say: "Wait a minute, there must be something I haven't thought of"—then immediately you leave that locality and you are attracted to another, which would perhaps say a larger truth representative of a larger community of life in the universe. It is also relative to how quickly you leave the body, but the most important is the intensity of belief—is there or is there not any flexibility?

DON: Jesus spoke of his Father's many mansions. Could we

take this to be a reference to the same sort of thing you were just talking about?

DR. PEEBLES: Exactly! Very good, Don, exactly. It is everyone marching to the beat of his own drummer, and that *is* the love of God. So whether you are the Baptist or the Buddhist, the atheist or the skeptic, or the believer . . . whether you are a criminal, in social terms, or whether you are law-abiding, each and every one of them contains their lessons to self-realization, divine realization, and it is impossible to avoid the pathway of God. It just—it does— you can hate God or you can believe in *no* God, and you still are creating very real techniques of thought that will move you closer to God.

Like, you know, if you take a rubber band and you stretch it from one finger to a finger of the other hand, you can seem to go farther and farther apart . . . but the farther you go the more tight the attraction, back to the source. You see?

Uh . . . Don, Linda, dear friends—if you would forgive us, we're going to leave this channeling. Our channel is—you've just got him so excited by your work, your book, and he is having difficulty maintaining. We can come, we work to some degree, but for the purpose of this book we would request total atmosphere through our channel. So I know that you will understand; we must leave. Please request a scheduling as soon as possible, and have no fear, there will be plenty and plenty of interviews with Spirit, and so you can relax about it. Our channel is —he's right here as I am talking, as a matter of fact, before we've even left—so God bless you, my friends; go your ways in peace, love, and harmony—and in your study, perhaps it is another book, but you will do a dissertation perhaps on the complexities and subtleties of channeling and more important, perhaps, the parallels as well as the ramifications to everyone's life. There are wonderful important parallels of breakthrough and insight for people. All right; God bless you both; we love you.

DON, LINDA: Thank you, Dr. Peebles.

[Immediately.]

THOMAS: Ohhh, God! I heard that.

DON: (*chuckling*) You heard it, eh?

THOMAS: Ohhhhh!

DON: We got some marvelous stuff.

THOMAS: Did you really? Oh, man, it was terrible. I just
kept . . .

DON: It was a lot longer than it seemed. We've clocked, uh,
twenty-five minutes.

THOMAS: Oh, that's good. Felt like—that's just me, that hasn't
happened in a long time—it was like I was having this
battle to stay. . . .

LINDA: Were you aware of the thunder?

(A brief but severe thundershower had moved directly overhead about midway through the session; very
unusual for this section of California.)

THOMAS: Oh, yeah, I think I do remember hearing the thunder.

LINDA: It really cracked. Rattled the windows, even. Cracked
directly overhead.

DON: Dr. Peebles reacted. He paused in the middle of a statement and said, "God *bless* you!" then went right on with
his statement.

THOMAS: Maybe that's what did it. I'm sorry.

DON: No, he said you're too excited about the book.

THOMAS: (*laughing*) Well, he ought to know.

DON: He wiped out my whole damn format again.

LINDA: (*laughing*) And left him sputtering for something to
talk about.

DON: Yeah; gee, thanks for your help there, kid.

LINDA: (*still laughing*) Don't look to me. I just sit there like a
dummy.

THOMAS: I'm sorry for the short . . .

Apologetic, see. This amazing guy is apologetic because he
couldn't maintain the trance during a thunderstorm—whether it
was inside or outside him—after sitting there for nearly half an
hour talking like God.

I think that is called humility.

7

Life

on Life

"The entire universe is a loving and living experience of divine thought . . . a fabric that is intermeshed with all things."

—*Dr. Peebles*

Thomas is quite sensitive to the understanding that not everyone is convinced that he is a genuine medium, that some—for whatever reasons of their own—prefer to believe that Dr. Peebles is either a deliberate concoction or some subconscious faculty of Thomas's own mind. There have been times when we wondered about that ourselves, but only very briefly and never with anything more than stubborn skepticism behind it. Actually it is much easier to believe in the genuineness of the experience than to try to refute it with convincing arguments.

The doubt remains for some, however, and this is sometimes very troubling for Thomas. He does possess a great sense of humor and is usually able to deflect the negativity with self-effacing comparisons between himself and Dr. Peebles. There could even be times when Thomas wishes that it were all coming from himself instead of having to share credit with another.

There are other times, however, when Thomas is clearly morti-
fied by something Dr. Peebles has said, *realizing* that some people
do give him all the credit—pronouncements on sexuality, in particular, as well as other subjects that seem to be very "far out." Like
the Yeti, for example, or the extraterrestrials and . . . well, you'll
see what we mean.

Thomas turned beet-red when he read the transcript of portions of this chapter. We can tell you one thing for sure: Dr. Peebles
is *not* a *deliberate* concoction of Thomas's imagination.

DR. PEEBLES: God bless you; Dr. Peebles here; it is a joy and
blessing when man and spirit join together in search of the
greater truths and awareness. Might I offer encouragement, my dear friends, as you strive to understand your
right to touch, to be touched—your right to experience
God within your own heart—to help the world do the
very same.

Greetings, my dear friends; you are gathered here
today to understand the nature of consciousness as a consistent activity within all life, human and otherwise, nonphysical as well as physical; to understand the purpose of
politics, of nations; to understand the sexuality, the drive,
the magnetism between all life; the illusion of separation;
for all endeavors of life truly reduce to a simple relationship between one and another.

It is the perception and the response that are subjective in nature that create the different experience for one,
and different for the other, from which each grows according to his or her own needs; for one person's pathway
of this spiritual maturity is another's distraction.

And so it will be the way of the world in the new age
that the differences will be celebrated rather than seeking
to change the very same.

We are very joyful with both of you in your work as
souls, for when you go to sleep you come over here and
you counsel, and our chore has been to help you hear
yourselves, to let yourselves be energized and moved in
your hearts, your souls.

Well, you have truly danced the dance of angels over
here; you have felt a new electricity, and you have declared permission to shout your truth, to sing your songs.
You have been an inspiration to us, and so we thank you
as well as acknowledge you for your courage. God bless
you both; and would you have question or comment?

DON: God bless you, Dr. Peebles, and thank you for that very warm greeting. As usual we are pleased, thrilled, and excited to be here with you. As you know, we have some incomplete business from the first session. We would like to return to that at this time. We were discussing the process of transition that we call death. What is that?—*really.*

DR. PEEBLES: All right. What you call death is birth into another reality, another experience—actually a greater reality—where all differences are celebrated, where the diversity of life is a support for true love of self and love of God . . . where God is seen as a composite of the entire color spectrum rather than only the blues, or only the pinks or the purples.

And so . . . on the spirit side, at death, each spirit begins to recover its ability to be alive in any environment rather than only a selected environment, such as the Earth. When that ability—or level of self-permission—is large enough, the spirit reincarnates according to its own path of growth.

Upon arriving in the spirit side, you encounter different zones, different localities, according to your belief system; according to the manner of your passing: was it very quick?—was it somewhat slow or very drawn out?—was it for the most part painless; done in your sleep, for example?—or was it through a very intense experience of physical or emotional pain?

All these factors lend to the locality and the type of helpers that you will see. Some people come into the spirit side and immediately need to go to a hospital—hospital of the heart and of the soul—where they are touched by at least three other loving masterly spirits who merely touch them and hold them as a child to the breast and comfort them till that spirit puts the head up and says: "What is this? Who am I? Where am I? What am I to do?"

Only upon the question is there a response from the celestial angels, from the divine force and from the higher teachers. There is always light and love available for those who come to the spirit—unless as we said previously, Don, unless the belief is so intense that there is no room for flexibility. Then one experiences what one insists on experiencing—and the universe, the entire universe, is so loving that it supports your desires rather than demanding that you change. For all things are contained within God.

The death experience is one of greater life, not of less living.

The death experience is one of greater light, not of darkness.

The death experience from earth is birth into a new permission to love and to be loved.

The death experience is in many ways for some a release from prison, from jail, into a true freedom of the mind, the heart, and the body.

The release through the death experience is an opportunity for increased communication, greater responsibility, and new depths of artistic expression.

The greater challenge—the more pain, my friends—is not from death from the earth side to the spirit. The greater pain, much greater pain, is from spirit to the earthly experience.

It is often with hesitation and fear—and trepidation, on occasion but not always—that a spirit enters—approaches the womb, and prepares to enter the womb. But then the warmth and the nurturing of the womb is so overwhelming that peace comes into the child, temporarily . . . but just previous to that, the death from the spirit side—ending, death is an ending, ending of the spirit experience—so that birth or beginning into the earthly experience, there is the greater challenge.

Coming to the spirit side, for the most part, with occasional exceptions, is a very, very pleasant experience. Do you understand?

DON: Yes, yes . . . that's very comforting.

DR. PEEBLES: This is part of the reason why many souls of their own desire really don't want to think too much about the spirit. There's a certain self-imposed closure in the mind, in the memory, so as not to remember the spirit, for that would be a distraction; for some people would want to leave Earth several times every year and return to the spirit; which does not serve them, you see.

DON: I see, yes. We have noted in very young children, especially from the age of three and back, when they are first coming into realization in their own personalities—that sometimes they make surprising statements that seem to be calling back some previous period. A little boy, for example, remembering a time when he was a little girl. Could that be, then, a valid statement by the child?

DR. PEEBLES: Correct. It is valid. It is not a symbol, not a translation; it is wholly and wholly literal. There is a very fertile ground of study for the philosophers of your day and age—to study these children and their comments, for they are not fantasy; they are not exaggerated; they are literal. It is at the age of five and six when they become fantasy; things get stretched out of proportion. But at the age of two and three, it is pure truth coming forward.

DON: We would do well to let our children become our teachers.

DR. PEEBLES: Exactly. Absolutely. This would be part of a new relationship between the child and the parent—where parents see themselves instead as host and hostess for another being who will create its own life rather than mother and father who must form the child as clay—and there is this desire to form the child through love, of course—but to form the child as clay, this is where the greater conflict and the falling apart of families comes forward.

It is to support the child, its desire to learn, to understand its own pathway; and it is the responsibility of a host and hostess to remind the child that responsibility for oneself is the technique. Responsibility for oneself is the greatest fear but it is also the greatest joy, the paintbrush of life.

And your challenge as the child is to accept responsibility as you grow into your maturing years, because you have rejected responsibility in past lives. There is no soul, my friends, who is reincarnated to Earth who does not have fear—some fear—of responsibility in their early life. That is why you are reincarnated. The state of full illumination and enlightenment includes, among other things, a great, great celebration for the permission to be responsible from the divine universe.

And so a child coming forward through the hostess and with the host—fundamentally, fears responsibility—and it is the host and hostess's job to teach them to *love* responsibility. Do you understand?

DON: Yes, I do. To go back for a moment to this death experience—and without getting too much into physics here—does John Doe release the body? Or does the body release John?

DR. PEEBLES: John releases the body. But now . . . there is an etheric envelope, an etheric vehicle that is finer than the physical body and yet still contains the spirit and the soul. If there is resistance to death in the personality of the soul, this etheric body can release the physical structure.

So, in some ways it is both. But overall it is the soul releasing the body.

DON: Are the terms *soul* and *spirit* interchangeable terms? Do they denote the same?

DR. PEEBLES: Yes. They are interchangeable. There are those who say otherwise, but they are interchangeable. They are the same. In fact, there is wisdom to understand that in your present state of being—*right* here, where you *are*— you *are* the soul. The soul is not floating around somewhere else in space. You *are* your soul. This is the composite of all of your experience.

DON: Of all the experience of all lives?

DR. PEEBLES: Right now; exactly. Not a portion of it. What you are right now—speaking—that *is* you. That's all of you. In your superconscious, your unconscious—what have you—are various details; but the conclusions are voiced in your attitude. You understand me. So it is important to see yourself as your soul. Literally speaking, your soul is larger than your personality. But there is greater value, there is greater wisdom in understanding that you, speaking, are your own soul.

DON: That's very interesting. So we always have the ability to reveal ourselves to ourselves. This same being, John, who has just died, can he be aware of events transpiring on Earth since his death? Can he see loved ones? And can he be aware of their reactions to his passing?"

DR. PEEBLES: "Yes, particularly for the first three months. Rarely is it longer than that. Often for the first three days the spirit is so involved with the total separation of the body—for upon medical death the spirit is not totally separate from the physical body. It can take some additional hours, or even up to three days, for a total release of the physical body, through the etheric; so the spirit who has passed can be more involved with self, the transformation, than with relatives. But on the third day, approximately— for example, at funerals—there is where the release has been completed, and the spirit often wants to bid adieu, or reassure those left behind—which is very difficult.

DON: Yes, I'm sure it is. Is there a period, then, on the spirit side which would roughly correspond to what we here would think of as a debriefing?

DR. PEEBLES: Yes, yes . . . self is spontaneously debriefed by self, and that can be very painful if the soul has left a lot of unfinished business on the other side, has come to the spirit side with very rigid attitudes, and so forth, but each and every soul who comes to the spirit side from the body is greeted by friends and family, a few or many. Each and every soul is greeted by a force of light. However, each and every soul has the freedom and the will to translate that as they choose.

So, look at the little miracles that you have in your own lives, as human beings on Earth, and remember when you chose to either disbelieve or simply ignore, or to downplay that light or symphony or that picture, that portrait, that theater, that ecstasy, that orgasm, that rapture and that pleasure of life—and through guilt, through self-punishment, through priorities of safety and sanctuary and so forth, you see it but you choose not to be touched by it.

So you see, we cannot literally take our hand of light into your heart and make it okay, even when you are over here. So we dance for you, we entertain you, we give you symphonies of life, and you have every opportunity to be thrilled to the core of your being, but it must be suggestive —it must be no more and no less than your own free will to translate as you prefer.

We are not dismayed by this reality. We are thankful and rejoicing for this universal truth, for this is what guarantees the light of life. Without that free will, you don't have life, there is no life. There's only movement. So it's to be thankful for that right, that permission and that power to be or not to be, regardless of your environmental circumstances, on Earth or here in the spirit.

Now . . . given the above, we do—according to a particular soul's plan—feel the joy of direct consultation and inspiration, so we'll wait. You know, sometimes in terms of time on Earth it may take weeks or months, sometimes years, before we have your ear—even with all that dance of the angels as you arrive over here—but as we have your ear, you will see us smiling, you will see us happy, you will see us embracing you, you will see us liking you—not just loving you but liking you—as you are, not as you could be. And that is what dumbfounds many spirits over here, particularly when they see their own sin as so great, which is what you term the debriefing. The pains and challenges of life on Earth are looked at in a very different light over here, and sometimes it takes the returning spirit a while to find that light.

But the options remain your own. For the most part, the soul recognizes—through that total unqualified support that we offer—recognizes a new hunger for life, a new desire to experiment, a new permission, then, to understand. With that understanding, however, there is not full healing. For there is a recognition that the understanding must be tested, must be extrapolated and repeated for a greater sense of self-love within.

It is not that you return to Earth to learn to become perfect, my friends. Let me repeat that ten times. It is to come to Earth to finally stop condemning yourself for what you think is lack of perfection. And, instead, translating that lack of perfection as the mysterious wonder of universal change, guaranteed eternally present. The state of perfection that you think you're supposed to have, that you want, would lock you into an immobility.

So the counseling is to forgive yourself—to lighten up, and not take yourself and life too seriously—and that's when you find a new desire, a new plan to reenter into life once again.

Do you understand?

DON: Yes, and that is beautiful. So at the time of death of the physical body, the Earth body, and the resultant transformation, release of the body . . . is this made easier through cremation?

DR. PEEBLES: Yes, and we highly recommend it. We strongly encourage the burning of the body as very healthy and as a wonderful experience that helps the passing, the spirit passing. You see? Also, the experience of a wake, for example, that celebrates death, this as well we strongly encourage.

Certainly the tears must be honored, for missing the presence of a loved one, but in terms of the loved one who has passed, you can feel good for them. They are much better off. They are celebrating their experience of love. They are being embraced in a blanket of love and warmth, probably beyond that of their experience of Earth.

So the wake is a celebration that the departed soul is well and that it is going on to a finer experience. It is also a "thank-you" to the soul for having lived with us and been with us. So the person who is on the spirit side, recently passed, feels so much better.

Compare that experience to John, on the spirit side, looking at Mary who seven months later is still crying her eyes out, day and night. And because he loves her, is he going to leave her? Probably not; he might stay around and still try to help her. And so Mary, in terms of loving John—if she really understood that—would stop crying, that's all, and feel that love she has for John, so he can go about his business.

DON: Actually that expression of love—the anguish—becomes a sort of a trap for the spirit, doesn't it?

DR. PEEBLES: Yes, yes, right. The question is where the love is directed. The love is supposedly for the person who passed, but it really appears as a sadness, not as an expression of love.

DON: Yes; a loss; a sense of tragedy. We probably should try to think of people who have died as having—uh, in the same sense that we send children to school away from home; they are still very much alive and functioning. Naturally, we miss them. But it is not a tragedy.

DR. PEEBLES: Exactly; yes; that's very good.

DON: Could you comment on the phenomenon in which those who have recently died are said to physically reappear to friends or family?—an actual physical appearance.

DR. PEEBLES: Yes. It is not that they are inhabiting their bodies again, but they are manifesting their etheric bodies that we referred to earlier, which can appear to be physical and can be touched.

This is consistent in the physics of death and of the universe. It happens even more frequently than is understood. Jesus, for example, was using his etheric body in a projection of his total and complete self, slowing down the vibration through thought and through will.

Now, this can take place not only through love but through great rage, or anger, or extraordinary emotions to slow the vibration down into an anchored locality in your physical world. And that's the etheric body.

DON: That would explain ghosts and uh . . . ?

DR. PEEBLES: Yes. Now, often the ghosts, however, are not the etheric body; they are the soul, they *are* the spirit, a little finer vibration. These are beings who have such . . . these are beings who don't have the certain flexibility that we talked about earlier. Their belief is so focused and determined on a given house or city, or a place in the forest, that that is heaven for them; they don't want to leave it.

DON: So we tend to create our own heavens by our beliefs too. And, uh, our own hells?

DR. PEEBLES: Exactly.

DON: Is there a place on the spirit side that would roughly correspond to man's concept of hell?

DR. PEEBLES: Yes, roughly speaking, yes. This is where those of like mind gather together to reinforce their anger. It's always an illusion of separation. The greater the illusion, the greater the anger. The anger is always predicated on some form of vengeance, of feeling rejected, not understood, not cared for, and so forth—so they gather together to justify and reinforce each other's anger.

And seeing others with their angers that just go roundabout, full circle, and are not released only creates more anger and more hurt, more pain. All understand eventually that this is not a technique for fulfillment. For they don't feel better, and they really do want to feel better. The anger is not the fulfillment. So they turn around one hundred eighty degrees finally and look in another direction, and there is the spirit of love who welcomes them and helps them to forgive themselves and forgive life around them.

DON: Wait a minute! The forgiveness is not from God but from self!

DR. PEEBLES: Exactly.

DON: So then in that spirit of self-forgiveness . . . ?

DR. PEEBLES: Yes; you see. They are sucked into a new vibration, a happier place of love.

DON: Is it possible for such spirits in this deluded, hellish reality to come through human mediums the way you are coming through now? Can that account for some of the phenomena such as so-called demon possession?

DR. PEEBLES: Yes, yes; that can happen. They do have an effect—it can be an effect. However, it is wise to understand that these beings you speak of in—roughly, hell—are no different from all of you on the planet Earth that have your moments of anger and rage in your lives, you see. It's no different; it's not worse; it's the same thing.

You watch yourselves as you go through your lives anyway, true? You go to work, you go out and walk, or you drive in your vehicles despite anger around you or inside of you; you live your life anyway. You should have that same attitude in your relationship with the spirit. There are spirits, many of them, who are very angry for a moment, but despite them, you should go on and live. It should be in your communion with God and the spirit that you let yourself reach out rather than use your fear of contacting an angry spirit as another excuse to stay alone.

DON: You are saying, in other words, don't be afraid to reach out to the spirit. Permit yourself to have intimacy with spirits and don't worry if you should get an angry one.

DR. PEEBLES: Yes, well, you would experience only a little bit of discomfort or anger from the spirit side, according to your need to experience that and, uh, also parallel to your physical life. If you are experiencing tremendous amounts of discord and anger inside you and around you all the time on Earth, you may attract that same energy when you are contacting the spirit. So from the spirit's point of view, those spirits who are frustrated—someone who is petrified of them makes them even angrier, because they are not feeling loved. See . . . imagine yourselves when you have been angry in your own soul—you were angry and you were furious—what you really wanted was someone to understand you; you were screaming for someone to listen to you and understand you, and it made you furious that no one would understand you. True? And instead, what does everyone typically do? They just put more distance between them and you, which makes you even more angry. So be not concerned about angry spirits.

Everyone has anger. Those of you who listen and hear and read these words: all of you have had anger. And when you had anger, did you not want people to stop and listen to you and care for you, rather than fight you? And so it is when you see others who are angry; listen; receive them, and their anger will be dispelled, and you will know love beyond your wildest dreams and imaginations.

DON: Yes; thank you. Well . . . it has been suggested by some modern thinkers—especially people in the earth sciences—that the Earth and its biosphere is, in their view, like a single entity, sort of a living system in which each constituent of that system is intimately responsive and, uh, interactive with the whole. Sounds good to me. Could you comment on that and perhaps relate it to the entire universe as a larger entity of somewhat the same nature?

DR. PEEBLES: Yes; it is what we call synchronicity and the oneness of the universe. In the Earth or in the universe or in the microbe or in the nucleus there is movement, there is motion. In that motion there is only change. And within that change there is always the return to the source; there is always the recycling, similar, extremely close in precise measurements, extremely close to a perfect circle but not quite; and so thereby becoming a spiral—figuratively, symbolically, and literally by measurement.

This is not only a three-dimensional but four-dimensional phenomenon and even beyond that. The spiral is the source of the greater frequency changes, such as black holes, which goes into the discussion of other dimensions, another reality, another universe; also internal combustion . . . ah . . . instantaneous or spontaneous combustion of an emotional experience, or a physical experience . . . uh, interdimensional travel, in the form of the spiral.

To resist change is to ignite pain and separation; to surrender and move with, and eventually to pilot change is to become the center of the universe rather than the periphery; the creator rather than the victim.

The entire universe is a loving and living experience of divine thought. It is a fabric that is intermeshed with all things. All particles are a part of this—and the science of the next century will not be priding itself on its great diversity, its great specialization, but instead will pride itself on a unified understanding. All the differences that have been found, or so-called discovered in your current century will . . . their source will be found to be common, into oneness, or a unified field, in the century to come.

So it is true that every movement in one part of the universe affects another part of that universe to some infinitesimal degree at least. And you are part of all life around you. Does that answer your question?

DON: Yes, yes, it does. And very beautifully answers my question. Linda would like to speak to you, Dr. Peebles.

DR. PEEBLES: Linda! This is a blessing! God bless you! I must say it's about time too. God bless you. You're invisible, aren't you? "Well now, Dr. Peebles, I'm talking to you now, aren't I? Take that." Bless you.

LINDA: (*laughing*) Yes. What can you tell us about our higher self and how we can contact or reach that higher self?

DR. PEEBLES: Ah, remember what we said about the soul? Who's talking right now? Linda? Or Linda, your soul?"

LINDA: O-kaaay.

DR. PEEBLES: Now I know it's more fun to think that it is Linda who is speaking and that your soul is somewhere else; thereby, there's some invisible hope that you are a larger being. And of course it is true that you are a larger being in your divine reality and source in God.

However, to become cognitive and active and participatory in your relationship to that greater divine being that you are, it is to see how you are doing everything you can do right now. That all the choices you are making now, Linda—conclusions, perceptions, and responses— are based on all your experience of your soul. And . . . you are doing the best you can and so is everyone on the planet Earth, no matter what their crime, no matter how barbaric their deed—which they—which you—must answer for and, in the karmic nature of things, will answer for.

Nevertheless, at the same time there must be compassion, for everyone is their own soul and doing the best they can—feels justified in everything they do. So, to come in contact with your higher self is to pay more attention to your own public and private personalities . . . watch what you do, and what you don't do . . . and that *is* your soul.

When you breathe that into your awareness as a practice, you will more rapidly understand the form of your soul, and how and where and why you do want to grow and accept change rather than fear it. And so . . . to contact your higher self is to love *you* as you are *right* now, whether that be invisible Linda, or whether that be the brilliant artist that you are, whether that be the great lover that you are, whether that be the little fraidy-cat that you are, whether that be the little—so forth and so on.

They're all part of your divine force; they're all wonderful. Loving allowance starts with this awareness. Loving allowance starts with the awareness that your higher self is you and . . . uh . . . that you have been doing the best you can, and thereby you will discover not only forgiveness, but, beyond that, loving allowance. For if you forgive, you will have had to judge in the first place, won't you? And to allow, you don't even start to judge. And when we say judge, we are speaking of condemnation. Certainly you must make decisions . . . that's how you grow. So the act of judgment is a tool that is greatly necessary and valuable in the Earth plane. But we are speaking of the historical references of religion . . . uh . . . judge not, common through all religions . . . which really means do not condemn. For what you see in others is within yourself. Do you understand?

LINDA: Yes. I do.

DR. PEEBLES: Does that answer the question, or do you wish to pursue it?

LINDA: No . . . I think that answers it.

DR. PEEBLES: You see . . . to feel that there is a higher self, I know, can feel so magical and exciting because now you can kind of forget your old self, can't you . . . go find your higher self. But to effectively transform yourself . . . you pull up your pants, pull up your boots, and tighten your belt, and stand tall and say, "All right, this is me! This is it!" and take responsibility for it, with allowance. And if you can't have allowance for yourself, then at least forgive yourself and the world around you. You understand?

LINDA: Yes, thank you. Okay . . . when does the soul enter the fetus?

DR. PEEBLES: Well, it can be anywhere from as early as six weeks . . . the great . . . the greatest frequency is . . . three months to fourteen weeks . . . and . . . sometimes it's not uncommon for it to be around the . . . oh, sixth month. We would make note that there are some human beings walking around on the planet that don't think the spirit has ever really come in all the way, quite a few, as a matter of fact. No, we tease a little. But, uh . . . it's most commonly between twelve and fourteen weeks to six months, occasional exceptions in both directions.

LINDA: Okay, uh . . .

DR. PEEBLES: Now, the soul, however, is hovering . . . is there . . . before and . . . leaves the body frequently after totally embracing the physical body. The soul is never fully inside the physical body while in the womb. The total, complete action of oneness takes place in the first breath upon birth. But between the third and sixth month, there is . . . oh, you might say, seventy-five percent inhabitation. You see? Nothing at all before that, just a hovering.

DON: What is the nature of life in that fetus, what is the biological constituent there? The life force then, we are saying, is not the same thing as soul?

DR. PEEBLES: That is correct. There is a life force that is the intelligence of the universe, within plants for example, within the biological activity of the body; it is not directed by an individualized soul, but it is the natural brilliance, the natural love transformation of the divine universe, again through the symbol of the spiral. So there is intelligence within the rocks and the grass, the air, and . . . the fetus, before habitation by the soul, and . . . when you grow a finger on your hand, and so forth and so on. But the biological activity is not necessarily directed by the souls, or directed by anything. It's just following a pattern of expression, a pattern of being, aliveness.

LINDA: Here in the United States the question of abortion is a strongly divisive issue. I was wondering if you could give us some insight.

DR. PEEBLES: Yeah, change the name! That will help a lot right there. Let's see here . . . well, it is true that all life has a right to thrive, and to be. It is equally true that all life is already in a process of being, and thriving. As you expand your concept of time, as a circle that does not quite touch itself but continues as a spiral, you'll begin to understand the past and the future as alive and living forevermore. In that higher view of experience, you'll recognize the presence and the reality of Spirit always and everywhere. You recognize that your day is the same as a lifetime. Your night is the same as a death experience. So when you live your life, when you awaken in the morning, you are in effect being born. When you go to sleep at night, you are in reality dying and leaving the body for a while.

Merely ask yourselves how often is it true that you just don't want to wake up in the morning. Or that as you approach awakening, and your eyes are open and you remember where you are, while so often there is relief, yet there are times when you recoil, afraid to meet the day at hand, preferring to be in a cocoon or to return to the dreams of spirit. So it is true with the spirit at the moment of incarnation. For the approximate time of three to five months presence within the womb, for the spirit it is the same as one night's sleep for you.

Consistently, there is a hesitation on the part of many souls. They hesitate. "I don't think I want to do this. I believe I would like to reevaluate. I don't want to open my eyes. I hear violence out there in the world. I hear argument between my parents. I feel a desire on my mother's part to kill a man near her. I hear offense through sound of discord and disagreement and disbelief and suspicion in the world. Why do I want to be born in this, thank you very much!" There's a hesitation. Well, that hesitation is in the mind of the incoming spirit but recorded within the physical experience of the womb of Mommy. This, to greater or lesser degree, has direct bearing upon the consciousness of Mother.

Now, in the meantime Mother is waking up in the morning, living an entire day which is like a lifetime, dropping dead at night, leaving the body and returning to the succor of dreams, and then deciding whether to be alive again. And life, while so beautiful, is often very difficult. For it is a school, and all souls incarnating are students, and you often feel that you'd just as soon grow tomorrow, thank you, not today. Merely look at your own lives.

So the mother—the reason for fear is, of course, the fear of responsibility. Underneath that fear of responsibility are the illusions of separation and the fear of intimacy. So the mother goes back and forth and back and forth— tremendous intimacy here, right inside of her, tremendous responsibility—she infers—with little knowledge or training or reinforcement from her environment that the child has its own destiny, its own will and plan before there is any language in the body.

So the mother goes through her cycles of nightmares and not wanting to wake up in the morning. So these two movements of consciousness reach out to each other and try to come together. More often, in the desire for abortion, it is the rule rather than the exception that there is agreement there—a real agreement, not implied—between the incarnating spirit and the mother, a change of mind— or an intention in the first place merely to experience some time in the womb, for reasons that are individual.

It is also true, however, that there are situations where the child does wish to come forward, and the mother—through a dread of responsibility, lack of self-love, anger at the world, and so forth—doesn't feel that she can be alive, and to allow the child to come forward would mean that she would have to come forward. So there is a desire to stop life before it starts. In that situation, we do support encouragement and counseling, support for the mother to open herself to the presence of this child. When that counseling is spiritual in nature, but in real and applied terms, you will find the mother changing her mind.

But, again—more often than not, the decision for what you call abortion is a cooperative decision. To leave life before it starts, as a baby, really is no different from leaving life after ninety years in the body, for from our awareness—and from the larger perspective—life is eternal. As our earlier words about villages over here, you've just decided—you've made a move to a new village and you've then decided you don't want to live there after all, now that you've come close to it and smelled the smoke.

So these are our thoughts, and we encourage those who contemplate abortion to understand it as an act of love, for all things are of God—to see it as quite possibly an agreement between cooperative souls for mutual growth, and we encourage sensitivity by all to the decisions made through prayer and meditation. But we also encourage those who demand and expect that all children must come forward—that you as well are demonstrating love. Both are right. Neither is wrong. God bless you.

LINDA: Thank you.

DON: Thank you, Dr. Peebles. Very good counsel. Probably won't reshape the battle lines or soften the rhetoric on either side, but perhaps we could hope for some common ground of sensitivity toward both positions.

LINDA: You mentioned—I guess it was in our first interview—that animals are guided by Spirit. Can you tell us more about that?

DR. PEEBLES: Yes. There is consciousness and individualized consciousness in many animal souls and species, and there is *general* consciousness within *all* life upon the planet Earth. Uh . . . the guidance system of the spirit is only a natural amplification of love, community, and family. When a part of your family goes somewhere else, you always stay in communication, don't you?—by letters or by phone. Even though you know that the person from your family must go on their own journey, travel where they must and where they want, you're always there to phone, or with a letter, or in dream-states and astral projection . . . because it's just love, nothing complicated about it at all.

And so when in a family—in the larger sense of the word, community—an individual member accepts the need and the joy of incarnation, the other members just stay aware of that and want to stay in contact with the individual. Some souls choose to become human, some choose to become animals. It's based on desire and on plans, and purpose.

Most animals do not become humans; most humans do not become animals; but it does take place consistently, nevertheless, although it is not the majority experience. And it is—although not the majority experience, it is of great value and it is often a wise decision to change species rather than maintain the same.

For example, in your biological sexuality and birth process, to intermarry into the same family and breed again and again, tends to devalue the wholeness of the personality intelligence, does it not? And so it is between species; exchange is not out of line, it is a broadening of an experience. It's nothing to fear. It redefines intelligence, redefines one's physical perceptions—where you look at trees and grass one way, you ought to try to be a *snake* and see how you look at grass and trees—an entirely different concept that goes far beyond words.

You might as well be in another . . . solar system, another galaxy, another universe, as to see rocks and trees from the human vantage point or from the snake vantage point. So, you don't need a spaceship to go somewhere else; just become a snake or vice versa, and uh . . . this gives you another sense, another rhythm, of God. That's all it is.

And each physical experience is very temporary. You know, the life in a human or an animal form is very, very brief. It's just the flash of an eye, from the higher perspective. So you should try to understand the transitory nature of life on Earth, that there is a larger expression and many opportunities for self-expression. And so, just as spirits help humans, spirits become human as if they are a family member going on a trip. So it is with those who choose to be the animal. Do you understand?

Now, it is the . . . it is possible for the soul to live two or three times in the same earthly time, context, so you can become a female in one incarnation, and in a different part of the planet be a male and be living two lives at once.

This doesn't happen consistently for everyone, but in some it does happen, um . . . with oh, advanced students, you might say, and there are those who live as an animal and as a human at the same time as well.

DON: This would be almost like a split personality from the earth viewpoint, a splitting off in spirit and becoming two individuals and not even necessarily two individuals in the same species.

DR. PEEBLES: Right, that's right. Sometimes the reason is that this advanced student, so to speak . . . I don't enjoy that choice of words, let's see . . . *brave* student, is uh . . . wants to intensely experience isolated introspection as the male, with no effect of the female inside. So most human beings or animals that walk around have both male and female inside—in the nuclear activity of their being, the vibration, the energy vibration. But when you split off into one male, one female, that's it . . . you're just totally female in that one person and totally male in the other, because you want to do that for some reason.

DON: Is it possible for the . . . say, for example, for a totally female spirit to find itself somehow in a totally male body, or vice versa?

DR. PEEBLES: Well . . . let's see. Not in my opinion. Not in the split soul; but in the typical rhythm of things, uh . . . one's self-image can be that of female, and for the most part, exactly for that reason, will understand the need to accept the male embodiment. So often one is in the male to learn about the male, and one is in the female to learn about the female. It's the simple truth.

DON: So would this partly explain, to an extent, homosexuality?

DR. PEEBLES: Yes. Homosexuality and heterosexuality both have a little to learn. And when we are speaking of sexuality, we are speaking of the nonphysical form, of internal attitudes—and of the internal attitudes, it is ultimately unavoidable and ultimately preferred and enjoyed to know self as bisexual. That is, attitude that in no way needs be expressed physically.

But as an attitude—to be able to hug a female and to be able to hug a male, and to not think of it as a sexual experience—but instead, a soul into the soul. You see? And the heterosexual who is proud of their heterosexuality—if it is a man, just loves women and can barely shake hands with a man, much less hold them—has something to learn, just like the homosexual.

If it's a male who prefers to hold males, and is angry

or uncomfortable or not attracted to the female, he has something to learn about the female, about self. Do you understand me?

DON: Yes. Is it possible that someone who is experiencing a sort of reversed role like that in the flesh has consciously chosen that as a means of working out some particular thing?

DR. PEEBLES: Absolutely. In fact, more often than not someone in that condition, in a condition of social bias, for whatever the reason be, in this case homosexuality, where the greater social attitude is one of rejection or confrontation, bias—it is always with intent and purpose for accelerated growth. That—in not only homosexuality, in anything—for example, uh . . . to be a black man in a white community, a white man in a black community, to be a woman in a predominantly male community, to be a woman in the Wild West of one hundred fifty years ago, for example, to be physically handicapped—all of these are intense choices for more direct growth patterns.

DON: That would certainly be a way of seeing another point of view most forcefully.

DR. PEEBLES: Yes, exactly.

DON: There was an instance some years back, during our great civil rights unrest in this country, where a white journalist found some way of dyeing his skin to look like he was a black man and lived as a black man in the South. The book he wrote, *Black Like Me,* was a moving experience for anyone who read it. We are experiencing this sort of thing without realizing it?

DR. PEEBLES: Exactly, *exactly* the same.

DON: We accept roles in order to learn.

DR. PEEBLES: Correct. There is no learning, except through experience. To learn in the mind is only a theory. Through experience is the growth, and so theory is only a tool; no more, no less. The nature of reincarnation, why one can in fact live *so* many lifetimes—hundreds and thousands—is because experience is the greater teacher. Everyone knows what they should do for the most part, but, uh, it's another story to do it.

So you see my point, however, is that when you choose a life, you theoretically know that the female is equal to the male, but you are not able to experience that in your soul. Eventually you are going to learn that; but by experiencing the female, or the avoidance of the female, uh, guarantees the impact that will invoke one into a different point of view.

DON: Sort of an acceleration of learning.

DR. PEEBLES: Yes. Which can be avoided, which many spirits avoid, which you are allowed in your free will to avoid. This is another reason why there can be so many incarnations to life. Many spirits will, lifetime after lifetime, do everything they can to avoid such experiences. Actually they are avoiding growth and trying to live in pleasure and safety. And the divine universe is such that . . . that is absolutely fine. But then, you see, there are still issues that have not been addressed.

DON: So for someone to be told that they are a very old soul, that is not necessarily a compliment.

DR. PEEBLES: Oh! Goodness gracious, absolutely, yes! Myself an old soul, I know. Formerly an old soul. No, really, my friends, an old soul is nothing more than a very *slow* learner. [Laughter.] Yes. You could use that as one of the quotes in the front of the book. Spirit told us to use this in the front; yah; take that. You can use that part too: "Spirit told us, suggested, to use this in the book."

DON: *(laughing)* Very well. We'll put it in the front.

DR. PEEBLES: In italics?

DON: Whatever you like, sir.

DR. PEEBLES: I tease.

DON: I love it. Uh . . . could we . . . ? Our scientists feel that the entire universe is evolving, uh . . . is there a parallel evolution on the spirit side?—a parallel that mirrors or somehow projects the physical evolution into our dimension?

DR. PEEBLES: Yes—well first, regarding evolution. Evolution is a reality. However, as your perspective becomes larger and larger, phenomenally large, then there is no evolution eternally. There is evolution over millions of years, thousands of years, over a few minutes. And, uh, this is part of growth, but in the true definition of evolution it is not a linear experience, from one to another, but it's part of that spiral that, again, is so large in scope that you can't see it, really, from the earth point of view.

It's like those lines in Peru—on the ground, you know, but you can't see them in any meaningful pattern until you get high above them—so with the spiral, the grand spiral, when the perspective is high enough, you see more and more that all shapes become spirals. Uh, in some sense.

The vibration, the energy frequency, rather, of matter is related to images, will, desire, self-image—uh, image of life and the relationship between the two. The frequency of that field of energy increases according to vulnerability, according to love, according to closeness, in attitude, according to acceptance, and so on.

That vibration becomes very dense as there is resistance and separation. Now the frequency of this energy must be so rhythmic that individualization is only temporary—and then you have union, union of two different points of view, two different bodies, two different nations . . . in the pulsations, the rhythms—and the mechanical physics that is physical now on Earth will become spiritual in the coming decades, will concentrate on where are the pulses?—where is the high point of the wave?—where is the low point of the wave? And instead of looking and studying the middle, you will see that high point of the wave and the low point of the wave as the entry places— the doorways, the windows—into multiple dimensions, into other aspects of the unified field that will go beyond the four fields currently defined in science.

Understand that your physical body is not solid but is porous and that it is a vibrational zone controlled by your image—your image of self and others. The mind, motivated through the heart, will increasingly become the pilot, the designer, the painter. People in the twenty-first century in much more obvious ways will truly be artists in their week of living, more so than in your current time or in your history, recent history.

This is where the study of physics will become an art form—nonphysical—a study of nonphysical reality much more so than the study of physical reality . . . and so the vibrational waves are controlled by will, images, feelings, intentions. Do you understand? Does that address your question, or . . . ?

DON: Uh, I think so, but . . .

DR. PEEBLES: We can talk about it more. We can pursue it.

DON: You have already gone way over my head to the point that I don't know what else to ask you about . . . uh, so . . .

DR. PEEBLES: Well, we're a little dizzy, too, yah, so it's all right.

[Laughter.]

DON: Is there something that we can particularly learn as human beings by a much closer study and affinity with various animal forms around us?

DR. PEEBLES: Oh!—goodness gracious!—yes! I would say from our vantage point, consistently, one of the first areas of healing, resolution for individual breakthrough, individual growth, and experience of love, and for planetary healing, is the relationship between humans and the rest of nature, starting with animals.

The relationship in the so-called civilized nations between man and nature is very incomplete. The true harmony and fulfillment that everyone seeks as nations, and as villages and towns and cities, will be through highly intensified, sophisticated study of that relationship, so that humans do not see themselves as the end-all of the universe . . . and as the—you know, truly, if one must be judgmental, there is nothing that comes close to the arrogance of the human being of planet Earth. And I'm talking about many other physical planets too.

The human being on planet Earth is really a sight to see! If we must use the word "tragedy"—the greatest tragedy is not among human beings but between humans and life elsewhere, and so this is what has brought on the great changes, and humanity has created this as a karmic experience—so the planet Earth is going to cleanse itself a little bit, take a shower, and humanity is going to be spanked a little bit, and they deserve each little spank—but it's nothing, it's not revenge, it's not anger, it's just a beautiful experience of love in the universe.

So there's much to look at regarding the human mind and the massive illusion of separation held by some. Typically, the more civilized the more separate.

DON: Such as the total separation from nature so evident in some of our large cities.

DR. PEEBLES: Well, yes, and it's going to catch up with the humans; what's going to happen, in effect. Now, I'm not talking about mass destruction. Life is going to go on, my friends, and you're going to love it. Life is a beautiful experience that you can enjoy and look forward to—you have much to look forward to in your century. However, there's going to be . . . uh, your weather patterns, for example, are going to break more and more records—in similar directions and in opposite directions—and it's going to make sophisticated societies pay attention to something besides themselves.

For example, the rain forests in South America are being cut away rapidly, and that affects the entire planet. Science knows it, so, uh . . . that's just one of many examples. Nature is going to spank the human being.

DON: There was something recently about holes in the ozone layer above the poles . . . scientists very much alarmed and . . .

DR. PEEBLES: That's just part of it. That is the part they can measure; actually that is the smallest part.

DON: You don't really foresee any great cataclysmic destructions of the Earth, then, but we are going to have to learn to cope with a new reality.

DR. PEEBLES: Yes. In other words, there will be required more and more money, more and more attention will be given by business communities and political groups to the relationship between man and nature. They're going to have to; and nature will cooperate to some degree, and you'll be able to work it out. There will be upheavals, there will be some earthquakes to be sure, and the eye of history looking backward—oh, two hundred years hence—will see it as a time of great change—but in your experience, my friends, of day to day, of waking up and going to work— it's fine, it's fine, life will go on fine, and you will be able to adjust. It's just that some social values will change and human priorities will shift a little.

DON: Somewhat in the fashion that priorities in the western world shifted as a result of our fuel crisis a few years ago.

DR. PEEBLES: Exactly, you're right, they are all blessings in disguise.

DON: Nobody really suffered but we thought we were suffering. Uh . . .

DR. PEEBLES: Linda! How you feeling over there?

LINDA: *(laughing)* Just fine.

DR. PEEBLES: God bless you! I just wanted to make sure you were still there! We love you so much!

DON: *(chuckling)* We have heard you speak to others regarding other intelligent species on Earth—that maybe humans take a little too much pride in that we tend to think of ourselves as the only self-conscious life on the planet. Can we talk about that?

DR. PEEBLES: Yes, well . . . the dolphins . . . whales . . . each individual whale and dolphin is a slightly different case, but overall the dolphin is—in the human concept of intelligence, which is limited—the dolphin is close, not quite equal to but close to the human being. However, there are some individual dolphins that are far superior to many or most human beings. More important, perhaps— the teaching of loving allowance is the greatest teaching for the planet Earth—and I'm not speaking of that in terms of addressing or listening to us, this source here— but in any words you want to use, in any language, in any religion, those parts of each religion, those parts of each philosophy that address in some way the concept of loving allowance. *That* is the lesson and teaching of Earth. And that, in many ways, is why anything comes to the planet Earth to learn, and the greatest teacher of that upon the planet is the dolphin.

The greatest experience of that is the dolphin. Their concept, their experience, as a community is such—they don't really need to change the human being, they just *allow* the human being and, uh . . . for they know, they have this intelligence that all will be as it will be, accord- ing to your growth, your karmic cycles.

So, for example, if a dolphin is captured, the dolphin won't necessarily be ecstatic about that experience, but will quickly surrender and become family with the captor rather than rebel. So the dolphin—not the clown but the teacher of laughter—uh, people walk away from watching the dolphin and they almost believe in God again, uh . . . they have been taught by a great master, although they might call the dolphin a clown.

So the dolphin is a great teacher, and a great experi- ence of allowance—that's okay, it doesn't affect them . . . and so, uh, another is a species that is not accepted by most humans . . . uh, typically called the Yeti. Ac- cepted or not, this is a real life form. They, as well, are extraordinarily gentle creatures and beings, and they, as well, are extremely intelligent and are, uh, teachers of al- lowance. From their perspective, as from the dolphin's perspective, the human being is the—in the literal term— can be a *vicious* beast—uh, to watch and listen to human beings talking about the beasts of the jungle is a little laughable . . . uh, so there are many different and new perspectives to see, for the human mind to see.

Pride in intelligence is perhaps one of the more subtle but consistent barriers to greater love among the civilized arenas of the earth.

DON: We see this also as intellectual arrogance.

DR. PEEBLES: Yes, correct; exactly. Which, of course, is demonstrated and experienced, cultivated inside one because one does not love self. One is afraid that one is not talented, and so a demonstration of intelligence is a technique of "trying to feel better than." If you feel better than, you might be respected. If you are respected, then you feel loved. But what everyone finds out in their own karmic life cycles is they'll be respected again and again; they'll achieve their goals and become very successful and life will respect them. And then they die lonely. They say, "Wait a minute, I guess maybe respect *isn't* love, so maybe it was a waste of time trying to be superior," and so forth.

DON: Where would we go to find the Yeti?

DR. PEEBLES: The Yeti is located in the Northwest United States, is located in the Pyrenees Mountains, in the great Alps, throughout Russia and Northern Europe.

However, you could have the finest sophisticated equipment and trackers; if the Yeti doesn't want to be found, you won't find him. The Yeti has a radar, you might say, far more sophisticated than anything the human mind has invented, and sees the human being just like the human being sees the cobra snake—as a great, great, vicious threat—uh, not with condemnation, however, but with a sense of sadness and understanding.

So now that isn't to say that the Yeti and the dolphins don't have something to learn themselves. They have some things to learn, and that's why they're on the planet Earth. So the Yeti will reveal themselves, they've done this a few times, not for earthly appeal but just because of certain individuals involved. Individual humans.

DON: We recently had a moving experience watching a television feature on the killer whale. It would appear that they are equal to or superior to the dolphin in many respects.

DR. PEEBLES: Absolutely, to a fine point. Well, that—it's really individual; right; correct. Some individuals—gray whales also. You will find a little more intelligence in some dolphins, but at that point you are coming down to individual souls. Also the bear is very intelligent, particularly the brown bear. The wolf is very intelligent. But then, of course, you have to define intelligence.

There are many definitions of intelligence. Sometimes human beings tend to define intelligence as almost related exclusively to whether one has a thumb or not. Because humans can build a building, because they have a thumb, thereby they are intelligent. It is not necessarily an intelligent conclusion.

Because the Adam's apple and the larynx work in such a way that you can create a vocal language, there's the understandable assumption that this is exclusively a demonstration of intelligence. However, this precludes an awareness of telepathic communion—but of course if you see telepathic communion as irrelevant or unreal, then it's a moot question.

As well, the intelligence based on the concept that the human mind can reason and deduce and deduct, uh—but you see, a greater intelligence doesn't have to deduct, there's no need to reason, for there is a more direct link to the source, and that doesn't mean death, does not mean boredom. Now, those who love to play chess, for example, working with their ability to reason, would take great issue with that, because they think it would be very boring. But those that—that's really because that pride of reasoning often means a person is very lonely, also, you see, and who really loves his reasoning power more so than the ability to be intimate.

DON: We don't deduce ecstasy, for example.

DR. PEEBLES: Right. And the greatest intelligence perhaps is union. Contact. Intimacy. Now, that's intelligence. And it's not a dead state; it is an active state of awareness, of experience, of giving and receiving, and so forth.

DON: We live in a much more beautiful reality than we can possibly be aware of, don't we?

DR. PEEBLES: Exactly. Yes. Life is beauty beyond beauty. If every human being would dedicate every day—well, no, just one day a week to discovering a greater awareness of the beauty that is right around you, been there all the time —uh, just ten percent more—we challenge you, humanity: One day a week can you find . . . oh, in *real* terms, just ten percent more awareness of the beauty around you; stopping and smelling the roses, in other words.

This can become a very sophisticated personal self-therapy, to help you week to week to week, where your day is dedicated only to that beauty. Now, with some repetition, the challenge is to recognize not only the beauty of life around you, but the beauty of yourself. For others it is to recognize not only the beauty in yourself—quit looking in the mirror now—but the beauty of life around you too.

And still on other levels it is not just the beauty of people who agree with you, and have similar points of view, and share your same color, but look at the opposites, the beauty in the other parts.

You see? Yes. Most humanity appreciates the beauty, it's, uh . . . it's the fear of change; it's the illusion of separation; there is the challenge. The smelling of the roses as well as your sleep states has helped you come alive again. All such appreciation of beauty is a recognition of Spirit.

All right, we're going to leave pretty soon. Would you have further questions?

DON: I think that about wraps us up for this time, Dr. Peebles. Thank you so much for coming again. We're looking forward to the next time.

DR. PEEBLES: All right. Linda! Anything further? Please! Please! Anything! Life wants to hear from you, Linda! They *do.*

LINDA: *(laughing)* I do have a question.

DR. PEEBLES: Life wants your work. All right? You hear us?

LINDA: Yes, I hear you.

DR. PEEBLES: And they want your work not just from that brilliant brain but they want it from your heart and soul. All right? So, let it out.

LINDA: *(laughing)* How many channels are you working with, at the present—working through?"

DR. PEEBLES: Ah, well, let's keep it in North America for now. That will keep it simple. I work around the world through various channels and in North America, let's see, there are twenty-five different channels I come through. There are others who are stretching for my presence and those that I work with and represent, and that's wonderful, but there's some more stretching to do before becoming effective channels.

LINDA: Do you find a somewhat different experience through each channel?

DR. PEEBLES: Oh, dramatic, yes; very different.

DON: Your channel is very important to how much of you can come through; is that right?

DR. PEEBLES: "Yes, or in many cases, what *part* of me can come through, effectively, for I do not want to overly influence the environment, but work *with* the environment, you see.

So, we love this channel. He has worked hard in other lifetimes and, uh—you know, when he was first working, over here, there was debate whether it was going to take place, and there were times when we were wondering if Thomas, bless his soul, was setting a record for pure stubbornness. To move him was to move a rock.

Ah . . . he is an exceptional being, an exceptional channel. There are other channels, however, I can come through with a little more scientific information and language that is difficult to bring through Thomas, because of certain fears and bias that, uh, impede the route and we will not interfere with that, you understand, we do not overpower.

There are also issues of . . . oh, maybe sexuality, for example, that I can bring through other channels more strongly, where it might be a little more roundabout through Thomas. However, there are many, many issues that I can bring through Thomas that are difficult or impossible to bring through others. You understand.

DON: Thomas has a very nice balance.

DR. PEEBLES: Exactly. Extraordinary sensitivity in a male being. Just like you, Donald, God bless you.

DON: Thank you, sir, very much.

DR. PEEBLES: All right. Go your ways in peace, love, and harmony. Life is a joy, particularly as you surrender to the delightful opportunities for growth. Let us say that again. [Slowly and precisely.] Life is a joy, particularly as you surrender to the opportunities for growth, each and every day. Though you may at first see them as pain or as struggle, these opportunities become *delightful* growth of the soul for those who take responsibility as creators of the struggle—never the victims of it—the pilots of change, never the passengers. As you then increase your communications with life around you, with respect, and as you make greater allowance for yourself and for life around you, recognizing all souls as creators and pilots of change, life then becomes a joy, a dance, a celebration of the divine in all things.

We love you dearly. God bless you each and every one.

8

On the Air

*"The human came forward . . . much
earlier than science has yet understood
. . . as the direct implementation of off-
planet beings, your space brothers and
sisters."*

—Dr. Peebles

As of the time of this writing, Dr. Peebles via Thomas Jacobson has had considerable exposure on the nation's airwaves, both radio and television, primarily in talk show formats as a guest. Needless to say, Thomas was usually presented with no great seriousness, often as an object of humorous curiosity and for entertainment value. But we were fortunate in tracking down the first broadcaster to bring this phenomenon to the attention of the public, more fortunate in obtaining a personal interview with Bill Jenkins, the irrepressible host of KABC (Los Angeles) TalkRadio's *Open Mind* show.

The transplanted Texan is tall and lean, bronzed and handsome, a veteran broadcaster who has experienced all the usual excuses to become cynical and hardened to the human situation yet retains a boyish enthusiasm and an undiminished zest for life. The product of a fundamentalist upbringing, he first told us about his reluctance to become identified with a weekly radio show devoted to a serious investigation of the paranormal and the occult, then he related his first meeting with Thomas Jacobson.

Thomas had been brought to his attention by a friend, and he'd set up an interview at the studio to determine if Thomas might be a suitable guest on *Open Mind,* a three-hour phone-in talk show aired live each Saturday evening. Bill had been busy screening some confidential material that had been supplied by another prospective guest—a man in North Carolina—which proved to be so fascinating that he'd forgotten about the appointment with Thomas.

So this is all amazing to me and I'm just trying to determine in my mind if I want to put this [North Carolina material] on the air, you see, to this large audience—they would think that Bill has gone really off his coot because . . . well, see, you may not always *believe* what the guest has to say but you can't just sit there and take potshots at him—at his academe, his research, his whatever.

What I mean is, how in the hell am I going to sit there and tell Edgar Mitchell that you didn't communicate mentally with somebody down at Cape Canaveral from space—I mean, give me a break! You know, if the audience wanted to do that, that's their prerogative, they can do that. I can't.

So that was all really kind of heavy on my mind. It was the first time I'd gone through [the material from North Carolina]. I hadn't talked to anybody about it. I had secreted myself back in one of the studios. I didn't want anybody to hear this information because it was very confidential. I didn't know what it was all about anyway.

Well, I'd gone out to get a cup of coffee—and there was [my friend] and Thomas. I had forgotten that I had made an appointment for them to be there at eleven o'clock. That's when Michael [Jackson] gets out of Studio D and goes over to Studio C. The idea was that we would then go into Studio D and Thomas would go into trance; you know, to show me [what he does].

So anyway we met outside and went through the usual tentative introduction sort of thing then immediately into the studio. We sit down and chat just a minute about innocuous things, then Thomas goes into trance; you know, mumbles this little prayer or whatever—and I am thinking *what the hell?*— then out comes this booming, almost comical, voice that almost blows me out of the studio—I mean, you've met Thomas, such a calm, quiet man—but then *boom!*—here's this . . . whatever.

He goes through this short metaphysical, uh, whatever that he goes through in introducing himself, this little preamble, then he gets right on my case.

He says—and I'm sitting there with eyes like saucers, I guess—he says, [mimicking] "Bill, I want you to know that we've been encouraging you from the other side." Like, "We've been working with you for a long time, and you're doing a marvelous job. There are a lot of us here (in the damned studio!) and there are some off-earth ones [here] too."

I say, "Some *what*?"

He says, "Off-earth ones."

"What's off-earth ones?"

"Why do you think you're so interested in the flying saucers? You think you did that because of your Texas boyhood?"

[Bill had previously worked on a documentary movie about UFOs.]

I admitted that I'd often wondered about that, and he said, "Let me tell you something about that spiritcom device [the North Carolina material] you've been working with, and George Mueller."

I am thinking *oh wow!* because I encountered that material just fifteen minutes earlier and—well, he told me all about Mueller and what a [character] he was—he was this, that, and the other thing, then he tells me, "Oh, by the way, they've lost contact with him for a while. He says he's moved to another vibratory level, which is one way to put it. And he's just having some instruction there."

But he goes on to say, "But actually they're going to regain contact with him through a trance medium in Colorado."

Then he starts telling me about my family, about Brandy —the dog—and all of this other stuff. I mean, he went into all kinds of stuff.

Well, you must know what this was doing to me. I had agreed to *see* the guy just out of courtesy, and now here he's . . . I mean . . . well, okay, I had invited Dr. David Viscott [who also does a show from KABC] to come down. He did. Right away Dr. Peebles says, "Oh, hi, David. You know we've been coming to you right along with that book you've been writing on spiritual psychology, and . . ."

Well, now David's eyes are *this* big, his mouth is open, and he is speechless—and if you know David, you know how unlikely *that* is. He has never mentioned this new book to anybody, not ever—you know, he's already got all of these best sellers kicking around and—but he's sitting there wide-eyed and speechless.

Dr. Peebles is saying, "You know, David, you ought to really go ahead and use some of that stuff on your show. We know you're concerned about what your peers will say and the religionists but . . . Would you have any questions now?"

But David is sitting there stunned and speechless—I swear to God, David Viscott speechless—he actually had paralysis of the throat, he didn't ask Dr. Peebles *any*thing.

So he just says, "Well, all right, good-bye, God bless you all," and Thomas breaks the trance.

Now, in that first session, he told me about the research I was doing, about the "channeling" I was doing—and that was the first time I could put a name to it, to my craziness—he used the names of my family, my dogs, he intimated a problem that my wife and I were having, he told me about a problem my kids had been having. As I look back now, I didn't know they were having that kind of problem at the time and he didn't exactly call it that, so I didn't tumble to it, but I know that was what he referred to. He told me about everything that was going on at the radio station—which is a real soap opera all the time, believe me—and how the show had developed because of the influence they [Spirit] had been giving me—that they were trying to work very closely with me but I wasn't listening too well and all that, and on and on.

So need I say that obviously Dr. Peebles went on the air the next possible air date. Which, sadly, was about three months later. That was the first slot I had open, the first time I could get him on the air. He was an enormous success. You know, I was a little worried at first—I mean, this is weird stuff, really, and we are talking wide audience, but God, he was an instant smash.

On that first show some of the promotion people were there, and you know we had the lights kind of low and you stay away from Thomas while he's in trance. But at a news break they turned up the lights a little bit so they could take some pictures—and Dr. Peebles got right on their case: "Don't you change the environment around here! Turn it back down! I'm really concerned about my channel, he's trying to stomp back in here anyway as it is."

Said, "We just wanted to take some pictures."

He says, "No flashbulbs!" Says, "Bill, you've got to tell these people this is something special going on."

I said, "Well, I really really think so."

I'd been listening carefully to the reaction of the people on the phone lines while we were on the air. You could hear them go, "aahhh aahhh" [sharp intake of breath] and you knew that he was hitting it right on the head.

It was interesting the way he does it, because he talks at many levels at the same time. If he is talking to someone else, I'm hearing *one* thing but you the person is hearing another. I remember we had a party over here [at Bill's home]. It was all the KABC people. Would you believe it was Christmastime and this house had eight-five or ninety people in it? It was raining outside, so it was all inside, and it was getting a little tight.

[Thomas went into trance and produced Dr. Peebles, who wowed the guests with direct interchanges].

Another friend of mine asked Dr. Peebles a question that night about their friend Nefertiti. Nefertiti was a dear friend of theirs and they had lost contact. So Dr. Peebles went through a whole dissertation on Nefertiti's character and the whole thing, and that they would never see Nefertiti again, that she'd gone off to do some other things that she wanted to do, and the whole stuff.

Now, *I* knew that Nefertiti was their *cat,* which they'd lost some time before that.

So I said afterward to these friends, "Well you know he can't bat a thousand."

They said, "Oh, no, he was right on target with everything he said."

His appearances on *Open Mind*—and there were many, I think maybe nine or ten—all of his appearances, that's when we had the most telephone calls to this station—you know, the busy signals—well, *Open Mind* always had the highest level of that, the busy signals. The line was always full. But Dr. Peebles aroused that audience more than any of the other guests, ever. So in that respect he was something else.

People want to run him for president. They *love* 'im. You know, you just—you just fall in *love* with this guy. I always felt sorry because I tried to devote a lot of time to Thomas as well —and Thomas is a very interesting and engaging guy and he improved, by the way, over the years, as himself, as he was learning to handle himself on the air, in his own processes—he became very engaging himself, in time. But during the first few appearances he was awed by it. Well, you know you've got this thing running around in your head, Dr. Peebles and . . .

But Dr. Peebles, you know, what a character, he just

wouldn't put up with anything. Like during the news breaks and some of those long waits, he would sometimes leave. He'd say, "I don't want to put up with this, watching you all go pee." He says, "I'll just be floating around; I'll be back," and he would just go off and leave Thomas sitting there.

But I think one of the most *dazzling* displays of the paranormal happened right on the air one night. The space shuttle was in flight. One of its missions was to deploy two different communications satellites, the Westar VI and the Palapa B-2. They had put up the Westar VI and they had *lost* it. It was gone. They couldn't find it anywhere. I mean, all of these sophisticated earth-tracking stations, the thing wasn't there. It was *gone*.

So during—I think it was the ten o'clock news break, as is usual I just toured back and went through the wire room—a routine to make sure that somebody hadn't shot Reagan again or whatever—and here was this bulletin that had just cleared the wire. They'd found the Westar VI but it had just been completely destroyed—you know, just in a thousand pieces, there in space, just total space junk. And NASA was at a loss. They couldn't figure out what'd happened to it; it was a total mystery.

So we came back on the air, and the first question—I didn't even tell Thomas that I had this bulletin—this caller said, "You know, Dr. Peebles, we've just lost one of our communications satellites that the shuttle crew deployed. What happened there?"

He said, "Just a moment"—the way he does, you know, where the hell does he go?—he goes somewhere to get the answers and he's usually back in a few seconds.

This time he came back and said, "You know, this is going to be really strange because some of the off-earth ones are tinkering with that satellite right now, so don't worry, it will be back."

Well, I'm looking at this bulletin that it's destroyed; right?

But he's still saying, "They'll find it. And not only that, they're going to send off another one and they're going to lose it too. And the off-earth ones are going to tinker with it and then they'll bring it back—and if your scientists are smart, they'll look and see what's going on there because they'll get a lot of information from what the off-earth ones have been doing with them when they get them back in another flight or two."

So I—very diffidently—read the bulletin. On the air.

So he says, "Ah! Well! Believe AP or believe Dr. Peebles, we don't care. We love you anyway."

I said, "Well, what about it? Are we to believe AP or should we believe you, Dr. Peebles?"

He says, "I'm just telling you what I've got here. But, Bill, Dr. Peebles can make mistakes too. But I don't think so, not on this one."

So the next morning I'm driving to work and they had launched the Palapa B-2. I said, "Ohhh, they're gonna *lose* it."

And sure enough by the time I got to work, been there about an hour, bulletin came in, they had lost the Palapa B-2 as well. Now they're *both* gone.

A day later they *found* them both.

They're both up there; they've got 'em tracked!

Two shuttle missions later they retrieved them. Woo! Let me get—let me read you a letter I received: "Dear Bill, I feel like I know you after listening to you on *Open Mind* for so long. My favorite was Dr. Peebles. I taped your session with him after the spacecraft blew up. I've worked at Hughes for eighteen years and I helped design and test Westar VI and the Palapa B-2. So I was very interested when they were recovered. I'm sending you a copy of an internal letter we got, December 7, 1984. Sure like to meet you" and etcetera.

The letter, the memo, to Hughes employees communications group, from an associate manager of the Commercial Systems Division: "We recognize that there is an intense interest in the two recovered spacecraft. Unfortunately however our recovery contract with the owners of the spacecraft severely limits our freedom to display the spacecraft or to discuss their condition. Accordingly, I ask your cooperation in observing the following conditions during the time the spacecraft are in our custody: there is to be no access to the spacecraft by anyone who is not an employee of Hughes, and there is to be no access to the spacecraft by Hughes employees who are not directly involved in the performance of the recovery services. In addition, all requests for information about the recovery or the condition of the spacecraft should be referred to the S&G public relations' etcetera."

But there it was, on the air, one of the most *dazzling* displays [of clairvoyance]. I'm looking at the AP bulletin that they blew up and, "Well, you can believe AP or you can believe Dr. Peebles. I don't care. I love you anyway."

Beneath a banner headline, the *Los Angeles Times* on February 4, 1984, reported that the Westar VI communications satellite deployed by *Challenger* was feared lost. A follow-up story on February 5 voiced the official fear that the satellite had blown up and disintegrated into space junk. "One theory is that it exploded as the onboard rocket was ignited."

Another *Times* story on February 7 reported: "A second communications satellite launched from the space shuttle *Challenger* sputtered and failed to reach its orbit Monday, stunning space officials with the third major setback of the mission.

"The satellite, called Palapa-B2 and owned by the government of Indonesia, spiraled up from the shuttle early Monday in what appeared to be a perfect launch, but then flamed out prematurely."

A story carried in the February 9 edition said that an investigating team was moving to impound parts of solid-fuel rocket propulsion systems from around the nation in an effort to determine what caused the two commercial satellites deployed by *Challenger* to sputter and go astray moments after being launched from the space shuttle.

A story in *Aviation Week & Space Technology* in its edition of February 13, 1984, reported that NASA was studying plans to recover the two useless satellites by the space shuttle during the next year.

Aside from a mention that the two satellites had been recovered later that year, we have found no further information on the Westar VI and the Palapa B-2.

But we'd already decided to believe Dr. Peebles.

9

The

Big Picture

"We encourage you to understand that sexuality is a wonderful experience of spiritual oneness, that all life is motivated by the drive to be together."

—*Dr. Peebles*

It is entirely characteristic that you never know where an interview with Spirit is going to take you. A seemingly very simple question often produces a startling and complex response; one thing leads to another and another and another until . . . well, you'll see what we mean.

Listen very closely, please, because the very foundations of human life on Earth are about to be discussed.

This is the voice of Spirit:

As we address you today, we would speak of the nature of love, the nature of romance and sexuality. We will encourage all of you to understand that the fundamental drive of the soul in the human sphere is to be one with life again. To be held by another person, to hold another person, this is the purpose of life, this is the drive. This is incorporated through all aspects of self, the mind, the brain, the physical body, the physical biological intelligence, and your physical sexuality.

It's all the same thing, part of a magnetic experience to be part of life once again. And when one surrenders to that intimacy, there is an orgasmic experience in the soul, thereby in the body. The orgasm is not the point, it is just a by-product of the ability to hold and be held, to be together in total union with another, union with the universe, union with God, union with all life everywhere; it is that moment of surrender that the greatest ecstasy of life comes forward.

We encourage you to understand that sexuality is a wonderful experience of spiritual oneness, that all life is motivated by the drive to be together. We encourage you to understand that romance is the dance of life, to understand that permission must be created from within, and not waiting for another person to create it for you. How can self create that permission to reach out and say, "Will you love me? Will you hold me? Will you ask me for my presence?"

How can you create that honesty with others instead of waiting for life to do that for you? There is the loneliness, there is the pain, there is the isolation from the great romance, the great passion of life. You simply do it yourself.

God bless you each and every one. Would you have questions or comment?

DON: Thank you for joining us again, Dr. Peebles. And thank you for that beautiful message. Linda and I are both very much aware of the magical quality of these experiences, but it still always surprises me when you open up by talking about the very thing I wanted to ask you about. I had thought to discuss human sexuality during this session, so how very nice of you to prepare the way for me.

DR. PEEBLES: Well, it is not that we anticipate you, my friend, it's just that you have channeled us, both of you, in your questions, you see. And you feel what we encourage you to think about, to ask about, and so we're just working together as a team. God bless you.

DON: That's wonderful. Whole new concept of teamwork.

DR. PEEBLES: We're proud that you hear us, that you capture those questions, some of them. You could've ignored them.

DON: Uh, probably not. But thank you. The question of human sexuality has for so long been such a troubling thing for people, and it seems that various social ideas and religious ideas have so manipulated our thoughts and ideas about it that . . . well, there's just so much confusion in the public and private mind about sexuality.

Certain religious ideas seem to be saying on the one hand that sex is sacred and divine, but on the other hand only if it is invoked for the reproduction of life—and then it becomes a sort of a duty. We're damned for doing it and damned for not. So we would like to have your comments as to the sexual confusion on planet Earth.

DR. PEEBLES: God bless you. In the nature of religion, often there is a desire to suppress passion, believing passion to be fundamental to crime and sin, believing that the purpose of life is to cleanse oneself of sin and thereby accept purity. To be pure, then, is to not have passion, for only passion leads to sin.

And, of course, really what takes place is only an experience of stagnation, a sterility—perhaps clean but yet figuratively dead. And so always there is the reincarnation, the desire to live again, in any plateau of time and space, so as to try to give self permission to experience passion as the touch of God rather than the curse of the devil.

It is in that passion that one is experiencing the natural magnetic drive to be with life, to be touched by life in any sense, and that touch is an electromagnetic activity of the soul that creates higher frequency, a vibration that becomes union, oneness in any sense, and this is where the great works of art and the great works of music, the great works of construction and composition in building and invention have taken place throughout history. It has been at that moment of being touched in the mind, in the body, in the heart, all of the above—intimacy, sexuality of the soul—when all invention and inspiration occur.

The fear of being overcome, the fear of sin and of evil, ironically dominate in the human spheres of Earth, dominate the desire for love, the desire to understand true kindness and compassion, where the great masters, all of them—Jesus, Buddha, and the list goes on—taught love and forgiveness. Nevertheless, the demonstration of human beings typically through organized religion is one of condemnation, fear, avoidance, protection, and greater and greater isolation.

It is a great paradox that some earthly religions strongly encourage greater separation rather than seeking to dissolve those separations, which is the true purpose of the study of God, or thereby, religion in human terms.

Sexuality is a beautiful experience—and in the finer societies, communities of the universe—including some historically upon your planet—some societies elsewhere in the universe, some in your own futures—it has been recognized as such and as a part of healing, as part of creativity and invention. In the future societies of Earth, sexuality will be something that is looked upon with reverence and respect, and with thanksgiving rather than fear.

There will be professionals, for example, currently called prostitutes, who will be looked upon with respect, the respect in these days of your society that a lawyer receives or a doctor receives, they will receive; for in their sexuality it will not be just the body. The greater concept of sexuality is inclusive always of the heart, the soul, and the mind, you see. This is what they will teach and manifest, demonstrate and inspire within others—spiritual sexuality, sexuality of the soul.

It is not the body that sparks the excitement, it is not the study of fine form of the physical that sparks excitement—it is that through that initial attraction of the body one begins to concentrate on another person, don't they, believing it to be the body, the physical male or female. But what you are doing, in a greatly accelerated way, is focusing on another person, another soul, another personality, another aspect of God, and the more that you hold your focus on God in any realm of Earth, the greater your excitement will be, the greater your passion.

It is true that crime is based on passion, but it is equally true, if not more so, that the greatest works of humanity are based on passion. So because humanity lives in illusions of separation, and thereby idolizes protectionism and safety, this is why issues of crime, of sin, of error and wrongdoing, of failure, tend to have a greater, a larger habitat, in the conscious attention of the mind. But that is a false concept, and it is only through repetition, practice, and continued experience that you learn that the same focus creates your reality. When most of your attention is on those issues, then you deny yourself greater attention on the great joys of life.

The nature of sexuality is a dance of God, and we encourage all who hear these words to surrender to your sexuality, to surrender to your contact soul to soul.

The diseases related to sexuality are not because of the sexuality itself. They are because of human fear, the human judgment, the human bias regarding sexuality— and that in turn manifests the diseases associated with the same, a reflection of the social mores and attitudes of your time. Do you understand me?

DON: Yes, I do. That latter part rather emphasizes the effect that fear and anxiety play in all areas of human health. The things that we feel so degraded by, we take into ourselves as ill health, don't we?

DR. PEEBLES: Exactly. Fear can be seen as a healthy tool, as it is by sociologists and psychologists, for example, but that is typically when your attitude is concerned with temporary well-being, when you are concerned with immediate survival, when you are concerned with safety—then fear is a wonderful tool. But in the ultimate growth of your soul, fear is—it is a challenge to overcome. It is a blockage, in a way, based on an illusion of separation. Do you understand me?

DON: Yes, I do.

DR. PEEBLES: It does not have to happen physically. Sexuality starts and ends in the soul. It is an illusion—an understandable one—that sexuality starts and ends in the body. For example, if a rape takes place. Now, it is certainly logical on the surface to believe that a man is driven by the physical appearance of the female counterpart, if that be the case. However, it is actually the soul, it is the spirit body, the astral and etheric vibrational field and how the man translates that energy into a subjective personal symbol that is the driving attraction.

The body, the physical appearance and all, gives the man—in this case, the man—permission to open up to that soul contact, but it is the soul contact that's already there, the soul activity of perception that's already at work. And so a man who is raping a woman feels the need to overpower her so as to dominate, and in that experience of domination to feel some sense of self-value, believing self to be empowered, uh, incapable of being loved by anyone except by overpowering them—believing love to be a result of respect—respect gained by fear, domination.

Sometimes, as to the female—you might not want to hear this—but sometimes the female who is raped has helped to create the experience. Again, though, not in any conscious, physical way—such as so-called invitation to rape—but in the way her own soul translates the call to sexuality. If there is a very low self-image within the female being, an image of inadequacy and smallness—although it can be hidden through temporary ego states and such—it can dominate the female as low self-esteem of the female self or principle, making the female inferior or smaller than the male—and so these two fit into each other. Both people create the experience, one with the need to love through domination, the other with the need to love through being dominated.

But, now, it is not necessary, in loving the many rather than the few, it is not necessary at all to have a physical experience with a second, third, or fourth party. However, if you spend your time denying sexual attraction and going out of your way to resist it, you are in part denying your God-self, so you acknowledge that physical attraction with the spoken word. You can acknowledge it with a compliment. You can acknowledge it with your eyes and you can experience it in your mind, and then go your way.

No, it does not require physical experience. Do you understand? If you become very mature in your being, you don't seek it yet you don't deny it.

DON: I see, yes. Much food for thought there. No need to isolate ourselves inside blocks of ice, trying to deny a physical attraction. Just acknowledge it and go on. [To Linda.] Did you have something you wanted to ask at this time?

LINDA: No, you go ahead.

DON: I've been having a bit of trouble, Dr. Peebles, trying to understand the relationship of soul to body. That is, the biological form that is energized by the life force, on the one hand, versus the soul, or personality, that indwells the body. We have been told what the soul is without the body, and I think I understand that, but what is the body without the soul?

DR. PEEBLES: It is nothing. There can be temporal movement, experience, excitement, as an electrical charge, through a body that is not inhabited. However, it is very temporary, and it extinguishes itself; the life force is gone.

Now, there are—for example—there are the concepts and fables of zombies—what are called zombies would be dead bodies that have been inhabited once again by a despairing soul, a soul in desperation or confusion. This, I suppose, would be possible. However, that also would be a very temporary experience.

When the original occupant, who has built and manifested that molecular form, has vacated permanently, then the body is quickly deteriorating into the fertile earth, returning to its natural state, the molecules, uh, disassembling themselves and rejoining earth.

The entire experience of intelligence comes from the soul.

Now, the brain, the physical brain, is similar to your computer of this day, computer technology. It holds information, it holds data, information; memories can be held and located in the brain. The brain is also a translator for language; translator, as a vehicle upon a foreign land, that is the brain upon the Earth experience. It is a vehicle to help you integrate.

The mind is dominant to the brain.

The soul or heart is dominant to the mind.

Does that answer your question?

DON: Partly. But I'm still a bit confused. In an earlier session we discussed the inhabitation of the fetus by the soul, and you stated that at the time of conception, the biological form that begins there is an indwelling general spirit substance or force—that which we identify as the life force—and then there is a moment in time when the soul indwells.

Then we discussed the process that we call death, in which the soul releases the body.

Is there a point somewhere between those two events, between birth and death—is there a point when the soul, the life force, and the spirit that produces the life force become almost synonymous, or do they indeed become synonymous?

DR. PEEBLES: Now . . . the soul and what?

DON: The soul and the . . . does the soul and personality—?

DR. PEEBLES: Ah, I see . . . uh, yes, in fact, it happens every week. It is a rhythmic activity, a pulsation throughout everyone's life; and part of the challenge of life is to become conscious of it, to become aware of it, cognitive rather than unconscious.

But in the natural state of affairs, it's taking place all the time, a union between the soul and the personality. And this is why we encourage people not to think of their higher self elsewhere, but rather to locate it in the frontal part of self—now, right where you are, in the front of your being, with your attention.

Yes, Don, they come into union, and this typically during daydreams or at the time of orgasm and afterward, in sexuality. It is during a climactic experience of artistic ecstasy, either as the performer or the beholder. It is accomplished during some small fragments of the deep sleep state. Yes, it takes place. The challenge, of course, is to make it consistent. You understand?

DON: Well, yes . . . so, at the time . . . when the soul releases the body, it is simply the biological form that then goes into decomposition; the spirit has also departed.

DR. PEEBLES: Yes, that is the word I was looking for—decomposition. Yes, correct, exactly.

DON: In, uh . . . I had another thought . . . we're not exactly . . .

DR. PEEBLES: Don, did you have feelings about that? What was your motivation? What are your feelings about the body decomposing?

DON: I have no problem with the body decomposing. But it is —I had another idea working . . . uh, I developed a theory many years ago that the personality that I am—me—I indwelled at the moment of conception and actually took over the mitotic division of cells and all that—and organized the body and I built it. And you said something in your last statement to the effect that this is what happens, yet I am still confused as to the distinction between the life force, the spirit, the vague spirit that comes in and starts the process going, and then the soul coming in at some later point and taking over and cooperating in the eventual development. Is this actually what happens?

DR. PEEBLES: Yes, the spirit and soul are one, as one. And coming into the child of the womb are very, very present, although not inhabiting for the first few months, but extremely present and *forward looking*. Whereas with death, well, I suppose you would still be forward looking but dropping the body behind you. There is no longer the drive to build it, but just to release it, and you're correct.

However, the self-image personality is imprinted for a time upon the cellular, molecular structure so that after the spirit has departed those imprints do remain, just like the stones called the . . . uh . . . fossils?—so yes, the entire self is in the microscopic aspects. However, with time it passes, it leaves completely, according to the attitude and locality of the spirit.

If the spirit stays bound to Earth, with anger and desperation or fear—well, that state of personality, that electrical state of personality in the cells, continues—and the body can even be used again, and brought up awake again to some state as the zombie. However, if it is a clean death, a clean departure, in about three days that imprint just disappears. Does that address?—is there more to your theory you'd like to talk about?

DON: There probably is, but I'm not well enough organized in my thought right now to pursue it; perhaps at some future time . . .

DR. PEEBLES: That theory would be more relative to other zones of reality. There are other places in the physical universe where the pieces can be picked up again in a very active way and reformed in their totally new experience, bypassing what is called birth and childhood, and perhaps that is what you were drawing upon, from other realities, but it's not really relevant, perhaps, to Earth.

DON: Well, now, in the evolution of soul—I presume that what we are going through here on Earth, in our recurring lives —and what occurs in the spirit world—is some sort of an evolution that we call growth and learning. But in the evolution of soul—did the first incarnations into physical matter occur with homo sapiens reincarnating as humans on this Earth or were there prior experiences with what we term lower forms of life?

DR. PEEBLES: Yes, it was previous, Don, and was as souls incarnated into physical forms nonhuman. The human came forward much later in the Earth experience, yes, though much earlier than science has yet understood, and came forward as the direct implementation of off-planet beings, your space brothers and sisters.

Now, of course that brings forward the question: where did *their* humanoid state begin? But relative to Earth, not only then but now, the soul does reside in many animal forms as well as in the human form. Do you understand?

DON: So homo sapiens is not really a natural product of Earth but it is an implanted species?

DR. PEEBLES: Exactly, right, correct. There are other—the banana, for example, came from another planet. It had nothing to do with Earth, didn't start on Earth; yes. It is perhaps the most wholesome food on the entire planet. You could live on water and bananas and be extremely healthy.

DON: That's why I love them so much.

DR. PEEBLES: Yeah. Smart man.

DON: *(laughing)* Very good. Well, now, that . . .

DR. PEEBLES: You see, there is such a thing as evolution. But evolution is not the cover, not the blue sky. Evolution is secondary to other laws of the universe. Evolution is a system that is true and valid, relative but limited.

DON: I see. It's sort of like a mechanism of change. It's like, God *said*—and evolution *does*. An unconscious force—

DR. PEEBLES: Right!—very good! That's very good, Don! May I use that in the future?

DON: *(laughing)* Yes, please do. Uh, so we've already partly answered another question I had in mind. The origin of a lot of Earth religions, some of our most hallowed religious forms, are actually the . . . memories? . . . of off-Earth influences in our lives?

DR. PEEBLES: Now, that's an interesting theory. Just a minute here. . . . [Long silence.] The, yes—the most ancient religions—that doesn't necessarily cover Christianity, for example—but the more ancient mystical religions, yes, are *loosely* the result of systems of thought and communication previous to the earth experience; correct.

DON: Uh, well, even Christianity—at least in the Old Testament, in Genesis, there are references to other beings who are having sexual contact with, uh, the early people, I guess—as a suggestion that they had some influence sexually on the human race and . . . and, uh, so this seems to be a valid idea even there.

DR. PEEBLES: It sure is. It happened again and again and again and again. Remember that your written history of only a few thousand years is just a piece of sand upon a beach. Human affairs on Earth have had so much other activity, and dominated by off-planet visitations and interactions. There have been societies that have gone on for thousands of years where there was a clear relationship between life on Earth and life from other realms; it was very clear. Well, this is what your world is returning to now—it's just in the very, very beginning; that's part of the Aquarian Age, where that will come forward again.

DON: Is there some connection, then, between this off-Earth influence—and I presume we are talking about physical entities, not from the spirit world but from some other physical vibration . . . ?

DR. PEEBLES: Yes, that's correct.

DON: So this is—would there be some sort of a direct connection between that fact and, for instance, the ancient Brahman idea that man came into being from the result of playful spirits who came in to sample our environment?

DR. PEEBLES: Yes, and what have been called angels—although reasonably believed to be spirit, or spirit teachers, at times—and they were, on some occasions—but often were actually the space people, your brothers and sisters from other physical origins. And you will find that in the writings of all of the older religions, that is consistent in all of them—even so-called myths and fables and the oral traditions from the oldest antiquity, in all lands of the planet Earth: it is consistent.

DON: They were trying to teach and lead?—encourage us to become more and more like them?

DR. PEEBLES: Right. They wanted civilizations that would be self-sufficient, knowing that in their matrix of travel and, uh, energy activity in the universe they could not maintain a hovering state around the Earth. They either had to be on the ground or go elsewhere. So they wanted people on Earth who would be self-sufficient. It was difficult, you see, because . . . to those who came to Earth, in touch with their totality, their intelligence, found Earth to be a foreign atmosphere, a very difficult atmosphere in which to maintain their state.

So they had to develop other physical biological systems that would fit, and prolong and reproduce themselves in earthly terms.

DON: And of course this also fit very well into the whole scheme—the greater scheme—the whole spiritual scheme of providing life forms of higher intelligence or higher reactivity that spirit could work through—that soul could embody and work through here on planet Earth?

DR. PEEBLES: Yes. Eventually science will see—and I believe some already know this—that . . . looking back in context of progression from one form to a higher life form there are many gaps. In fact, there are reversals. And that's because of interaction from off-planet sources.

In current times these space people are making visitations—over the last thirty-five years, in particular—and some of their work is—what they are doing when they work directly with physical human beings—these are souls who are part of their family, in their ancient past, and they are unlocking memories. And so the various devices—implements, instruments, and the electrical insertions that have been noted—part of it is unlocking some of that memory. This is, uh, in preparation for greater collective public conscious integration again—with very little panic—with more fascination and love and sharing, you see.

DON: Could this be why some contactees experience such confusion and even fear as an aftermath of a close encounter of that kind?

DR. PEEBLES: Yes, because in their conscious mind—they are living, remember, on the Earth in illusions of separation— so they feel violated, feel raped, feel taken over—and typically, as with most humans, feeling like a victim, not aware of how they invoked this in their dream state, or from other times and places.

There have been many who have enjoyed the experience. But, again, because fear and pain tend to dominate attention—look at your news media, for example—then that is what the public hears most about.

But it is the fear, through illusions of separation, not because they are being hurt; it's because they are resisting the experience in their conscious selves.

DON: I am beginning to get a big picture here that the . . . this whole concept of the illusion of separation is much bigger . . .

DR. PEEBLES: It's fundamental, oh, yes, everything is based on that.

DON: . . . than most human beings would come to think it is. You're talking about, now—the entire universe is really a single, living system. . . .

DR. PEEBLES: Yes, exactly.

DON: Our aliens, our UFOs, our spirits, you yourself, me myself, we are all one and the same thing happening, going on, all in—

DR. PEEBLES: Yes, and not only are all planets part of the same system, all systems part of the same galaxy, all galaxies part of the same universe—but everything is part of every-thing else—and what you think is a difference, eventually you personalize, identify as an aspect of self. Then you have less and less need for protection, and more ecstasy of union.

DON: So these off-Earth beings, who really seem to have a much vaster technology than we have here on Earth and have been in a self-conscious form for eons longer than we have, they are still at a level of physical incarnation—bound to the physical realm, that is—still working through the physical—

DR. PEEBLES: Learning, yes. Correct. In many cases it is a karmic bond and this is why they are here again, for they take some responsibility—to their credit—for having mo-tivated these illusions of separation, and this is what began to form the Earth as a school concentrated on separation; they were part of creating that, so they're here trying to meet their karma and to reverse that.

DON: Earth, then, is a very *special* school. It's not just like all the other—

DR. PEEBLES: No, no; yes; right.

DON: There are very definite—it is like, you have a university composed of many colleges—so maybe one college is law, another is medicine, another is—Earth is the college of separation, you're saying.

DR. PEEBLES: That's right; exactly.

DON: Aha. Okay, so . . .

DR. PEEBLES: That's why when you are finished with the in-carnations of Earth, thank your blessed soul there's still more growth, more schools to go to. For the university is *every*thing, it's the entire universe.

DON: Good, uh, choice of derivation there: universe, univer-sity.

DR. PEEBLES: Why do you think?

DON: Language is, uh, a symbol of, uh . . .

DR. PEEBLES: Exactly. So your university of life . . . master-hood is loving learning rather than resisting and fearing it, never believing that you've learned it all.

DON: I think that would be death in the true sense, having nothing left to learn.

DR. PEEBLES: Very good, Don; yes. Relative, right, to the local . . . and the human concept of death in a negative con-text, right. It is believing that you are complete, fulfilled. See, death has terrible connotations for the human mind.

Some who will be listening to these words? And so we must take care to clarify which manner of death we're talking about. Because when *we* are talking about death, we're talking about the beauteous experience, the doorway of change—that is a beauteous experience—but in the literal concept of death as a total ending, yes; that is the isolation, loneliness, that can be created by believing you've learned it all. You are truly alone then.

We have so many spirits come back over here who believe they're finished. Because they think they've learned it all. What a shock! They go through major trauma, and they have to have much counseling and love and help before they will give themselves permission to come into the body again. They are *stunned.* They feel like they're almost starting over again because for so many lives they were trying to be above it all. Now they've got to go back and get in the mud, and that's just too terrifying at first, you see.

DON: We humans seem to have a penchant for that. Uh, the idea that *now* we know it all, at various plateaus in our lives—such as, say, starting the first plateau at the age of about six or seven—suddenly we know everything; even Mommy and Daddy are stupid, compared to us—then we do it again at twelve or thirteen; junior high syndrome. Seniors in high school are probably the most fearful and honest because suddenly it dawns that they know nothing whatever and it scares hell out of them, but then again by the second year of college, it's all-knowingness again.

DR. PEEBLES: Right, and some never graduate from that. It is the loneliest isolation the mind can find. Believe me, I know, because I learned the hard way, too, just like every other human being has to learn, through experience, through being present with the truth—and being present with the truth gives you to understand how much more truth there is to be learned.

Because love, in the illusion of separation, love is believed to be achieved—oh, semiconsciously, subconsciously, unconsciously—is believed to be achieved by gaining the respect of your peers.

But that's not love. It's valuable, but it's not love. And so—for example, in the concept of evolution, there are many, many spirits, Don, who have been of the animal community, who will never need to be human beings.

DON: Really?

DR. PEEBLES: That's right. That's another assumption—yah, see—that there is still a higher form, to become the human being—no, they don't *need* to, they don't *need* to go through that particular bias, that particular limitation. In a different sense of intelligence, they're beyond it and they haven't regressed to that state.

If you think about it from a different point, Don, you'll recognize how separate humanity is.

That's not because they're smart.

If humanity were smart, they wouldn't be so separate from everything.

It's that pride of intellect—and because of the illusions of separation—remember, that's an unconscious drive through everything, Don—that human beings use intelligence, the concept of intelligence, to separate, to justify their separation which they feel is sanctuary and safety. And there from that place of isolation they don't have to feel guilty, and can feel good about not treating life very well, around them.

Just as a human being who, in their particular lifetime, has murdered someone, they were able to justify that for a moment by feeling so separate.

So it is with human beings who feel so separate from the rest of life that there is no care for the feelings of life elsewhere, beyond humanity. And, uh, if you could try to recognize intelligence not as an idol, not as the God of all things, but rather as a tool—uh, and a challenge, to be sure. There are those souls who lived in the animal experience with a certain type of intelligence, a very real intelligence, who have learned the *real* lesson, which is to touch and be touched, to be close, to be part of all life, to work with life rather than against it.

DON: In that sense, then, our great strides in technology are taking us farther and farther into the illusion of separation?

DR. PEEBLES: Some of them are, yes, absolutely. Some are doing the opposite, Don. But many, perhaps even most, are taking you farther into separation; correct.

That is why so many mystical, religious, visionary beings have predicted a calamity, because it—it's just coming to a head.

But . . . it's our opinion that the good will of mankind is superseding, now, the technological pride. And you can have the technology—but only as a servant, not as a God.

DON: Yes; I guess that's our big problem. Maybe, uh . . .

DR. PEEBLES: That's what happened to Atlantis.

DON: Oh! It is?

DR. PEEBLES: Yah. We'll talk about that another time.

DON: Uh . . . okay. Uh, so . . . if we do have more contact with off-Earth beings who are obviously so further advanced than Earth in technology, things of this nature— that is likely to be a rather humbling experience, would you say?

DR. PEEBLES: Oh, absolutely. Humble pie, as they say. That will be good for humanity; right.

DON: You know, Doc—the further we get into this—this—it's, uh, it's so amazing, there are such depths . . .

DR. PEEBLES: But, now, the human mind, I would like to add, Don—the human mind does have—in the human concept of intelligence, which is rather fairly accurate—does have a mind that is more powerful than the animal, that's true. But what we're saying is: is that really that important? How relative is that? And in fact, the way of human beings, typically—with exceptions—is to separate, because of that intelligence, rather than the intelligence being a servant to help you come closer to life.

Now, obviously there are many exceptions, and in current time—and in ancient history—increasingly there are communities and collectives who are working together with that harmonic of using intelligence to come closer to life instead of more separate.

All right, we're going to leave in a little while. God bless you.

DON: I have one other idea here that I would like to pursue before we close, if you will. You have mentioned a couple of times to me personally that I am undertaking a work that I could have left to another lifetime.

DR. PEEBLES: That's right.

DON: I had open-heart surgery in 1979. During that process I experienced something similar to what others have described as a near-death experience. Could we talk a little bit about the near-death experience?

DR. PEEBLES: Yes, of course. It was a death experience, Don. Wasn't near-death; it was death. And if you had not chosen to come to the body, you just would have kept going right where you were, with what you were experiencing, and there were spirit beings coming closer to you—and there was the enormous, enormous power of light through every fiber of your being; you became aware of the voices behind you, that it would be wise to return rather than do it later—and you could have chosen to do it later. We did not insist that you had to come back. That's how you remembered it, perhaps; but it was your choice. You said, "Aha, I see what you mean; I agree."

In doing so—the reason you did so, Don, was because you changed your priorities—here on the spirit side. You said, "Ah. I did what I did and it was good and it was an act of love. And now I'm gonna be even more direct about my agony and ecstasy of love, and I'm going to accept the minister I am—and I'm not gonna have to camouflage it anymore—and I'm going to, uh, *thrust* myself into the vagina of life with all the male of my being, and I'm going to let my seed into the entire Earth so that children may be born with greater permission to love and be loved; I'm going to help humanity—of the western hemisphere, in particular—redefine the male so as to allow gentleness in the male instead of fear it, to revere the sensitivity of the male rather than hide it or pretend it's not there"—and that's exactly what you are, is extraordinary sensitivity and gentleness in a very strong male—and that is a very high spiritual teaching that you are going to bring forward—and, of course, of the spiritual philosophies and psychologies you are going to be a forerunner—and it is you, Don, who is going to be thrust into the public eye, in the years ahead, as a spokesperson—and you had to decide if you really wanted to do that or not.

Because when that option became clear to you here on the spirit side, you were shown pictures; you saw little movies of other lifetimes where you did something similar and you regretted it, because life tried to hurt you, and sometimes loved ones turned against you, and sometimes it appeared that your choice created pain for loved ones, and—but you met that, and you said, "Ah, I see. All right, well, everyone around me is the creator, too, as well as am I, and I must speak my piece, I must express it to the world and then allow the world to respond as they will."

And you said, "All right, I'm ready, let's go!" And you clapped your hands together and dove right back into that body. You understand me?

DON: Yes; thank you, Dr. Peebles. I'd like to close on that note. Thank you very much.

DR. PEEBLES: God bless you. All right, my friends . . . Linda? Any communication? We sure would like to talk to you. How you feeling over there?

LINDA: I'm feeling great! Thank you, Dr. Peebles. We love you.

DR. PEEBLES: All right, we'll let you off the hook there. God bless you. We love you very much. Go your way, we love you—both of you, all of you, go your ways in peace, love, and harmony—we're with you, and when we leave this channel, remember: [With incredible feeling.] we're still here. God bless you each and every one.

LINDA: Thank you.

Thank you, indeed, Dr. Peebles.
We have the big picture now.

10

Principles of Spiritual Psychology

*"We give you these three great principles
. . . and first among them is the principle
of Loving Allowance for all things to be,
in their own time and place, beginning
with your own self."*

—Dr. Peebles

*"There is probably at least a little bit of
truth in everything you have ever heard."*

—Dr. Peebles

The human instinct for religiosity is like a flowing stream, tumbling and rushing down a mountainside in its race to the sea. Every now and then it encounters a level place and collects into deep pools, but the movement continues through the pools and on toward the sea unless something occurs to block the flow and contain it in a static condition—for example, if an insurmountable dam is built, either accidentally or by design. But then the stream will merely cut a new bed and go around the obstruction, for it will not be denied its access to the sea.

If the stream is the human religious instinct, then the pools represent the various religions and the sea is God. A dynamic pool is one that remains open on both ends so that the stream may continue to flow through it without obstruction. Thus the pool is continuously replenished and refreshed, the water remains clear and clean and healthy, a positive life environment is maintained.

But the obstructed pools lose their viability relative to the strength of their dams. Those with the weakest dams will sustain themselves the longest because the flow continues over or around the dams. Those with insurmountable dams are in the greatest danger of becoming isolated and static. If the backward pressure is strong enough, the stream could thus become diverted somewhere upstream and the pool will become stagnant and eventually it will dry up and totally cease to be. The stream itself, of course, continues the plunge to the sea.

The great religions of the world today can be seen as viable pools or lakes through which the human search for God is finding satisfying expression. And, of course, the human landscape is littered with the dry beds of other religious notions that found themselves outside the flow toward God.

The strongest, the most persistent, and the most profound teaching that we get from Dr. Peebles has to do with the value of the diversity of God's expression: all is contained within God; therefore we encounter God (perhaps without recognition) in every activity, every locale, every thought and deed. *God cannot be avoided* because everything we encounter with the mind *is* God. Thus our stream rushing to the sea is a stream of consciousness, and the religious instinct is no more than some dim recognition within ourselves *that we live in God* coupled with the desire to express that recognition.

Should it then be so remarkable that we define God to ourselves in terms most familiar and most closely connected to ourselves? Neanderthal and Cro-Magnon man, themselves intimately immersed in nature, recognized God in their immediate environments and *expressed* that recognition in appropriate terms. Bronze Age man, flowering into creative capabilities, recognized God as the great creator and again expressed that recognition appropriately. Warrior tribes revered God as the great conqueror, the Age of Wisdom saw God installed as the great thinker, and so on through the development of human consciousness and cultures.

We find God where we are, because that is always where we apprehend Him. Which is why today we have a Baptist God, a Catholic God, a Buddhist God, et al. These are merely different aspects of the one God, as perceived by different people in different places. Often, of course, these aspects take on territorial significance, exclusivity features, competitive traits. Each man's God is the only true God, in that reading; all others are false Gods.

Listen to Dr. Peebles: There are no false Gods. Each God *is* God—and even that which is not perceived as God is God. "All issues are resolved therein."

It makes sense to me that a billion Christians cannot be wrong, that half a billion Moslems cannot be wrong, that even a mere seventeen million Jews cannot be wrong. None are wrong; all are right; each defines God according to his own apperception of God, and *all are contained within God.*

So what is the issue? If a Christian feels closer to God through the crucifixion of Jesus, why should anyone wish to deny him that path? If a Moslem finds his identity with God through the example of Mohammed, let's cheer him on. It's a huge universe, after all; surely there is room in it for every conceivable aspect of God as well as every conceivable religious expression. It makes no sense for any human to attempt to confine God within any small pool of thought or faith, to shape Him into *our* image, to dam the flow so as to contain it regionally and deny access except to those who come to drink from our shores and on our conditions. God is beyond any conditions set down by the human mind, and is immediately accessible anywhere to any seeker. To dam the flow behind any bulwark, however well intentioned or conceived, is to frustrate for a moment the whole grand plan of human life on Earth.

The impulse for diversity, so obvious in the most casual inspection of nature, is a movement toward maximum expression of all that God is. To live to the point, to be present in that multiplicity, to celebrate the differences and embrace the diversities is to join that flowing stream of consciousness and move with it toward the ever-waiting sea, sampling along the way all that God is on that mountainside. Even the stagnant pool eventually finds its way to the sea, because to "dry up" is simply to be taken up into the heavens and again "rained" onto Earth, there once again to join the flow. No one is lost, forever left behind; we all end up at the same place sooner or later.

Loving Allowance is an all-embracing concept. It encourages every expression of mankind, applauds every movement, deifies the human experience as a consequence of the diversity of God's expression on Earth, links every man, woman, and child on the planet in mutual love and respect—*and it celebrates our differences.*

Dr. Peebles seems to be telling us that *our differences do matter* —but in a positive, not a negative sense. One point of view always amplifies another. One attribute always strengthens another. *Sameness is stultifying.* Roses are beautiful, but their beauty is enhanced by the contrast with other flowers; would we want all flowers to look like roses? Is the presence of God better expressed through sameness or through diversity? What if every human being looked exactly like every other human being? What if our appearance never changed between birth and death? What if humans were the only form of animal life upon the planet? What if the piccolo were the only musical instrument, and Brahms the only composer ever to have lived? What if every human being knew only how to build houses and none wished to farm or develop technologies or play music?

We are *enriched* by our diversities, and each of us enriches the world by our own differences, our own thoughts, our own priorities, our own talents and interests and skills. *So why do we lay so much store in finding others who are exactly like ourselves?* Why do we "put down" other people for what they do or say or think or feel? We need it all, folks. We need every expression the mind can conceive and we therefore need to applaud the differences.

That is what "loving allowance" is all about. To love God is to love everything, for everything is God.

There are those, of course, who will not agree with us that everything is contained within God, for obvious reasons. Some simply do not believe that there is a God, by any name. Roughly six percent of Americans, as revealed by a recent Gallup study, are totally atheistic. For these, the universe merely appeared from nowhere for no reason and is headed nowhere, mankind with it as incidental baggage. It is a depressing view, but in loving allowance it must be seen as a necessary view for some people for some reason that is valid to their own journey.

The great majority of Americans appear to believe in a loving "father" God with whom some form of a personal relationship can be achieved, usually through prayer and devotion. Many of us will then resist to some degree the notion that God is All, depending on how literal is our interpretation of holy scriptures and biblical creation doctrine. It can be a difficult bridge from "God the Father" to "God the All, Including Me," since most of us have been encouraged by our religious practices and beliefs to view ourselves as separate from God and unworthy of God unless and until we are raised by grace and made worthy.

Some twenty million Americans, though, seem somewhat ambivalent in their concept of deity, allowing that probably there is some higher power but unsure as to just how that translates into the human reality. There can be some difficult bridgework here, as well, from an impersonal and distant, or unknowing and uncaring, natural force or power to an intimate and all-encompassing being who interacts spontaneously and continuously through and with every particle in creation.

So it is not our mission here to attempt to sway or convert the reader, whatever his or her particular religious orientation. We are not presenting a new religion, but rather we hope to add some dimension to the metaphysical reality from which all religions are drawn. We say that all are true, and right, and proper for the time and place in which they are being experienced. Dr. Peebles loves us all, supports us all, encourages us all to be more and more present in our own truths.

But we also feel that we are presenting deeper truths, new insights into old truths, and a correlation of all truths that have brought mankind into his present state. We do not suppose that everyone will be entirely receptive or comfortable with all that we bring forth. We bring it forward for your consideration only because we feel that it may bolster your own truth or provide some new perspective. We presume that you are present with us now *because* you do not feel that you already have all the answers to the mysteries of existence. Well, neither do we, but we do feel that we have uncovered a few answers that could redimensionalize your own quest—and we offer them here not to supplant your own deep-felt beliefs but to strengthen and illuminate them, if only by contrast.

This view from Spirit agrees with all points of view, if only for a moment—embraces all diversities, excludes not a single atom or quark or widget, person or thing; loves all, *is* all, contains all, is contained by all, gives rise to all and is raised by all. It is a total view, a universal view. It has at its center the theme of immortality that *begins* with the reincarnation scheme but then *evolves* into higher states upon states without end: to live again repeatedly and eternally, without sin or guilt, regardless of errors, ignorance, attitudes, misconceptions, prejudices, foul deeds, beliefs, doubts, fears —to live again and again, in God and as God, fully developed in the mind of God and now realizing the many aspects of that fullness through educational roles in living—forevermore, throughout all time and space, the child of God already God but learning how that came to be, both in spirit and in flesh.

This is not a religion. It is a metaphysical principle glimpsed and implied in all religions but fully expressed in none. All religions are right and valid in their own place and time, yet also all religions are incomplete. *No religion on the Earth today fully celebrates the true glory of God in His multidimensional aspects and intimate interactions with the infinity of being.* I can say this without fear of error because no human brain can conceive or contain or even translate such all-inclusive knowingness. *Not even the angels in heaven can do so.* No man has ever apprehended all that God is. We apprehend God in pieces, even in our most inspired moments and through our most revered revelations. Those who would attempt to contain God and bind God and form God in some human image and reserve

God through a select creed or covenant may be right for a moment, but the larger truth will overtake them here or hereafter, so we might as well try to open ourselves to the limitless possibilities here and now.

How do we test religious ideas when all purport to be the divine word of God? We might begin by asking, how large is it? How inclusive is it? How beautiful is it? How loving is it? How rigid is it? How ugly is it? How confining is it? How petty, mundane, regional is it? Find the truths that make you as large as you can imagine yourself to be and reject all else as dry pools along your stream of consciousness.

Then make loving allowance for all things to be, in their own time and place, beginning with the self. If we can do that, then we are already halfway home.

There is room enough in most religious beliefs to admit fresh inflows of inspiration from the spiritual stream. All religions have God as their centerpiece, and all attempt to define the relationship between God and man. All or most advance some concept of immortality. All or most attempt to provide some path or vehicle or mode by which humans can personalize God in their daily lives. None, however, appears to offer any clear picture of who or where God is, exactly what immortality entails, or how God manifests direct influence upon the humanly affairs of Earth. So there remain many vague areas of considerable importance in every religion that could benefit from a uniting vision.

The vexing problem for all who would attempt such an integration of viewpoint will be found in the need to separate the core of their faith from the structure that contains it. The religious edifice is itself not divine. It is built by men, not angels; it suffers from the same bureaucratic inconsistencies as any human collective undertaking and so is confused, not direct; it stands rigidly behind ramparts built for the protection and maintenance of those who built it, not of those who worship there.

So, yes, it can be difficult to separate the core from the structure, and we do not even suggest that you attempt to do so, only that you try to place the conflicts in some perspective and to remember that we deal here with metaphysical principles, not with competitive religious fundamentals.

There is no reasonable need for any of us to lock horns on such issues.

As a perfect example of loving allowance, we wish to share with you the fruits of a recent conversation with the Reverend Dr. Robert H. Jacobson, head pastor of the Church of the Palms in Sun

City, Arizona. This is what he told us about his feelings for his eldest son, Thomas:

I would like to say that there is a common bond between what he does and what I do in the Christian ministry, because we both believe that the spirit lives on after death, just as I believe in the risen and living Christ; so, who knows what spirit may exist. What I don't understand, of course, is how one communicates with the spirits of another life, but I can't dismiss the fact that some may know how to do so even if I don't.

There have been various junctures in history where various Christian leaders have felt that they have had communication with the spirit world, and so no one in the Christian Church can take the position that it cannot be the case. We have to let that be an open statement.

But as I said, we have this common bond that we both believe that the spirit lives on beyond this life. As far as my relationship to Tom, one thing I'm quite convinced of is his absolute integrity. His integrity is above reproach. In fact, there have been times when his devotees have tried to form an organization and make him their guru. He has refused to do so, because it is a temptation to power, and he's recognized that.

I have great respect for the fact that he has just consistently done what he knows how to do. He has taken a lot of guff from fundamentalist clergymen, and he has had the courage to stand up to them, and I admire that.

So there's no question on my part about his absolute integrity about what he's doing.

He purposely makes himself vulnerable to other people, and if they want to laugh at him or give him a bad time, he permits that to happen and he just laughs right back.

Many, many people who have been on the frontiers of new discovery have had to take a great deal of guff from an unbelieving public. I have encouraged him to go on with his work. I support him in what he does, and you don't need to hesitate to quote the fact that I support him in all that he does.

As I say, I don't necessarily *understand* everything that takes place, but that doesn't mean that it's not an authentic experience.

Of course, we have gone in different directions, and Tom has had a more unique road that he has followed than my other two sons, who've had a more conventional approach to life—but that sometimes is often true of the person who's on the frontier.

He sometimes laughingly refers to himself as the black sheep, but that definitely isn't the case. It's just that he follows a different star than my other boys do. The more you get to know Tom, the more you realize what an extraordinary insight he has into people—and, uh, where it comes from is a fascinating question. I take no credit for it at all. I think it has to come from another source.

After talking with this delightful man, we would take issue as to the matter of "credit." The father is clearly reflected in the son. And we are given hope that the religious structures of our nation are perhaps in better hands, here and there, than we had dared hope. One becomes weary of denunciation and negation in religion. It is refreshing to find love and unity, allowance for other viewpoints, respect and good will.

Dr. Peebles regards this planet as but one of many "schools" in the dense universe in which souls matriculate for intense learning experiences. Earth is the school of living relationships and all human activities upon Earth ultimately resolve to that focus. We are not here to become holy or spiritual per se, but to experience the illusion of separation from God and from one another so as to study and eventually understand how it is that each soul is both unique in its differences yet intimately one with the all.

That is what we are here for.

If that sounds too simple, just consider for a moment what the *lack* of the art of relationships has brought to the planet; think of all the bloodshed, pain, poverty, injustice, hatred, and terror unleashed upon Earth during the time of man. All are evidence of our sense of separateness from one another, either individually or in clumps—and even the holiest of causes often proceed as though God is not present upon this planet or else is present only within the cause. Competitions between individuals, families, tribes, and nations—often accompanied by hatred and violence—bear little testimony to the universality of a loving Spirit that permeates all and binds us all together as a living unity.

So just how simple is it, this living course in relationships? How different would the human world of Earth be today if we'd all graduated from the School of Relationships in prior incarnations and were here now for postgraduate studies?

It is not so simple a course. To graduate, we must first experience God as a living presence upon the planet, as nature and through nature—and that includes you and me—and as a spiritual presence that rejoices in all our unique contributions to the collective. We must recognize God through every disguise, in every plant and insect, in every sunrise and moonrise and every darkness, in every word and thought and deed, within the gaze of every man, woman, child, and animal upon Earth; we must feel His presence in all work and play, in all manufacture and commerce, in song and dance and every artistic expression, in sexuality as well as spirituality, in every apprehension of the mind.

No, it is not an easy school. And there is nothing simple about our mission here.

Dr. Peebles comes to us as a graduate, and he brings three "simple" tools as aids to our studies:

- The first is Loving Allowance for all things to be, in their own time and place, beginning with your self.
- The second is Increased Communications with all of life everywhere, and with respect.
- The third is Self-Responsibility, for you are the eternal creator of your own experience, never the victim.

We create our own reality, he reminds us, through the way we choose to perceive the world about us, and then through the way we react to those perceptions. Is the glass of water half full or half empty? Is it a cause for rejoicing or for anxiety? Is the world a fearful place filled with uncertainty or is it an exciting place brimming with delicious mysteries?

Increased communications, with respect, may help us discover the truth of our created reality and encourage us to create a larger reality, but it all must begin with loving allowance for our own failures and frailties along with the realization that all are students and therefore all are prone to mistakes and weaknesses, for which allowance must be made.

Evil, as a force or power, is notably absent from the world according to Dr. Peebles. Whatever devils or demons may exist are created by human consciousness in this school of hard knocks—and everything that we perceive as evil is ultimately resolved in Spirit as an errant aspect of consciousness.

Sin, too, is seen as a peculiarly human preoccupation. No soul is judged except by itself, no failure great enough to separate the soul from its source in God, no error strong enough to disrupt the unity of being except in individual consciousness for a moment.

This is where loving allowance comes into play. We are here on Earth in human form to learn how our unique differences contribute to a perfect whole in the spiritual unity. First we must become convinced of our own unique worth—not through piety or some human standard of perfection but through the simple recognition that God reveres us *exactly as we are.* We don't have to earn that. It comes with the territory. We would not even *be* unless God loved us as part of himself. Our task is to see ourselves as God must see us. To do that, we must first recognize our own value. Then we must look at the other person and try to see him in that light. Who are any of us to denounce or condemn anything that God has wrought?

In speaking to us of crime and punishment, Dr. Peebles meticulously makes the point that only a very subtle movement of the soul marks the difference between a murderous act and a saintly one. Both are motivated by the same desire for love and acceptance. One is expressed negatively, the other positively, but both are a movement toward God *because all movements in the universe are God moving upon Himself* and no other movements are possible. In the very next movement, vis-à-vis the murderer and the saint, the polarities could be totally reversed *but the movement will be the same.*

In this view there are no murderers per se, and no saints. There is no death, no failure, no sin, no error; all movements of the soul are seen as growth and all paths lead to God.

So how do we apply that to the human situation here on Earth? I believe that we first need to realize that we all are in this thing together, that we share a common bond and a common purpose— that we are all "family," in other words—and that we all are trying to work through certain self-imposed problems toward a common goal. We need to have compassion for one another, we need to support one another, and therefore we need to stop condemning, stop competing, stop isolating, stop warring, stop resenting, stop hating.

Think of what would happen in a world where all the business community sought to make available the very best products and services for the very fairest profit, where the same merchants sought to cooperate with one another toward the maximization of that goal rather than trying to corner the trade, where all workers refused pay not diligently earned, where all citizens were as concerned for the well-being of their neighbors as for their own, where government sought only to serve the common good without thought of personal power or enrichment, where every person was valued and recognized and justly rewarded.

Utopia, you say?

Is there something wrong with that picture?

If not, then I say let's make Utopia our conscious goal on

Earth so as to have more resonance with the goal in heaven. Maybe then the school of Earth would not be so difficult for graduation. Realistically, I don't expect anything like that to happen during our lifetime, but I guess it could start in pieces.

It could start with loving allowance, increased communications, and self-responsibility.

Recently I overheard a man complaining that Dr. Peebles speaks too generally and doesn't give us step-by-step instructions toward enlightenment. Actually, he does do that in direct one-on-one encounters, when he's asked to do so, but again, some people simply don't get the message because it's not the one they wanted to hear.

Some of us will not wish to hear about loving allowance, either, because it takes us too far away from our points in bias from where we view the world. We wonder how to show loving allowance for Communists who wish to bury us or terrorists who wish to blow us up, for neighbors who willfully abuse us, employers who harass us, murderers who stalk our children, or simply the guy on the freeway who's driving like a lunatic.

Increase your communications, assume your own responsibility for helping to create the situation, then look at it again from the godly point of view.

I won't guarantee that you will like what you see, even then, but maybe at least you will see a more compassionate response from yourself and learn something valuable from the experience. Maybe you will even touch the face of God through your increased sensitivity and resonance, and maybe you will hear the cries of a soul in self-imposed torment who wants only to be loved, and touched, and held in value.

Perhaps that soul will be your own.

Never mind, because all souls are of God and all are trying to find their way back to the center of God.

With loving allowance, maybe we can join together and discover God at the center of us. And when that happens, you see, we graduate and leave the school of Earth for the undergraduates to worry about. They'll work it out, each in their own time.

So, as Doc likes to say, "Lighten up a little and enjoy the experience."

Experience, I take it, is what it's all about.

Karen is not her real name, but by any name here is a woman who not only knows what makes the world go round, she helps it get there. As a departmental director within a powerful federal agency in the nation's capital, her work places her in steady contact not only with scientific and management minds at a very high level but also with members of Congress and other high government officials.

Karen's formal training and experience make her an excellent communicator, as Linda discovered when she interviewed her by telephone on June 26. Although she spoke freely and gave full permission for the use of her name herein, we have chosen to disguise her identity and actual role in Washington to protect her political vulnerability in a highly visible job.

Here is the transcript of that very interesting interview, for your consideration:

LINDA: Could you tell us, just in your own way, how you became interested in Thomas and how that interest has impacted your life, if at all.

KAREN: I became interested in channeling as a result of several past-life regressions that I had undergone under hypnosis. For me, visualization such as is necessary to receive information, if you will, from your higher self or the spirit plane or however you want to term it, was such an arduous task that when someone mentioned channeling it seemed like a way that I could understand information from another dimension in a form with which I was comfortable—actual language. So, because spoken words are used in the communication, I became interested in finding a channel through whom I could work to get the same kind of information—but in more positive form—about my life, my previous lives, and where I am on my spiritual evolution.

Well, Thomas came to my attention through a friend here in Washington. So I called and set up a telephone session with Dr. Peebles. Now, at the very first interview with Dr. Peebles I was absolutely astounded at the accurate reading that he had on me and the obvious fact that he knew exactly who he was talking to; that each person I mentioned, he knew exactly who I was referring to. Just the accuracy, the crispness, the wonderful way he has with words and his sense of humor and the kind of coloration that he is able to give to the spiritual quest was just absolutely fascinating. As for impact: the main impact is that it goes a long way toward answering the questions that we all ask. Why are we here? What are we doing? What is it all about? What's it mean? What is God? What is the universe; is it the only universe? It is such an expansive experience to begin to understand that we human beings are all here on the planet generally on our way from one time and space to another time and space. So just the wonderful sense of continuity and the sensibleness of it all was very striking to me.

LINDA: That's beautiful, yes. So your experience with Dr. Peebles has been entirely on the personal level?—you haven't had any professional interest or . . . ?

KAREN: I have not; however, my expectation is that I will build toward applying the knowledge that I am getting through Dr. Peebles in that direction. I am surrounded by a scientific and technical work force. I'm trained in science communication. That's what I like to do and now, as I read articles about the search for life elsewhere in the universe, and searches for solar systems around other stars, questions about cosmology and the formation of the universe and the big bang theory and so on and so forth, I view all that very differently now and I'm thinking about how to integrate the experience that I'm having with Dr. Peebles into my work. So, you know, I'm very intrigued with what the future holds. But no, I haven't asked any questions about my work. I asked some health-related questions which were interesting, just in terms of my physical body and a friend's physical body and the information was very useful.

LINDA: Yes, we have found that he can be very helpful in that area too. We've been doing in-depth interviews with Dr. Peebles all this month and it has just been fascinating for us. Some of the stuff we are getting into is just awesome.

KAREN: Are you doing them in person and sitting in on them all?

LINDA: Yes. What an experience! You come away talking to yourself and wondering what in the world!

KAREN: Yes, it is fascinating, isn't it? You know what it is?—I think it's very self-affirming. It gives you a real sense of purpose and a real sense of community and one really begins to acknowledge the predominate commonality of human existence. You find that you don't focus on all the differences in human beings now, you focus on the similarities—or at least I find that happening to myself. It's very uplifting. It's very expansive, very uplifting.

LINDA: It certainly is. We're just hoping that we can carry that feeling into the manuscript—you know, help our readers get that focus. This has all happened just since the first of

June. It's just . . . it s all happened so fast. I don't know where we're getting all this energy, but I'm sure we're getting some help from somewhere.

KAREN: You're probably getting some help. The other thing that I would say, that is very interesting, is that it seems to me that more and more, every way I turn, there are more people interested in this kind of phenomenon. The other thing that one really learns very quickly, as you probably have, is that the old—is it Buddhist?—the maxim that when one is ready to learn, a teacher appears, so people who are not at a point where they are seriously considering questions about their selves and their own niche in the larger consciousness are not going to entertain notions of channels, spirits, guides, and such, let alone reincarnation. And people who *are* ready for that are very interested, even if they're skeptical. That's okay, you can still be skeptical.

LINDA: Right. Okay. Thank you so much, Karen. Your work sounds very interesting.

KAREN: Yes. And it's sometimes very interesting to consider where a lot of the members of Congress and senators may be in their own personal spiritual evolution, which was something I had never really thought about before I started doing the work through Thomas. Oh, another thing . . . after every conversation with Dr. Peebles I have ten times as many questions as I went in with. You're not in the mood for something, or he'll make a reference to something and you won't catch it at the time but you'll listen to the tape and you'll go ahhh . . . you know—and the other thing is that at each successive listening of a recorded conversation with him, you get more and more and more, again based on your own ability to absorb the information.

LINDA: Right; we've found that too. I think when you are in session with him you are so subjective, so it takes a little time to sit back and . . . as you say, as you listen to it again you hear all kinds of things that you weren't aware of the first time.

KAREN: Yes, and if you listen again in three or four months, you get whole different shadings, and in six months—as your own maturity, as your own evolution continues— you're able to hear even different things.

The other thing that Dr. Peebles does—I don't know how you work this in or whatever—but we all have spirit guides and we all have connections to our higher selves, and what conversations with Dr. Peebles do is get you started on figuring out how to do it for yourself. One real benefit that I've noticed is with this business of being open to help, being receptive to help, and understanding that the truth is inside oneself—and when you hear something, you know it for the truth. It's not that Dr. Peebles says something and I think—I wonder if that is true or not. As soon as he says it, I know that it's true. There's a resonance in your deepest, most fundamental core that says, "Yes, this is valid information; this is what I knew about it," even though you may not have been able to articulate it before.

LINDA: Right. We experience that continually. It's been so nice talking to you. We'll keep in touch. Thanks again.

Linda thoroughly enjoyed her conversation with this delightful lady. And we are getting the feeling, dear friends, that Dr. Peebles is pulling a lot of people much closer together. That, you know, is not even half bad.

One of the least understood theories of immortality among Western cultures is that involving reincarnation, or many lives in different bodies. There is much resistance to the idea, in fact, and that is understandable, given the spiritual climate in Christianized countries. It is not our purpose here to proselytize, but since it is a fundamental theme of Dr. Peebles's, we feel that our readers should be aware that the belief in reincarnation is not limited to the continent of Asia nor is it confined to any one particular culture or religious faith.

The following expositional essay is quoted from my own novel, *Life to Life.*

My hero, Ashton Ford, is speaking directly to the reader here:

I am aware that the idea of recurring lives in this same system sounds crack-brained to many people. But it is an idea that has been with us since prehistory, and it has been entertained or embraced by some of our greatest minds. Virtually every primitive culture has some version of reincarnation at the center of its religious thinking. It is a global idea, existing wherever mankind is, throughout Africa and Asia, Europe and America, in all the island nations, wherever man has paused to wonder about his origins and his fate, seeping into his art and literature, his sciences and philosophies. Longfellow's famous *Song of Hiawatha* embraces the idea in the farewell speech:

> I am going, O my people,
> On a long and distant journey;
> Many moons and many winters
> Will have come, and will have vanished,
> Ere I come again to see you.

Hiawatha was an actual figure in Indian lore. He was also known as Manabhozho and was a messianic figure for the Indians, who expected him to return to life at some time with great power over the final fate of humankind. The speech quoted is a dying farewell, in almost the same spirit as Jesus' Last Supper and Kahlil Gibran's *Prophet.*

Though once thought to be an idea peculiar to certain Asian religions, modern scholars have discovered that the idea had wide currency throughout early America, both North and South, and even the Eskimos have a reincarnation tradition. Similarly, the ancients of Europe—from Scandinavia to Italy —believed in reincarnation and the idea persisted into the Christian Era. Indeed, scholars can point to many examples of early Christian and Jewish thought centering on rebirth, also among the Greeks and Romans—most notably Heraclitus, Herodotus, Socrates and Plato, Aristotle, Cicero, Lucretius, Ovid and Vergil, and the Emperor Julian.

But that's all primitive stuff, you say; enlightened people of this modern age cannot be expected to swallow that stuff. Well, maybe not, but here are a few who have tasted it: Joseph Addison, Louisa May Alcott, Hervey Allen, Honoré de Balzac, James M. Barrie, Arnold Bennett, William Blake, Johann Ehlert Bode, Napoleon Bonaparte, Bernard Bosanquet, Francis Bowen, Sir Thomas Browne, Robert Browning, Pearl S. Buck, Sir Edward Bulwer-Lytton, Luther Burbank, Samuel Butler, Tomasso Campanella, Thomas Carlyle, Edward Carpenter, Edgar Cayce, Gina Cerminara, James Freeman Clarke, Samuel T. Coleridge, Sir Humphrey Davy, Charles Dickens, Emily Dickinson, John Donne, Feodor Dostoevsky, Lord Hugh Dowding, Arthur Conan Doyle, John Dryden, Thomas Edison, T. S. Eliot, Queen Elizabeth of Austria, Ralph Waldo Emerson, Henry Fielding, Gustave Flaubert, Henry Ford, Benjamin Franklin, Frederick the Great, Robert Frost, Mohandas K. Gandhi, Paul Gauguin, David Lloyd George, J. W. Von Goethe, G.W.F. Hegel, Heinrich Heine, Herman Hesse,

Oliver Wendell Holmes, Victor Hugo, David Hume, Aldous Huxley, Julian Huxley, Thomas H. Huxley, Henrik Ibsen, William James, Mary Johnston, James Jones, James Joyce, Carl G. Jung, Immanuel Kant, Søren Kierkegaard, Rudyard Kipling, Joseph Wood Krutch, Leibniz, D. H. Lawrence, Pierre Leroux, G. E. Lessing, John Leyden, Charles A. Lindbergh, Jack London, Henry Wadsworth Longfellow, Maurice Maeterlinck, Gustav Mahler, Norman Mailer, John Masefield, Somerset Maugham, Herman Melville, Henry Miller, John Milton, Friedrich Nietzsche, Eugene O'Neill, Edgar Allan Poe, J. B. Priestley, Ernest Renan, Jean Paul Richter, Rainer Maria Rilke, J. D. Salinger, George Sand, Friedrich Schiller, Friedrich von Schlegel, Arthur Schopenhauer, Sir Walter Scott, Ernest Thompson Seton (founder of Boy Scouts of America), William Shakespeare, George Bernard Shaw, Percy Bysshe Shelley, Robert Southey, Edmund Spenser, Benedict Spinoza, Robert Stroud (Birdman of Alcatraz), Alfred Lord Tennyson, Henry David Thoreau, Leo Tolstoy, Voltaire, Richard Wagner, Walt Whitman, John Greenleaf Whittier, Thomas Wolfe, William Wordsworth, William Butler Yeats . . .

Thomas Carlyle once said, "Every new opinion, at its starting, is precisely in a minority of one." That "minority of one" may always seem kooky to the rest of us. But 'taint necessarily so.

It may seem a very long list of names, but please believe that it is a minuscule sampling. Scan the list and you will note captains of industry, great thinkers and doers, noted writers and poets, educators and scientists representing the very cream of Western intelligentsia who have turned to reincarnation theory as the most sensible model for human immortality.

There are many excellent books on the subject, available at any decent public library and from booksellers anywhere; if you don't see any, just ask (because you may not see it on display, depending on where you live).

Our favorite is *Reincarnation: The Phoenix Fire Mystery* by Joseph Head and S. L. Cranston, with a foreword by Elisabeth Kubler-Ross, M.D. We highly recommend this excellent book.

11

The Dance of

Consciousness

DR. VISCOTT: *JUST BEFORE THOMAS*
WENT INTO TRANCE AND BEGAN TO
SHUDDER—JUST THAT VERY MOMENT
BEFORE THE SHUDDER, THERE APPEARED
ABOVE HIS HEAD WHAT LOOKED LIKE A
WHITE PUFF OF SMOKE. WHAT WAS
THAT?

DR. PEEBLES: *SOME WOULD CALL IT IN*
DIFFERENT WORDS. BUT THEY SEE THE
ENERGY OF DR. PEEBLES, WITH SOME OF
OUR FRIENDS HERE, COMING INTO MY
CHANNEL AS HE QUIETS DOWN.

The human body, like all biological matter, is embedded in a "living wave" of electromagnetic energy, the dimensions of which exceed the physical matter that is produced within it.

Please note the subtle distinction in that statement. The body does not produce that wave energy. It is the wave energy that produces the body.

You may have not heard it put in just that way before—and perhaps the statement will be challenged by people with a better grasp of physics than mine—but the implication seems unavoidable in any application of wave theory (which has dominated the study of physics for the past fifty years and more) to the study of biological phenomena.

I need to elaborate a bit on the idea. In my novel *Eye to Eye,* I stated:

Entropy: the word was coined by a nineteenth-century German physicist, a man named Clausius, to describe a thermodynamic principle in nature: the observation that a certain amount of energy is unavailable for useful work in any system undergoing change. The universe itself is such a system, and it has been postulated and experimentally demonstrated that entropy (disorder, useless work) always increases and available energy diminishes at a steady rate in our physical reality. What this means, essentially, is that our universe is steadily decaying and has been doing so since the big bang, which supposedly began our race through space and time. There will come a time when it all runs down, when there is no further energy available for useful work—such as star-building and the formation of dynamic matter. Our *entropic reality*, then, appears to be a dying universe in which the natural tendency is toward further and further disorder.

Upon this scene strides man, carried on the back of countless generations of other life forms from the amoeba to protoman. The miracle of life is that it is here at all. Life gathers together, unto itself, the energetic particles of a decaying universe and infuses them with *purposeful* activity. That is a powerful idea. Even the lowly amoeba is a majestic miracle of purposeful activity when considered in company with a band of lifeless molecules. The molecules are steadily decaying and giving up energy while the amoeba absorbs that energy and grows with it.

Consider, then, that the amoeba is built of essentially the same particles of matter that builds the lifeless molecules. They all started together in a star, somewhere, the erupting product of nuclear fusion and the building of complicated atoms, flung out into cold black space to drift and coagulate into congealing lumps of matter which somehow in time found a space for itself in orbit around the star that built it—and the same debris that built the decaying molecular planet built also in its dust—or vapors, whatever pleases most—a vehicle by which quite another force, not encountered in any free form anywhere in creation [or is it?], began purposeful activity.

That is what life is. And that is how, to the best of human understanding, life began on this planet.

That understanding, however, is woefully inadequate at the present stage to answer the deeper questions about life. It does not answer, even, nor attempt to answer, the question of how "purposeful activity" arose in a lump of lifeless matter. Many scientists today would avoid the question by saying it is not in the province of science to answer such questions. But it definitely is within the purview and the province of science to ask as well as to answer every question bearing on the nature of this reality we all inhabit. So don't let them get away with that.

One scientist who did not try to get away with it was . . . the late astrophysicist Gustaf Stromberg (1882–1962). It is a pity that this man did not have access to recent findings in the still-infant science of microbiology. The postulates he did come up with, while microbiology was still a primitive science, would have been Nobel prize material had he not been so far ahead of his time. As it were, he was largely ignored or pooh-poohed by his contemporaries who perhaps were embarrassed by this scientific lapse into what surely was regarded as mysticism.

But Einstein himself wrote a glowing cover blurb for one of Stromberg's books, *The Soul of the Universe,* in which he sets forth a brilliant theory of life processes.

Stromberg, you see, though an astrophysicist, apparently became intrigued by what was happening in microbiology during the second quarter of this century. And he was fascinated by the research being done into basic life processes, particularly that having to do with the embryonic development of a living creature, or embryogenesis. Considerable spadework had already been done by various eminent biologists, including De Beer and Huxley, to show that embryonic development occurs within an "organizing field" and the German biologist Gurwitsch had published a study in 1922 in which he stated: "The place of the embryonal formative process is a field (in the usage of the physicists) the boundaries of which, in general, do not coincide with those of the embryo but surpass them. Embryogenesis, in other words, comes to pass inside the field. What is given to us as a living system would consist of the visible embryo (or egg, respectively) and a field. The question is how the field itself evolves during the development of the embryo."

Gurwitsch's "field (in the usage of the physicists)" is an electromagnetic field and it posits the existence of "an organizing field" of electromagnetic energy in which the embryo is embedded.

Stromberg envisioned "living wave systems" which he christened—are you ready for this?—*genii.* It is patently unfair to do so, but I will try to sum up, for quick consumption here,

Stromberg's conclusions by quoting a single paragraph from his book, *The Soul of the Universe:*

"Matter and life and consciousness have their 'roots' in a world beyond space and time. They emerge into the physical world at certain well-defined points or sources from which they expand in the form of guiding fields with space and time properties. Some of the sources can be identified with material particles, and others with the living elements responsible for organization and purposeful activities. Some of them exist in our brain as neurons, and some of them have a very intimate and special association with their ultimate origin. They are the roots of our consciousness and the sources of all our knowledge."

That said, I need to talk about the human aura, long felt by most people to be no more than the imaginative product of neurotic people and would-be psychics, and I want to tell you flatly that every object of the physical universe does indeed project an aura, or something that is called the aura.

There is nothing mystical or even psychical involved in seeing an aura. It is a matter of pure physics, not psychics, and anyone can do so if they know how to go about it. I cannot offer any laboratory findings to back me up in this, but let me tell you what I think the aura is.

The aura of any physical object will be found in that space surrounding the object in which collide the outer edge of the electromagnetic field of the object and another electromagnetic field produced elsewhere. For convenience, let's shorten the term to merely call it an energy field—and understand that every object however small or large in space-time is embedded in such a field.

The natural assumption would be that the object produces the field. But it can also be argued without violating the tenets of field physics that the field produces the object. The logical extrapolation of that idea gives us invisible organizing fields that are responsible within them for material particles that are produced and/or collected in specific patterns that materialize as physical objects, and that is the story of all matter in the space-time dimension.

I believe that these guiding fields are more rightly properties of the so-called spirit universe, in which Dr. Peebles assures us that one and all we are embedded within, as well as everything that we can see, touch, smell, hear, and taste.

This may seem a long way around to discuss the human aura, but it is necessary because it is also my belief that what we see as the aura is actually the interaction of the etheric body with the natural environment—most commonly with light. But the interactions between two etheric bodies have also been demonstrated through the process known as Kirlian photography, developed by the Russian S. Kirlian in 1939.

That same interaction (between two bodies) can be "felt" by sensitive people who are seen to react to the "vibes" of others, even from across a room.

To see the human aura with the naked eye, one must rely on peripheral vision. I do not know with any certainty why this is so; perhaps an ophthalmologist could help us understand it. I have heard it suggested that in the early conditioning or early attempts to see auras, it is necessary to "fool" the direct vision by lulling it in a fixed stare, allowing the photoreceptor rods used for peripheral vision to dominate the field of vision. I do need to say something here, also, about the so-called "fixation reflex," which perhaps has the largest bearing on the matter. If you are gazing straight ahead and a bright light appears in the periphery of that field of vision, your eyes reflexively turn to fix on that light. You have to resist that automatic reflex because to gaze directly into an aura is to see it instantly disappear, which is why we do not see them without a bit of practice. Perhaps this is because the optic rods that provide peripheral vision are stimulated by this very fine energy while the cones (which provide focused vision) are not, or perhaps it is a matter of synchronicity as suggested just above.

If you are interested in seeing auras, try practicing in private with a friend (we do not recommend this with strangers in public) in an area of moderate lighting before an uncluttered background— preferably a bare wall of a color for good contrast with your subject —light-haired person against a dark wall, dark-haired person against a light wall. Fluorescent lighting especially helps the novice, but once you get the hang of it, you'll be seeing auras everywhere you go whatever the lighting conditions—but there does have to be some light, because it is the light-energy interacting with the etheric body that produces the visible phenomena.

Begin by picking a spot on the wall about six inches above the subject's head and stare fixedly at that spot (no blinking) until you begin to feel a bit of strain. Then let the gaze crawl slowly down the wall until you encounter the aura. If several tries are fruitless, start again at a spot twelve inches above the head and repeat. If you are patient, you will eventually spot the aura. It will appear as a sort of luminous silvery shimmer like a corona above the head, and as long as you do not focus the eyes directly into it, you should experience it as a band of light raised two to four inches above the head. Look into it and it's gone. You can use that as a test to see if you really have the aura or if you have a ghost image imprinted on the eye. Ghost images will move with the gaze; the aura disappears if you look into it or too far off it.

If you try and try again but do not succeed, it could be because you have been looking into your subject's aura all the while. It is exceptional, but some individuals have quite powerful auras extending five to ten inches (at times) above the head—and some people who are experiencing strong emotional states will "pump" an aura a foot or higher off the head.

Don't expect to see colors unless you have a strong subjective sensitivity to emotional states.

I have told you all this primarily because I want to talk about Thomas Jacobson's aura—and I want you to believe what I am saying about that.

That was one of the things that had us so bowled over during our first session with him in April. In his normal state, Thomas has a rather normal aura—a softly mystical light raised about four inches and extending from shoulder to shoulder. It varies a bit in a sort of a rhythmic pulsing while he is inducing trance. This could have something to do with the internal adjustments he goes through, beginning with a relaxation routine and concentration on the breathing. After ten to fifteen seconds of this, he appears to already be in a light trance with the body processes greatly stepped down; the aura dims a bit and recedes a bit; then the pulsing begins, with the aura growing steadily brighter and expanding gradually to a strong corona extended six to eight inches. After several minutes of this, Thomas is breathing so lightly that you can just barely detect the movement.

But when Dr. Peebles arrives, the diaphragm seems to explode upward; with that same movement the aura flares dramatically to engulf virtually all the visible space above his head and often billowing out to a diameter of several feet from the waist up. We have also noted (a) zigzag stovepipe auras that disappear into the ceiling and (b) rather ragged and imprecise inverted-pyramid auras sometimes alternating with the expanded aura (and we have no explanation whatever for this).

At a recent public session in an auditorium, Linda and I independently sketched the same effect: an inverted pyramid more than twenty feet wide at the top and extending to the ceiling, with the tip seemingly concealed inside Thomas's head.

We have also noted full-body auras extending from members of the audience who have gone to a floor microphone to converse with Dr. Peebles. At times the effect is most remarkable, with the luminosity appearing to swirl away from the side of the body like a sheer white garment lifting with the wind. This phenomenon disappears the moment the person steps away from the mike.

We have cause to suspect that even individuals who are conversing via telephone hookup from across the country would reveal a similar effect if we could see them, and we feel that the greatly enhanced auric activity could account for the "electric feeling" that is so common an experience for those "in touch" with our good doctor.

He has told us, you know, that we are being "lullabied" while he and his spirit crew are present. I have to feel that this crew is interacting with us in very subtle ways. And obviously the entire phalanx is working on (or through) Thomas. It does not seem possible that the effects noted could be solely the properties of Thomas's own energy field.

Perhaps this could account also for the physical and emotional letdown experienced by Thomas after trance. If our theory is correct, it would be difficult to understand how he could feel any other way after such an incredible mingling of energies.

He always returns like a shy little boy who has been surprised while joyously riding a pony that no one else can see. The eyes are clear but also clearly embarrassed and wondering, the voice a bit muddled as though just awakening from a night's sleep.

Picture yourself nodding off at a banquet table, then jerking awake with the napkin in your mouth and wondering what else you'd done to make a fool of yourself while asleep in public. That will give you some small appreciation of Thomas coming out of trance.

But it is the coming-out aura that truly tells the tale. It is soft, and golden, and rides the shoulders like a halo.

And that is the only time I ever envy him.

It would be understatement to introduce David Viscott merely as a genius. He is that, certainly, but also so much more. The word *genius* defines but a state of intelligence. Dr. Viscott is a self-realized genius. He is not only an inventor and innovator but a whole moving process of self-discovery and then dynamic communication of that discovery; he is knowledge, knowing that it is, and he is life, living what it is. He is a self-realized man continually finding new depths to be realized. It is perhaps, then, a natural consequence that he is also a brilliant and highly successful psychiatrist.

Now, he does not walk on water.

But it might be difficult to convince the millions in his national radio and television audience that this is not so.

David is a channel and a psychic. I have even heard him admit it, though not in so many words, over the air. He discusses the process in terms that cannot be mistaken by those who understand that language, while insisting that what he is channeling is "my highest energy." But he downplays that dimension of his talents, preferring to tell us that we all are psychic, despite the sure and certain knowledge by those with whom he is conferring that he touches their innermost selves, and he appears to be denying that he has any access to knowledge that we all do not have within ourselves. He seems to believe that what occurs within himself is primarily a matter of teamwork between the two hemispheres of his brain.

I would not argue the point with a self-realized genius. I would reply only that it appears to me, then, that David Viscott's brain—totally encased, as it is, within its fortress of bone—has some mysterious and magical connection with my brain and your brain as well as everyone's with whom he is processing information. I simply cannot otherwise believe that if you call him on the telephone and tell him that your hand hurts every Monday, he can then get you to divulge the information that you detest your job, when you never really knew that yourself until that moment of revelation.

Allowedly, there are subtle techniques of deductive skills at work there, also, that explain much of his success in psychiatric counseling—but just simply to know David Viscott is to know that there is more to the story than brilliant deductive techniques alone.

A resident of Los Angeles, that is also his media base. His KABC TalkRadio *David Viscott Show* is aired nationally and has a listener base of several million in the Los Angeles area alone. A few years back, he had a Saturday night show at KABC immediately preceding Bill Jenkins's *Open Mind*.

Bill Jenkins himself has already told us about the first meeting between David and Thomas Jacobson. The second meeting apparently occurred on December 10, 1983, when David moved from his studio at the conclusion of his broadcast that night and joined Bill and Thomas for the first hour of *Open Mind*.

The three discussed mediumship in most specific terms—with David very interested and asking probing questions of Thomas regarding his early development as a medium. When Thomas later went into his trance and produced Dr. Peebles (on the air), David had the first question for the visiting entity. It was a personal question having to do with David's short-term future. Dr. Peebles addressed the question at great length, painting a future of great challenge leading to even greater realization of career.

David's response: "I have a lot of affection for you, my friend. It is remarkable how you speak to that hidden wish that I have to be meaningful to a lot of people and help them with a better, more honest, and open life. I have a feeling of solidarity with what you say."

We had the feeling, there, of a great meeting of minds.

The Doc replied: "God bless you. You will find that your life personally, intimately in your private thought, will confront the issue of vulnerability and exposure on a public and private level. This was an important decision for your soul, for in the distant past you have been in a similar position as a great healer, revered, who was quite inaccessible in private. You will find that there must be a merging of the philosophy with the life demonstration, privately as well as publicly. You're working nicely on that already; it's one of your personal creeds and teaching, of course. And yet it does remain part of your continued growth. You will be called upon by many, high and low; you'll be called upon to be the master teacher, you'll be called upon to be the Christ energy, as well as many others —and your need, of course, is to help everyone understand that *they* are the Christ energy. God bless you. David, you do that *very* well."

Bill Jenkins commented: "He was obviously speaking in the terms that we know you and the audience knows you; you're very well known in Los Angeles. But it seemed to me that he was speaking very very intimately to you, there, as well. Am I correct? The things that are foremost in your mind that you don't really share with us? You want to air yourself a little bit here?"

David Viscott very soberly and with obvious strong feeling replied: "My goal is a simple goal, and it's to make my own life the model of everything that I preach and believe. I have no dark closets in my life; I'm exactly what I seem to be, and I'm the same way on the air as off the air."

JENKINS: I can attest to that.

VISCOTT: I don't claim to be special; I claim to be what I think everyone is when they try to be giving—and to try to come from love is the constant struggle of my life and to be giving of what I know, and to try to help other people make their lives an example of the best they can be. If we all did this, that's how the New Age would be ushered in. Not that there would be anything magical or mystical or spiritual in that, it's just that we would be living up to our potential. If we could all do that, the world that we seek would be here.

I've always seen my goals since early childhood, when the only vision I ever had was a voice that said, in the second grade in Miss Donnelly's class, it said, "Someday, David, you will tell people what they really feel inside." I was very shaken by that, but that is precisely what I have done my whole life—whether it was my mind synthesizing my belief at that early age of eight, or not, it's how I've tried to live my life, and I live my life this way because I feel best living this way, and it's where I feel most honest—and I think what I've *heard* is, again, a reinforcement of that belief. It doesn't come as new knowledge—although the extent to which it is mentioned are things I've thought about, not in anticipation but in understanding how people tend to distort constantly what they hear, and to lionize a person who's in the public eye, and how I always try to make them understand that they're the ones who're in control; I'm just living my life —why don't they live theirs?

JENKINS: So Dr. Peebles was pretty much on target with you, then, in a very very close way.

David Viscott's voice was tinged a bit with awe as he replied, "Yeah, it—it's a bit freaky, folks."

Another meeting was on May 12, 1984, when David stayed over at KABC to guest on *Open Mind* for what Bill announced as "a special, special night indeed" with Thomas and Dr. Peebles. Another guest, via telephone hookup from Franklin, North Carolina, was George Meek, inventor of the "SpiritCom" and head of the Life Beyond Death Research Foundation.

Before Thomas went into trance, George Meek came on to state: "I had a private session with Thomas and Dr. Peebles about two months ago, and I was most impressed. I've studied mediumship abilities in many countries for the past fourteen years, and Dr. Peebles is one of the most knowledgeable and enlightened spirit persons I have talked with."

JENKINS: I noticed from the transcript that you sent me that most of your questions were very, very scientific and—

MEEK: They were, and it's very rare indeed that such questions can be asked of a spirit entity. Of further interest, Bill, when I returned to my offices here in North Carolina from guesting on your show several weeks ago, my secretary told me that at last she had started to catalogue my library, and she'd come across a book that Dr. Peebles had written in 1869. It has been published in several languages. My English language edition had been re-published in New York City in 1903—at which time Dr. Pee-

bles was said to be eighty-two years of age. It is titled
Seers of the Ages—with a subtitle, *Spiritualism Past and
Present.* As revealed in the book, Dr. Peebles himself was
highly clairvoyant and skilled as a medium, which helped
him in his writing and his lectures.

JENKINS: So he has stayed true to form.

MEEK: He certainly has. The publisher's preface reads, "Dr.
Peebles is distinguished as an author, orator, physician,
and traveler who has circumnavigated the world four
times. His name is recognized in climes all over the globe.
His kindness and benevolence are too well known to bear
mention here." The author's name is shown as J. M. Peebles, M.D., Ph.D., and inside his first name is given as
James . . . the book itself is a monumental effort to trace
spirit communications from the beginning of recorded history and in all areas of the globe. It is a masterful job.

Later, with Thomas in trance, Bill Jenkins wanted to follow up
on that directly with Dr. Peebles. He suggested, "George, what did
you find about him?—and perhaps Dr. Peebles will go ahead and
'fess up as to who he was."

Meek, by telephone from North Carolina, replied, "Well, the
most important thing is that I came across this very wonderful book
called *Seers of the Ages,* or, *Spiritualism Past and Present.* It is by all
odds one of the most remarkable books that I have come across.
The places, uh, the reality of spirit and spirit communications from
the earliest of recorded history."

The Doc replied: "Yes, this is my writing literally; however, I
cannot take full credit for it, in that I entered into trance states, of
automatic writing, of inspired writing, and ponderance in the
meditational state. It was a collective effort by several dozen others.
Many of the individuals mentioned in this book simply spoke directly to fill in some of the details that I never would have had time
to research myself, as well you know from reading the book. However, we have a great desire here not to put attention upon my
personality, for as I speak as Dr. Peebles I bring forward other
aspects of other personalities as well, and we believe that the content of what we speak is the relativity. So, with your permission,
and with respect, we would request that you minimize attention
upon a former lifetime that is no more. I have even in the past, with
some occasions, denied my reality as a personality so that we could
have best attention on spiritual matters. God bless you. But I like to
play, if you want to talk about it. So, uh, God bless you."

JENKINS: *(chuckling)* George, d'you have other further questions?

MEEK: Just one quick thing. Dr. Peebles speaks about the many many wonderful people who helped him; I wonder if he would, for my purposes, identify Aaron Knight [Spelled it out.], the person to whom there was a personal greeting written in the opening pages of *Seers of the Ages.*

DR. PEEBLES: God bless you. Aaron was one who facilitated my channel. Aaron was a medium who was never understood as a medium. He was almost taken off to the insane asylum a couple times, for example. However, due to the influence of some of his friends—in Parliament, for example—he was not carted away. Due to my great joy with that state called craziness, I found a friend. He helped me to feel safe within myself. He helped me to create environments, using plants, using certain air waves, using coloration schemes that greatly helped amplify the channeling.

This is something, George, as you continue to prove the reality of the spirit, that you and others will find grateful celebration and joy in the creation of environments for channeling by everybody. You're doing such a good job! God *bless* you.

JENKINS: Does that answer your question, George?

MEEK: It certainly does. Thank you, Dr. Peebles.

Earlier during that same show, David Viscott again got a crack at spirit when Dr. Peebles came forth. Here is that exchange:

BILL: Dr. Peebles, welcome back to the *Open Mind* show, and we're delighted to have you. We have some friends of yours—on the line is George Meek, talking to us from North Carolina, and Dr. Viscott is here.

DR. PEEBLES: Hello, George! I was just visiting with you just a little while ago. God *bless* you, David.

DAVID: Can I ask you a simple question? The strangest thing happened—I don't know whether anyone in this room saw it, but just before Thomas went into this trance, and began to shudder—just that very moment before the shudder, there appeared above his head what looked like a white puff of smoke. What was that?"

DR. PEEBLES: That was *meee.*

DAVID: Has anyone ever seen that before?

DR. PEEBLES: Oh, yes, many people see that. Some would call it in different words. But they see the energy of Dr. Peebles, with some of our friends here, coming into my channel as he quiets down.

DAVID: The appearance of it was just about . . . an area maybe a foot and a half square, like a little piece of white cloth was waved, and then suddenly descended into you; you shuddered, and then the voice came.

DR. PEEBLES: Yes. Thomas disassociates off to the right of the physical body—to his right—I come forward through the upper back, through his solar plexus, and down through the crown chakra. If any of you in this room would put your attention, your eyesight, off my channel and look with your peripheral vision, some of you will see glimmering purples and violets, for example, around the throat and shoulder areas. God bless you.

Later during that show, Dr. Peebles did a past-lives sketch on David that included a Druidic influence as well as many others.

Bill Jenkins was the first to comment on that. He said, "David, you've been around."

David replied in very subdued tones, "You know what's really strange? The home we lived in just prior to moving out to California was owned by people who were Druids. What I had uncovered on the property was a lot of their symbolic materials and went about restoring them, just because I seemed to have an affinity for it."

JENKINS: Now you understand.

DAVID: Yes.

DR. PEEBLES: It's all true, my friends. Just surrender to it. Goodness gracious.

Later, after Dr. Peebles had departed and Thomas again was present, Bill Jenkins remarked: "David, it's good to have you here—talking to David Viscott—whose opinions on matters such as this we have the highest kind of regard for. I know this is the second or third time you've seen Dr. Peebles. What is your candid reaction to this? Are we experiencing some sort of an act, or is this really going on?"

Viscott replied: "Well, the thought I had before you asked the question, in looking at this, and in reference to the way he was reacting, is that the sensitivity of the entity is just—without making any judgment about its reality—or the other-statedness of Tom's consciousness—is that the sensitivity of the reality, and this is just forgetting Thomas, is very very high. It's higher than Thomas's. I'm sorry, Thomas, but it is—well, you know, you look at him and he's different. There was an aura around Tom's head during this whole thing. And it's not there now.

"I realize my own credibility—and I'm talking to my people as well, but I wouldn't lie to you; it's just, what I see is what I see. And now the aura is not there. Tom came back during the break. Then when Peebles was returning again, there was a fragmentation of the aura. It wasn't like the first time. It was just like little pieces of energy floating by—not enough to say that you actually saw it, but at the moment you saw it and thought about it, suddenly Peebles is back and tells us he's been hovering around. That was the feeling I had about it. And now what am I thinking?—I'm thinking that this is an extremely sensitive entity whatever its origin. Whether his reading of my life as a former Druid or a great warrior is only symbolic, it is a read which has an extremely high accuracy.

"Now, the man who called in [During the show.] with a career problem—I mean it was in the voice: if he'd called my show, I would have said, 'You're going nowhere right now, aren't you, pal?' I mean, it was right in the voice. But there was something that Peebles could see beyond that, without any person adding anything to it, which was more than I would have risked, with my sense. If I were more open, I would've risked more, but there is a higher sense of knowing, but it—but there is something . . . just *weird* about this, everybody."

All three men laughed about that, then David added, "It's very difficult and I'm normally a clear person, and I'm having trouble with this—because it's your darned reality box, Bill—and it's wanting to maintain, you know, what I'm here for—which is clear and untainted; [I don't want to be] leaping over into anything. But something happened here that is not quite right."

Three years later the experience apparently is still "not quite right" to this brilliant mind—but it would seem that David Viscott is still mulling the possibilities. Here is a statement that he gave us:

> Mediums are always a fascination because they illuminate a part of consciousness we cannot study objectively. Without speculating on the source of Dr. Peebles's energy, the manifestation itself is entertaining, often illuminating, and usually outrageous; another piece of evidence for a case which has not yet been decided definitively.

Thank you, David. We appreciate your candor and your courage. God keep.

DR. PEEBLES: God bless you, Dr. Peebles here. It is a joy and blessing when man and spirit join together in search of the greater truths and awareness. Might I offer encouragement, my dear friends, as you strive to understand your right to experience wisdom within your own heart, as you strive to understand your right to experience the divine of your own very soul.

You are here, my friends, to understand the nature of your own reality, your own consciousness, your own creative craft, through thought. You are here to understand will, as the motivator, the bridge between your soul and thought. Thought, in and of itself, is as nothing, as dust in the breeze. It is, in fact, the will—the desire of your soul to be, to be seen, to be heard, to be felt, to be known, to be identified; to be experienced as alive, as relevant, as real and present, in any aspect of the divine universe.

It is the nature of consciousness, then, to experience attention, to gain the attentive attitude of one or more beings around you, and through that attention to validate your own reality, your own right to know thyself. And so it is that the ego is not only relevant, but critical, as a vehicle upon the school Earth to understand your image. For only through accepting your ego can you feel the motivation to identify your image, and through identifying your image, to know God; to know the divine. Through the forgiveness of yourself—through error, the forgiveness of error, of failure, of all events of trauma in your life, there you will see your image in the nature of God. For God does demand nothing of mankind and of you, but only to sing the praises of your being, your own communication.

My friends, you are gathered here to understand your right to communicate with spirit, with God, with the magic of the universe. And through the written word that you are bringing forward, you will inspire millions of people to come forward into a personal experience with God. God does not wish to be an eternity of time and space away from you, but rather to be experienced within each of you; not only one of you, but all mankind everywhere is the master, Jesus, the Buddha; He is within everyone all of the time.

It is the awakening, to become consciousness, to accept that grand responsibility fearful to the human mind only because of the limited concepts of judgment. God and all life is so loving that there is no concept of failure, of death. And so to accept the divine within yourself is only an act of great beauty, of great love.

God bless you each and every one, and would you have questions or comment?

DON: Thank you, Dr. Peebles. It's such a pleasure. You have been such a major force in our lives and we do thank you for that. Earlier in these sessions you made reference to the process or a reality that you termed the constant metamorphosis of God. Could you elaborate on that for us, please?

DR. PEEBLES: God bless you. God is all things, and God is consciousness—God is aware and active in the universe and throughout all time and space. Each and every human mind, mind of the animal, natural intelligence of the plants, and of the entire relationship of universe, are particles of this mind.

Each and every experience of life is an episode of movement—and through movement, unavoidable change, turning—in place, or around and with another. And so you have the solar systems, you have the galaxies, and you have the universes, each related to each other. You have the molecules, the electrons, and so forth, all related to each other.

Related, relation*ships,* this is the nature of all things. It is the turning—the turning within, the turning without —that is the revelation, the discovery, the doorway and the window to the greater power—in any context, in any definition. The ability, then, to create change as one turns is to discover a larger experience of self, of life, and of both. The greater you discover of life and of yourself, the greater you discover of God. To experience change in your life is to grow, to go beyond what was safe once upon a time.

And so it is movement, it is metamorphosis, a constant change. The universe has never, ever been the same. It is always different—even with the repetitions, even with the rotations, the revolutions, precise and similar. There is constant, constant change.

This is the greatest joy of the divine experience to the universe—to be aware, to be conscious, to be participating with that change. On the contrary, the greatest pain in the universe is to resist the very same.

So metamorphosis of self is to understand the metamorphosis of God. To embrace metamorphosis rapidly and with celebration, one must, of course, embrace the metamorphosis of yesterday. But here, where the system of judgment of human kind—amplified by the illusions of separation—tends to see failure and condemnation of experience, elimination of the presence of various people and souls from your presence for their failure rather than compassion and reeducation; here is where you are denying metamorphosis. You are denying that another person, no matter how grave their error, in your peer group, has the ability—in fact, the unavoidable reality—of changing that, always eventually to the opposite—to total love and compassion.

And so, more so erroneous than that being who's being gravely judged are those who are judging, who are staying in a solid place, without change, with only very subtle metamorphosis. These are the ones who will have less love later on, while this being—the one being judged—will have greater love. And so, it is the swinging of a pendulum, the ability to experience the passion of self, for behind the passion is truth and honesty, insight.

To avoid that passion—in other words to resist the will, to camouflage the will—is to reside only in the mind as if it in turn were the source, as if the mind were the divine. It is not. It is an extension, an amplification, a beautification of the divine—but it is not the source.

The source is in the will—or if-you-will, it is the heart. God bless you. Do you understand?

DON: Yes, I do. Would it be improper, then, to think of the living soul, the spirit—the individualized spirit and soul—as being somehow in a relative position of great importance to this constant metamorphosis? Is God becoming realized in His true self through our own metamorphosis? Would it be improper to look at it that way?

DR. PEEBLES: No, it would not be improper. I would explore an alternative word to *becoming*. God is already complete. For God has total concept and celebration of change, brought forward through self, toward God. So, there is no —there is no concept, no consideration, no doubt, that the universe and life and humanity will change. It is impossible not to change. It is only possible to resist the change. And so God is fully realized, no matter how grave the error, Don. No matter how difficult the experience, no matter how black the failure of human consciousness,

God is realized, nevertheless, *in* that experience. So even when one totally, totally resists change with some success for a moment, he is nevertheless still contained within God and God is fully realized. Does that answer your question? Was that your intention?

DON: I think it does. I'm still having a little bit of trouble with the concept, perhaps because it has long been my feeling that the relationship of man to God—and saying that man is any self-conscious life spirit or life force—is somehow more important than most of us have stopped to consider.

DR. PEEBLES: I see. All right, let's take a look here. . . . Well, I understand why you feel that way, Don, and you do so with accuracy. For in a very real sense, all of God is within each and every being; each and every essence of life, all of God is within.

With each utterance, with each movement of your being, you *are* making a major statement in the universe, and having a very real synchronistic effect upon the entire universe. And so to take greater responsibility for that effect is an act of extraordinary love.

Yes, the human mind—the mind of any consciousness in being—would be wise to understand that it is large, that you are mammoth, that you are huge, that the size of your soul is far beyond that of your largest city upon your planet. So the answer is yes, Don, but also the answer is that God is complete—is already complete, is total. Everything is contained and taking place in God, no matter what takes place—World War II, Hitler, Genghis Khan, and others—no matter what takes place, it's still within the context of God and it's still part of an overall experience of growth and love and completeness. You understand me.

DON: Yes, I do. There is no way, then, that all of life could combine to frustrate God.

DR. PEEBLES: Correct; exactly.

DON: God could never go insane because of all this errant consciousness running around.

DR. PEEBLES: Exactly. You see, it would be of some value for spiritual scientists of the decades ahead to look closely to your criminal systems, for example, rather than avoiding them—rather than dealing with the sweet and subtle psychology of human beings with some career difficulties in their lives. Deal with some of the great traumas of your societies and the difficult questions, including crime and punishment.

And referencing our earlier statement, the higher teachers—the masters—looking upon mankind, would often perhaps have more favor with a human being who sins greatly and creates a crime against society in their passion—honest passion albeit a massive illusion of separation, and then a crime. This person perhaps is succeeding more so than some people that would condemn that soul to an eternal hell, that would presume to be very separate and who would remain frigidly detached and separate—not out of love but out of cold separation from love. Do you understand? They will tend to stay that way, while the person who through honest passion betrayed another will more rapidly explore the heavens of love.

Can you follow my thought? I am having—there are difficult words here, subtle meanings, and I am having difficulty with my channel. But do you understand?

DON: Yes, sir; you are coming in loud and clear. But, uh, you surely are sensitive to the understandable fears and confusion in the minds of good people who with all their hearts and minds and souls wish to be forgiving and wish to be understanding, yet . . .

DR. PEEBLES: Oh, absolutely, of course, yes.

DON: Yet in the case of very heinous actions on the part of some individuals who, for example, repeatedly have committed the same crime, have been given therapy, have been imprisoned, only to be released and come out and repeat the crime—maybe it is a crime against little children, where one is committing all sorts of heinous tortures against little children . . . our pain in trying to deal with this, and trying to see the full picture, yet what do we do to protect our children?

DR. PEEBLES: Yes, well . . . the concentration—again, because everyone is living in shared illusions of separation—the understandable concentration is on protection. Within that context, it's certainly understandable. In containing and taking that person away from society, that is right action; perhaps a certain person doesn't deserve to live in society.

So, first we want to support you in that. There is karma. Everyone must meet their karma. So it is right action for a person who has betrayed and separated from their self-chosen society to find oneself contained by that society and imprisoned.

That's right action, in many cases. However . . . what takes place then? Does society not then betray itself? More enlightened societies will eventually have different approaches for these vexing social problems. For example, the use of theater, of minigovernments and politics in which these beings will be allowed to gather with those of like mind and be given exactly what they think they want. Their own way, for example, but in a very limited environment, so that they can experience the fruit of their own labor, which will be agony, through letting them accomplish what they think they want.

This will be part of revolutionary therapy. It will become understood through a spiritual consciousness that there is great love in this person, that life goes beyond this life and beyond your society, and you will become concerned with the soul—your own soul and the soul of another, for that being is your brother, is your sister.

So education and therapy will be given much more emphasis. But now we don't mean to say that there is softness of a feather across the face of this person, but rather that they grow from meeting their karma in a more clear, educated way, where they have to take responsibility.

There's no question, Don, that the criminal you speak of—the heinous criminal—has the greatest illusions of separation of perhaps anyone on the planet Earth. But there is also a certain poignant and relevant power in the honesty of the passion that goes beyond the theoretical sermons of some of those who condemn that soul.

There is something to learn from this being, who can be as equally, extraordinarily charitable, magnanimous with just the right certain movement inside. That is not likely to take place in the present prison systems of your planet the way they are; rarely do.

Whereas for those that have condemned a soul, it is a lot more than a little movement, for they are concentrating on condemnation, which is a movement away from love rather than toward love; do you see? A crime of passion, however heinous, is most often a misdirected movement toward love, although it may appear on the surface to be the opposite, in which the being is enraged, for he or she is seeking love and understanding but cannot experience that.

So, it's difficult; it's complex. But the therapy, the restitution we are speaking of—there must be karma, there must be responsibility, and they do have massive illusions of separation. However, it behooves you as a society as well as a soul to treat these beings with the respect that they have not shown another—and to discover God within; that is the great challenge.

Can those who are proud of their human mind—of their Christian or other religious love—can you discover that love? Do you have the love to discover that love within an enraged being?—and to resurrect him, as all the great masters have been resurrected?

There is the greater value to your society. For then through education and communication the people of society will become inspired that there's always hope, uh—as well as responsibility but there is always hope—and that there is forgiveness, there is compassion here. So I can be more honest with my environment, I can be more integrated with my society, for if and when I err, I must meet my karma but it will also be with compassion. Do you understand?

DON: So perhaps our greatest concern should be to not condemn ourselves through condemnation of others.

DR. PEEBLES: It is automatic, Don. It cannot be avoided. For the cold condemnation is a conscious separation from God.

DON: As you spoke, I was thinking of Robert Stroud, who came to be called the Birdman of Alcatraz. He was condemned to Alcatraz prison for life because of violent crimes. Yet he went on to give the world a great understanding of birds, became a leading authority on the subject. This was a resurrection?

DR. PEEBLES: One of the notable exceptions, yes, of your prison systems. And I tell you, Don—in social terms of your planet—if one wishes to compare, sometimes the more dangerous people are those who have no passion, who are not alive.

DON: I know what you mean, yes. Could you tell us more about the will and the movement of the heart?

DR. PEEBLES: All right, just a moment . . . [With precision.] The physical brain is a translator, extremely sophisticated translator, but *no more* than that. And I say that without qualification. Behind the brain is the mind, that is creative and subjective in nature and is able to go beyond language to form symbols. The force behind the symbols that the mind begins to design and expand upon, that force is the will. Without the will, there is death. Without the will, the mind is irrelevant.

So the will is invoked by heart or soul; we use the two interchangeably. Without heart there is no soul. The heart-soul has feeling, has desire to be manifest. I believe we said it completely in our opening statement. To be manifest is not possible until you have a reflection or echo. And so a second being was born, a third was born, and it is only through that reflection or echo which you can experience that you are made manifest.

If there is no echo, there is no being and no life. Now . . . the principle of one and another—one and then two —is an echo that helps one be evident; to *be*—to be aware of self, to be alive, to be in reality. However, even with the second state of being it is still insufficient, for if it is only one, and if it is only two, there is no change. There are only two echoes.

So this is where the principle of three—where three or more are gathered, for example—comes forward. For then you come into community, into the trine and the principle of three, which is change. You can call it, in some aspects of itself, evolution, if you wish. You can call it, in other aspects of itself, death, if you wish—or birth— so forth and so on.

So . . . those are some thoughts.

DON: If my heart center is closed, I am closed to my *soul,* then, my real connection.

DR. PEEBLES: Yes, because they are the same thing. And if those are closed, your mind can be very operative but it's irrelevant. Whatever success you create in your society on any level, with the mind but with your heart closed, will be very short term—insufficient, uncomfortable, etcetera.

You know what, Don, I'm going to leave pretty soon here.

DON: We thank you for being with us.

DR. PEEBLES: All right, my friends, go your ways in peace, love, and harmony. Life is a joy only as you surrender to the delightful opportunities for growth.

Certainly in the pain and paradox of daily life, forgiveness of self, forgiveness of others, will help you to relax, to lighten, and not take life too seriously; yet on the other hand, please honor your tears, and it must be with sincerity and seriousness that you enjoy the episodes of life as opportunity for change and thereby growth and then conscious oneness, enlightenment, with the divine.

There *is* such a state, my friends; there is enlightenment; you will obtain it.

All of you gathered, all of you listening to these words and reading them, are approaching that state . . . *rapidly.*

God bless you each and every one.

Linda and I had been working night and day for nearly a month. Two days after the session reported above, I had a strange dream during a midday nap. It was very vivid, and I can recall it now almost exactly as I experienced it.

In the dream I was asleep and dreaming—so I guess this would be a dream within a dream. In the interior dream, I was having a trance-channeling experience with myself as the channel. In the exterior dream, though, I understood that I was merely being given a demonstration of how the process works, and I was very interested in that, marveling at it.

The interior dream had me in total darkness; I could see nothing in that dream; however, I was experiencing pictures within that dream that I understood through the exterior dream to be images superimposed from somewhere outside myself but not emanating from the exterior dream.

Is this hard to follow? I was dreaming that I was dreaming. In the dream most distant from my conscious self, I was acting as a channel from the spirit world. Someone I could not see was asking questions of me, and I was answering them—but it was not *I* who was really answering; I was merely providing a *brain* that could respond to both the questions and the answers.

Now, in the outer dream—the one closest to my conscious self —I understood that I was receiving instruction about channeling— and I understood that the inner dream was playing out in extreme slow motion so that I could follow the process from my observation point in the outer dream.

Here is what was happening inside that dream within the dream. I was asked a question but I do not remember now what it was—so let's invent one for illustration: what is love? I made space between myself and the question, conscious space, pushing it away from me. As I pushed with the mind and made space, a word from somewhere outside me slipped into the space. Let's say that the word was *love*. As that word slipped into the blank space, I uttered it. In the utterance, I also pushed it away in the same direction as the question. As I pushed the word away with the mind, creating space again, another word fell into the space and I uttered it (for example, *is*) and in the utterance again pushed it on ahead, creating space for the next word (to complete our example, *God*).

In the actual experience, though, it was a complicated question with a complex answer, and I just kept uttering and pushing, uttering and pushing, as one by one the words of the answer fell into place in the space I was creating for them, but in very slow motion.

I was marveling at this in the outer dream, realizing that I was speaking of things that I knew nothing whatever about in my own knowledge.

The dream awoke me from my nap, and I discussed it with Linda. We had dinner with Thomas that evening. We discussed the dream and I asked Thomas, "Was I being shown the basics of channeling, in a very elemental sense?"

Thomas told me, without even thinking about it, "Oh, no, you were being shown a very high level, very sophisticated process. You would use that method in full consciousness. I mean, not from a trance state but from your conscious state."

Well, I am still thinking about that.

Still wondering, also, just what the hell consciousness is, anyway, and wondering if it is something I have or something that has me.

Whatever, I have decided to dance with it.

It has got to be the most exciting tune in town.

12

≈

One on One

---

*"It is our joy to be with you and to learn
with you. For what is life, if not a
sharing?—and what is love, without
growth? To be with you is both our
greatest recreation and most powerful
growth."*

—*Dr. Peebles*

Dr. Peebles is at his best when directly counseling an individual.
The wit, warmth, and wisdom are always there, always helpful and
eye-opening, usually entertaining—and much of the personal advice
could apply to many of us. So the book would not be complete
without a sampling of his direct manner.

The material in this chapter is transcribed from recordings of
Thomas Jacobson's weekly radio show, *Journey to the Heart,* on
KFOX, Redondo Beach, California, during which Dr. Peebles takes
telephone calls from the broadcast audience. Some of the questions
are quite personal, so all names have been changed in this transcript.

SANDRA: Dr. Peebles?
DR. PEEBLES: Hiiii, Sandra. God bless you, my dear.
SANDRA: Hello. This is the first time I've heard you and I'm

very excited to talk to you. My question is: my life just seems to be stuck. That's the only word I can use to really describe it. Things don't seem to be working out. The energy that I put out doesn't seem to be coming back to me in the way that I would like it to.

DR. PEEBLES: God bless you, Sandra. Well, you're a beautiful soul, and you are properly trying to take responsibility in your life. You *are* trying to be the creator rather than the victim. You *are* trying to create your own reality, your own experience, and we tip our hat to you. Actually you're doing a very good job. However, as you communicate with people you've forgotten a little bit about the student inside of you. In your desire to be the mature being that you are, you have lost sight at times, my dear, of the child within. And you feel embarrassed and apologetic about the child within your being—the universal child, within you.

So our invitation is to return to the child within you without apology, to return to the child within you with that same excitement that you've just expressed, for people's response to you—the response of human beings around you, particularly when they criticize you, particularly when they have points of view different from your own. How else will you grow, my dear, other than to receive and harvest those different points of view?

You've received lots of those over the last year or so, and sometimes you've translated that as lack of understanding of your own self from others, as people not caring about you—when, in fact, Sandra, it was just your self not *really* caring about their different points of view, and breathing it into your own being.

You're very talented, you're very artistic, you are a vulnerable being, but you're afraid of your vulnerability.

Point two: In your fear of vulnerability, you've spent much of your energy, Sandra, trying to be careful, trying to maintain and build your self-image through an element of protection. So, free yourself. Look forward to that shock to change rather than fearing change—life will become very colorful, beginning now, beginning tomorrow morning. Each and every day, you start the day: "Hello, life, here I am. Tell me what I don't know about myself. Go ahead, criticize me, I look forward to it."

You understand me?

SANDRA: Yes, I do.

DR. PEEBLES: Does that help you at all?

SANDRA: Yes, it does, it really does. I didn't even think of that. I've been meditating on it for quite a while, but . . .

DR. PEEBLES: Well, remember, too, you're doing a very good job because you are trying to take responsibility. We've watched you and we're very proud of you, my dear; keep it up. It's just that in taking responsibility, don't isolate yourself again, and in trying to create your reality, my dear—*all* of you listening—that only happens through harvesting, integrating the different points of view around you. That is how you create peace on Earth and peace inside of yourself, not trying to get people to agree with you. You understand me.

SANDRA: Uh-huh, yes, I do.

DR. PEEBLES: Yah, bit of the preacher in Dr. Peebles, isn't there? Yah, I like to flap these lips on my channel, you know. It's fun to talk in the human body. God bless you.

SANDRA: Thank you.

DR. PEEBLES: All right, Sandra. God bless you.

JACK: Thank you for helping us. Dr. Peebles, twelve years ago my wife's mother died, and since then has been—shall I say—around us, on and off, in a negative way. I was wondering what we could do to learn what's going on or to help her go on *her* way.

DR. PEEBLES: All right now, this is who speaks here now? This is Jack?

JACK: Yes.

DR. PEEBLES: And your wife's first name?

JACK: My wife's first name is Tammy.

DR. PEEBLES: And her mother's first name?

JACK: Lois.

DR. PEEBLES: All right; just a moment. [Ten-second pause.] Yeah, Jack, you're feeling her around you right now? Your —yah, she says, "Who's that talking about me over there?" All right, just a moment—yah, just a moment. [Fifteen-second pause.] Huh! All right. Yes, I agree. She is a reality, she is *in* your reality, and she is projecting her point of view frequently.

Now, from her perspective that's all she's doing. Because she feels that love is discipline, is control, is helping people do what's right, whether they like it or not . . . helping people, trying to invoke cooperation in people to do the proper thing, to do the right thing. You know, that's an impossibility, there's no such thing, so she's guaranteed frustration and anger; so she's angry.

On the spirit side she feels like she didn't complete her life, she feels like she's wasted her life, she's angry because she feels no one cared about *her;* she thinks that she was just constantly helping other people and being strong for them, especially family. She saw herself very much as a family being, dedicated to family. She doesn't feel it was returned to her. Well, this is because, Lois—she's listening to me—Lois, these are because of *your* illusions of separation, and your not taking responsibility. Your desire to create love through cooperation is understandable, but now you will create love through enjoying the different points of view that come to *you,* Lois.

So she hears my words; she is around you; the spirit, uh—she's turning around, and she's gonna become more aware of her own teachers now.

You will light a candle, and in that candle you will express love for Lois. You must understand that from her perspective, Jack, she's not being negative. She feels she was not loved and understood, and she's still trying to make everyone do what she thinks is right—which, of course, is just doing what *she* thinks should be done, just what *she* believes.

So, she's going to change that point of view even as I speak. You can look forward to a withdrawal of that energy as you light this candle and both you and Tammy together and in separate moments, talking out loud to Lois and saying, "Well, you know, Lois, I recognize that part of me is that way, too, and so I have understanding and compassion for you. And come to think of it, I've learned from you because of it. So I am told by another spirit that the teachers are around you, so perhaps you can join them as we will seek to join *our* local community on earth." You understand me.

JACK: Yes, Doctor, I certainly do.

DR. PEEBLES: I believe that will be a hundred percent effective.

JACK: Thank you very, very much, Doctor.

DR. PEEBLES: God bless you, my friend.

ELAINE: God bless you, too, Dr. Peebles. I would like to ask about transmigration, coming back as animals. I just can't accept that in my mind. I wanted to hear what you have to say about it.

DR. PEEBLES: Yes. Well, it s true, it's absolutely true; however, there is a little bit of dogma in some of those books you've been reading. However, you are also correct, too, my dear, because there are human spirits and there are animal spirits who *don't* change. There are many, many human spirits who have never become an animal. Many, many animal spirits who never became and never will become a human.

However, there are many who have done both. It is simply an act of choice. It is usually, I might add, a *mature* choice, giving you a larger, more rounded perspective —not only of intelligence, but of the *true* nature of love.

For, you see, in the animal community they *do* have a *soul,* and they do have intelligence—no, they don't have the ability to articulate, to do much deductive thinking and reason as you understand it—but, you know, I wouldn't become too proud of those particular faculties. They really aren't the point. Love and enlightenment is not accomplished through knowledge. It is accomplished through love and intimacy.

So next time you're around an animal, not only look into that animal's eyes—let the animal look into your eyes and feel the loving spirit that has so little demand inside. Your heart will relax and you will understand a new consciousness. You understand me.

ELAINE: But we do have a choice. We're not forced to reincarnate as animals, like these people that have done mass murders of animals, they wouldn't be forced to go back into an animal, then.

DR. PEEBLES: No, they wouldn't, but it would be strongly suggested to them, for maybe a few hundred years. You see, on the spirit side you have a higher perspective as an individual. Eventually you will see that you want to do something, that you *have* to do something, and eventually through your free will you decide, I'm gonna do it.

So someone like you just mentioned who's been cruel to animals—on the higher perspective will say, "Goodness gracious, I see what you *mean*—they are a living, breathing soul; they have feelings and emotions; I didn't know that, I thought they were a biological robot here for my pleasure. So now I *want* to understand them, and I *will* become an animal because at this moment of my higher perspective I don't feel that pride, I don't feel like I would be a lesser being." Do you see?

ELAINE: I feel that I'm a little bit higher intelligence, that . . .

DR. PEEBLES: Ahhh, there you go, now, see—

ELAINE: That's wrong?

DR. PEEBLES: Well, it's not wrong but, you know—animals, my dear, some animals—not all of them—all animals have lots to do, also, in growth—they're not perfect—in the formal sense of the word, but there are some animals— like the dolphin, for example, and there are others, who actually really are your teachers, my dear. They are teachers not only in their experience of loving allowance, teachers of allowance, but they have a larger intelligence in many ways.

    You see, if you'll think about it, with a higher intelligence why would you have the need to deduce anything? If you see something and you understand something, then why would you need to break it apart and analyze it? You see what I mean?

ELAINE: I do.

DR. PEEBLES: And the human intelligence prides itself on that ability—well, you know, it's a valuable tool but it's not the highest experience in the universe. Not at all.

ELAINE: I see.

DR. PEEBLES: Food for thought, eh?

ELAINE: Yes, it is, Dr. Peebles, and thank you so much. Love you and love your program.

DR. PEEBLES: God bless you, my dear.

MARK (announcer): Interesting points there. I like that. So many times, Dr. Peebles, we feel that we're better than something because we're smarter or we're more intelligent or we feel something along those lines.

DR. PEEBLES: Exactly, Mark, well said. It's not only between species but between individuals, as you've inferred. So there's one human being to another, thinks he or she has a high IQ and thereby they're superior—*hog*wash! That's what I say. God bless you.

MARION: I talked to you about a month ago, Dr. Peebles, and I have to say you were completely right. You told me to have my mouth checked for an infection. I had just been to the dentist a little before that so I knew there was nothing wrong but . . . well, there was, and if I hadn't taken care of it I would have had a *very* bad infection in my gums that would have probably caused the loss of some teeth.

DR. PEEBLES: Give yourself the credit, my dear. It was you who asked the question and you who followed up. God bless you.

MARION: I didn't ask; you just told me. Anyway, thanks, and now I'd like to ask you about—I'm in a relationship and it's been back and forth and I just don't know what to do anymore. Do you feel that what I'm doing is okay, or . . .

DR. PEEBLES: Do you feel free to give a first name of the other party?

MARION: Oh, yes, uh, Bill.

DR. PEEBLES: All right, just a moment here. [Pause.] Well, you know, you must, of course, follow your own heart, Marion, and you're to understand that you could pay more respect to your own feelings—not only your feelings of fear but the feeling of curiosity and attraction to be with this man.

I would suggest this relationship is not complete, it's not over, there's a little more exploration here, and that you are worthy of each other's further attention. I would say that the main problem here, really, is that you have hesitated in expressing yourself with him. So ask yourself how can I be much more honest, much more quickly.

Now, I know that later on—hours later, weeks later —you're very honest, but I'm talking about right now, in a given subject or exchange with Bill, how can you be very honest and then—point two, of course—allow him to respond the way he wants to. And then you won't feel that you're in prison, you won't feel like he's controlling you and denying you and holding you back. It's only yourself, my dear. You understand me?

MARION: Yes, I do, Dr. Peebles.

DR. PEEBLES: What do you feel about that? What you gonna do?

MARION: Well, I'm just going to have to say my feelings at the time instead of just never saying anything until—just like you said—until a week later. You're right.

DR. PEEBLES: Yah. You see, really the value is not in the *discovery* of truth—because actually everything has some truth somewhere—the value is in the *process* of seeking truth. The value is in the exchange between you. That's why the delayed communication is very unfulfilling and frustrating to *all* concerned. You see?

MARION: That's true.

DR. PEEBLES: Yah. So just let it out and let him come back the way he wants to. And when he comes back the way you don't like, you just let it out again, exactly what you feel. See what I mean? Don't try to be loving and spiritual! Just be honest, and you'll automatically be loving and spiritual. You understand me.

MARION: Yes I do, Doctor.

DR. PEEBLES: God bless you. It's a good relationship. Don't you leave it yet, there's more to explore.

MARION: Oh, thank you, Doctor. Bye-bye.

PAUL: God bless you, Dr. Peebles. I've had this feeling for six or seven months now that there have been spirits around me, and lately when I've been meditating I've been seeing a gal in a white dress but I haven't been able to make contact with her.

DR. PEEBLES: All right, just a moment here. [Pause.] Hah! All right! The name she wants to present to you, for you personally, is Stori—S-T-O-R-I—and she by intention she relates that to story S-T-O-R-Y so that every time you call upon her, you will immediately invoke the experience of a story inside you.

She says whenever you have a problem, whenever you have a challenge or a confusion or a hesitation, call upon her by name, call upon Stori, and she says immediately you will begin to see a series of memories or pictures and feelings in your being. Pay attention to the story that develops very quickly in your mind and heart, and she says contained in that story, in your case, is always the answer, and that through that repeated practice and study you will understand the master that you are, the insight— you know, she says you have such great insight for other people, that you are a caring person, they come to you for your points of view; you give them not only a mental theory, you give them your heart, and she wants to compliment you for that.

She's a great master. You are honored to have her around you. So, she says concentrate on the story inside you as you call upon her by name, and you will be able increasingly to give yourself the counsel and the love that you have given to others. You understand me.

PAUL: That sounds very nice. Thank you.

DR. PEEBLES: Does that help you?

PAUL: It helps me very much.

DR. PEEBLES: Other humans can be jealous of you, having Stori around; she's quite spectacular, she's something, she's a beautiful lady—elegant, she's enlightened, she has no more lifetimes on Earth, she understands the relationship between ego and humility—and both belong inside of each other—and she balances to take heaven with Earth, the left with the right, the black with the white, the up with the down; she creates balance, and that is her teaching to you, through a story. God bless you.

PAUL: God bless you, Dr. Peebles. [We use Paul's real name here because he brought the tape to us when he heard that we were writing this book. Paul is a writer, too, and works with *stories* all day every day—but he was just another voice on the telephone when Dr. Peebles gave him this.]

PENNY: I've been out of a relationship for a while and I was just wondering if you had any insight on whether I might meet someone soon.

DR. PEEBLES: Well, let's see, uh . . . would you join me tonight for a little dinner and wine? Uh, yes, if I were still in the body I'd knock on your door tonight; absolutely; you're a delightful lady. Just a moment here. . . . Well, the truth of it is, Penny, the man—goodness, yah—man's gonna have his hands full with *you*.

You're a powerful being; you are full of love and light; but also you have some fears, like all human beings —and sometimes, you know, Penny, you put great emphasis on protecting yourself and you are tired of doing that, that's all. It's a new cycle.

You're tired, you're bored by it, and you're ready for a little interaction, a little intimacy—and we compliment you for it. So, let that be clear inside of you; vibrate that in your being. You're gonna have men responding to you— maybe some women too—you're gonna have people who will want to be with you, and your job is to [very deliberate] not look for the perfect one.

But just remember that you're not trying to make a life decision. You're just gonna dance. You know, just the dance of life. You're just gonna touch and let yourself be touched. You have many relationships in front of you. I know that you want a permanent long-term relationship, but that will happen only through the ability to create change in relationships and to be with the many rather than the few.

PENNY: Do you by any chance see anyone coming soon; and, if so, do you have a name?

DR. PEEBLES: Well . . . if I did, I wouldn't tell ya anyway, but we'll take a look here. That would take the fun out of it, Penny, you know, that's all part of the challenge of life to create your experience. Now, just a moment . . .

Well, you gonna open yourself up?

PENNY: Yeah.

DR. PEEBLES: So are you going to go outside of your place of living?—go out to the world?

PENNY: Ohhh, that's a good one. How did you—?

DR. PEEBLES: Yah. You just can't sit and wait for the phone to ring, you know. I know you're very good in mental telepathy, but some of the men are a little slower than you, you know. So let's see here, just a moment . . .

You got to get out there and dance. Not only figuratively but in fact. You know?

PENNY: Uh-huh.

DR. PEEBLES: Move your physical being, shake 'em up a little bit, you know, shake up the men, get them excited, uh . . . you know, use your sexuality instead of being afraid of your sexuality. That is a *spiritual* activity, to create greater intimacy between yourself and others. Do not let sexuality, as it has in the past, become a frustration like a thorn in the side. Sexuality is a beautiful experience when accomplished with respect, a beatific and divine experience that inspires people to touch each other. Otherwise you'd all just lie in your beds reading books all the time or watching television. So surrender to your sexuality. Go outside your room. Men will respond to you—yes, you'll see a little *fire* in their eyes, and there's the challenge— will you withdraw again because of the fire?—or will you *become* the fire? You understand me.

PENNY: Yes, I do, Dr. Peebles.

DR. PEEBLES: And when you become the fire, you're not gonna feel less spiritual; you're gonna feel *more* spiritual, *more* loving, *more* alive. You understand me.

PENNY: Yes, I do, and I thank you very much.

DR. PEEBLES: I would say that by next, ah . . . when are you going to start all this energy?

PENNY: *(laughing)* I'll try to go out today.

DR. PEEBLES: All right, good girl! You're a fast study, aren't you? Yah, all right, let's see—I would say you will have a date before next Wednesday. So call us back, let us know.

PENNY: I sure will, thank you.

DR. PEEBLES: You'll probably have two or three—so get ready, you're gonna be busy. God bless you.

PENNY: Thank you, g'bye.

Some of the material within this and the next chapter has been added as the book is being readied for publication, almost two years after the original manuscript was completed—sort of like a post-script inserted into the middle of a letter. We feel the need to tell you this because of the time frames involved in several of the pieces, where obviously we have been tracking the results of the interactions between Dr. Peebles and the individuals whose experiences are related herein over a much longer period of time than was required to produce the original manuscript.

Actually, we could fill another book with the personal testaments and transactions that have been gathered, but of course we cannot print them all, and there would be a considerable redundancy if we did because there is something of a common effect shared by all who directly experience the loving touch of Dr. Peebles, regardless of age, sex, educational background, or social status —to the point that we have had to constantly remind ourselves that each human being on the planet is absolutely unique, that therefore each effect is unique *no matter how "common" it may appear on the surface.* Still, there are correspondences shared by all, so it is our hope that the selection of personal testaments printed here will strike chords within many of our readers.

We spoke with Ruby Totter, a resident of Buena Park, at the Gathering Place in West Los Angeles following a public session one evening, and she told us: "This is all just so beautiful. I always envied the people who had access to Edgar Cayce. Now I feel so lucky that I am living in the same time, space, and community with Thomas and Dr. Peebles."

Beauty, see. Many, many people spontaneously speak of the beauty of the experience and the privilege of this kind of contact with spirit.

Mark Jungheim of Burbank stated: "Dr. Peebles and his philosophy have made a large impact on my daily life." This is a common understatement often encountered from those who never miss a public session or radio broadcast. *Impact* is the key word here, a sort of shaking out of priorities and a different orientation in life.

Gretta Axt of the South Bay area put it this way: "It is highly enlightening and totally uplifting. You know, you can feel the presence when you're there with Dr. Peebles, more so in a small room in private consultation. I have tried to describe the feeling to people.

When I left, it was like my feet weren't touching the ground, and I felt ten years younger, and the weight I'd been carrying on my shoulders was no longer there. It was a wonderful feeling and a wonderful experience."

Not everyone is able to put it into words as definitively as Gretta has done, but many to whom we have spoken have mentioned the "lightness" and the wonderful feeling of youthfulness and freedom following direct contact with Dr. Peebles. We have actually seen this effect at every public session, so startlingly visible in the faces and postures of those gathered together in spirit. One very elderly lady who walks with some difficulty told us: "I can just barely get in here every week but I always feel like I could dance all the way home."

That's how it is to dance with angels.

Many people, of course, come to consult Dr. Peebles on various personal concerns, and for these the effects are usually quite specific. Alicia Marion of San Diego gave us this testament:

> Dr. Peebles helped me to open the doors to my inner self —a self long ago locked away and forgotten. He taught me to become as a child again, to open to life and love and joy—that being vulnerable, honest, and present would give me back to me. He showed me that the soulmate, the partner, the friend I so desperately searched for was myself all along. Thank you, Dr. Peebles, for putting light upon a darkened path to allow me to see that I am, and have always been, truly loved.

Millicent and Marc Keagy, mother and son, also from San Diego, gave us these written statements. First, Millicent:

> I feel happy to encourage any person to hear Dr. Peebles. His wisdom is of such great value in general—and, in particular, he knows each of us and will give information to each that only Spirit *could* know of. It seems that this is his way of letting us know that he understands things that are meaningful to us in a personal sense, while the general audience will hear it in an impersonal sense, so our secrets aren't displayed to the world, only to each of us individually. I can't say enough of the wisdom of Dr. Peebles and wouldn't hesitate to suggest that any person would be greatly helped by hearing him.

Millicent obviously was touched by Spirit's gentility and sense of propriety, and she felt him inside her in a highly intimate and personal way—which, also, we have found to be a common effect.

Her son, Marc, is a handsome and intently serious young man who was touched in a more specific way:

> Contact with Dr. Peebles has cleared an earlier confusion of nebulous concepts, the sum of which never equaled a coherent whole. Now I understand that the incoherent sum is in fact *me*, and that I must reach consciously toward an expression of the whole.
>
> In that reach, I am in combat with the illusions of separation so often cited by Dr. Peebles as the source of all confusion. I am so involved in the process of dissolving the illusions of separation now that I tend to think of Dr. Peebles as me and myself as Dr. Peebles. This is the deeper teaching, I feel.
>
> The wisdom and personal insight given me by Dr. Peebles has given a new focus to my life. He planted the seed and now I am germinating it with courage and hope, allowing it to grow as it will into the fullness that I can be. What a relief it is to bid adieu to the confused pieces of myself that were proliferating for so long.

Something that is of more than passing interest here is the fact that Marc Keagy had not directly experienced Dr. Peebles as of that writing and had never met Thomas Jacobson, but had gained his insights as a result of listening to tapes of recorded sessions and via a subsequent telephone session with Dr. Peebles. This, also, is a common feature of the Peebles effect—and please note that both mother and son, a generation apart, were identically touched by the "wisdom" of this enlightened spirit.

Another San Diego resident, Nita Reynolds-Jodzio, frequently makes the long drive to Los Angeles to attend the public sessions at the Gathering Place. She has also had private sessions with Dr. Peebles and is an alumna of *Journey to the Heart,* Thomas Jacobson's powerful workshops in transformational spirituality.

Nita is delightful, a bright and sparkling tribute to the power of spiritual psychology. A few years ago she was a "mess"—diagnosed as a manic depressive and still "psychotic" after twelve years of intense therapy. Nothing seemed to help, not even in the short term, and her life was an endless nightmare. Then one day a friend took her to "see" Dr. Peebles, and what she "saw" was Nita. It was a truly transformational experience that led to her total recovery and . . . well, let her tell you herself:

> There are those rare moments when an extraordinary event or person is instrumental in changing the course forever

of one's life. For me that was Dr. Peebles. After years of depression, despair, and endless unsuccessful therapies, his insight enabled me to heal at last . . . to feel alive, to be excited, to feel inspired and—most precious of all—to bubble with laughter, often. My suffering has truly ended. Thank you, thank you, thank you, Dr. Peebles.

It is very difficult to look at Nita now and imagine that this bright and bubbling thirty-four-year-old art teacher could have ever known what "suffering" is. She is a delight and a joy at any gathering—and we, too, thank Dr. Peebles for her lovely presence.

Jefferson Lanz has become a fixture at the weekly public sessions in West Los Angeles. Young, handsome, energetic, he has done some acting and is a talented writer, teaches aerobics, and is into many things. Jefferson is one of those sparklingly blithe spirits who never seems out of place, never meets a stranger, can always be counted on to add a bit of life to any gathering. He has had at least one private consultation with Dr. Peebles. Here is the way Jefferson sees his communion with spirit:

The impact Dr. Peebles has made on my life is enormous, but the biggest area of change has come from my search to improve relationships both personal and in business.

I have been seeking answers to why my career goals are not being met when all the right stuff is in place. I believed that I had the proper training, mental outlook, good attitude, and determination, but something was missing to get the ball rolling.

"The question I posed to him [Dr. Peebles] dealt with charisma—what is it and how do I develop it? I believe that people who have it seem to draw everything toward them. Dr. P. agreed, but what he said in response was that thinking you have it rather than just letting it be can actually turn people away; like a magnet—which can both draw things in and, with a reverse polarity, push things away. Further, in order to be more charismatic and draw things toward me, I must let my natural charisma come forward rather than portray it. For when it is portrayed or put on, people see through that and they say "why bother?"—and the results then push them away. Since relationships are an exchange between two people and money is only an agreement of exchange, by pushing things away it will cause me to exchange more slowly and therefore the money and job security doesn't happen.

As usual, Dr. P. seemed to have the missing ingredient to

the recipe. Since that time, I have been working at letting people see the real me. By letting them see both my hopes/desires *and* fears, I am allowing them to be more a part of my life and hence draw them closer. It has been a difficult road because in the past I have thought that my "colorful and entertaining" self could be a turnoff to them and hence the reason I would lose out on a job. But in reality, those fun aspects would draw people in and when they got too close, I would give them what I thought they wanted—which wasn't right—hence, I ended up pushing them away.

Now that I have granted myself permission to be me, whether everyone likes it or not, things are starting to happen. More job opportunities are presenting themselves and rather than be forced into a situation, I can choose. Because Dr. P. opened my eyes to things that were already there, I am eternally grateful.

Jay Halford presents an interesting contrast to our friend Jefferson, almost an alter ego personality. Jay is a study in stoic strength, a chiseled figure in stone who rarely displays emotion even when emotion seems appropriate, yet who possesses an irrepressible sense of humor and a merry laugh, an engagingly dry wit, and an almost sardonic sense of the ridiculous. He is your patented "strong man"—but beneath that visage of stone dwells a gentle poet and a warmly sensitive nature. Jay has become one of our very best friends. We love him like family and feel honored by his friendship. He is not an easy man to "know," but to know him is to love him— and that may seem surprising to some who know him by his record only. Jay, you see, has had trouble with the law, and he has served time. That was many years ago—he is in his mid-forties now—and he got off to a rough start in life, but he does not try to alibi it or make light of it. He was prominent for years as a guiding force in felon rehabilitation and stands today as a model for those who have been in similar trouble. He is now a journalist, poet, aspiring screenwriter—and he wrote this piece for our book:

This marvelous medium, Thomas Jacobson, in tandem with the wise and wonderful Dr. James Peebles, creates a living flesh-and-spirit catalyst for transformational growth. The operative principles offered *do* work when earnestly applied, and there is a palpable love that emanates from both Dr. Peebles and Thomas.

In 1987, just prior to the observance of the Harmonic Convergence, I chanced to hear Thomas Jacobson channeling

Dr. James Peebles on KFOX radio. I was immediately struck by his power of insight and genuine compassion as he probed, counseled, and inspired troubled souls seeking guidance.

Immediately I resolved to attend a public channeling session at the Gathering Place, and for the next months I closely scrutinized this wonderful phenomenon of spirit possessing flesh and commanding the undivided attention of a roomful of strangers and admirers.

My earlier life of violence and imprisonment had prepared me to recognize a scam, but my "mean-streets smarts" and intuition told me that this fusion of Thomas and Dr. Peebles was genuine and positive and alive.

I can relate to Dr. Peebles's own history of some three hundred and fifty lives on this planet, learning and relearning the lessons of spirit and consciousness. He has inspired me as perhaps no other entity could. I love, respect, and honor this brilliant soul and his teachings.

Following my release from prison in 1963, I had become active on the political left and, subsequently, developed an elitist, "servant of the people" mindset. I believed that I was better than others—different, handsomer, more creative, tougher, and brighter than anyone else. My life was confrontive and I battled all who dared to differ with me. It was an ages-old impulse that came easily and quickly, and it had gotten me into a whole lot of trouble.

In one of my private sessions, Dr. Peebles identified for me a life in Greece several thousand years ago where I was a prominent military authority. In that life, I was responsible for the deaths of many who resisted my desire to impose Greek culture upon the world. "You weren't cruel, just convinced," Dr. Peebles advised me, but intuitively this cut me to the quick and I wept, for I recognized that Grecian experience as the genesis of my intolerance of other points of view during this lifetime—and the recognition came at a very deep level of cognizance, so deep that there was no mistaking the carryover into this life.

Dr. Peebles has inspired me to embrace life as a creative adventure for which I must take full responsibility. His sage advice has enabled me to focus my understanding that relationships between people are what life is all about, to trust myself, to be vulnerable, and to believe in my destiny as a writer and a healer. He has helped me understand the tumultuous journey of my soul on Earth and how, in this incarnation, I have come to specifically reconcile the subjective with the objective—to synthesize the two into a harmonious world view of self, people, and external events.

Unlike other spirit teachers who inspire with aphorisms and general information, Dr. Peebles is specific and personal, and he comes into your very soul. He elaborates the three principles of loving allowance for others and self, increased communication with respect, and total self-responsibility for our own lives—past, present, and future. As he is wont to say, "We are the pilots, not the passengers, of our ships of life."

Some religious reactionaries may wish to link spirit channeling with the would-be dark forces, but from my experience I see Thomas as elegant—with true surrender—and Dr. Peebles as illuminated, with real love and wisdom—and I celebrate the great and glorious God who permits us an interface with the sea of spirit that permeates our porous lives as human beings on Earth, ever available for our inspiration and guidance but *nonintrusive*—we must ask, and then it will be given. Contact with spirit is my proof that I am not alone in a world of shared illusions.

Very powerful stuff, isn't it? But that is the kind of power we have come to expect in the vicinity of our "interfaces" with the spirit world, and we thank one and all for sharing their impressions with us.

Now we will take you a step further, into direct interaction and a follow-up critique by those served.

We first met Lee and Carol Chaifetz at the Gathering Place during the early summer of 1987. They were in regular attendance throughout the time that we were developing material for the book and have been ever since. It has been another common experience that so often our interest in Thomas and Dr. Peebles has brought us into contact with very likable people, and many nice friendships have thus been engendered.

We liked Lee and Carol immediately. She is a strikingly beautiful television actress (you can see her on daytime TV most any day of the week) with a warmly vulnerable personality, very friendly and direct in manner, easy to know and be with. Lee is a writer. He has the physical frame of a football lineman, big and powerful but not at all threatening, a genial and outgoing gentle bear who loves intellectual discussions and obviously spends a lot of time inside his own mind.

We spent time with this engaging couple most every Thursday evening for more than a year, often going out with them at the end of the evening for coffee and dessert en route to our respective homes, yet we never got to know them really well during that period and never saw them at any other time. Their interest in Thomas and Dr. Peebles seemed to center on the general phenomena itself, but occasionally they would ask questions related to career and other routine personal matters—and at coffee afterward, the mood was usually light and the discussion more chatty than substantive.

Then came the evening of July 21, 1988. Carol showed up at the Gathering Place without Lee, and she was the first in line to speak with Dr. Peebles when he threw the discussion open for questions from the floor.

Here is the transcript of that exchange:

CAROL: Hi, Dr. Peebles, this is Carol.

DR. PEEBLES: Hi, Carol. God bless you, my dear.

CAROL: God bless you too. My husband, Lee, who I know you know, was admitted to the hospital yesterday and the doctors say that he has one of the forms of leukemia and so . . . well, what we're wanting to know . . . it seems—I don't know, maybe we're wrong, it seems like it's pretty bad, but we haven't gotten all of the results back. We want to know what the source is, what the lesson is to be learned, and what we need to do. And by what we need to do, I mean do we go with the medical treatments, do we go to a holistic healer or . . . I guess we'd really like to know if this *is* his time—and, you know . . . so we'll know how to deal with it.

DR. PEEBLES: All right. Just a moment here . . . [Thirty-five second pause, perhaps the longest ever recorded during one of these sessions.] God bless you. Lee, you are a beautiful soul and you are a *great* soul. Part of you understands this and part of you disbelieves the same. For you have a great fear of responsibility. I speak not of the day-to-day affairs of mankind, but fear of responsibility in applying your own self—intimacy, Lee, between you and the world around you.

You are—as a soul, as a spirit—in frequent discussion with us over here in the past year or so. And in this discussion you have understood greater clarity of anger, anger within your own being directed at your self, feeling and believing that you have wasted so much time, and disbelieving that you can, in the body, truly love your intimacy, creativity, through your own power.

You are then in fear of total application in this present life. Part of you wants to leave and start over again, not as an escape but out of fear that you are repeating old errors and that it would be better to end this present dance with your karma and try again in a different body.

However, your work as a spirit is far from over in this lifetime, my friend. Yes, this particular disease has some hold inside of you. I would suggest that this hold is somewhat firm and that this disease is responding to your own request and requirements, Lee. You will find that the days, the weeks, and months ahead will be the most powerful, meaningful, and beautiful of your entire present lifetime. Reflection, reevaluation, life decisions—your healing in the body with leukemia is related to a series of decisions —decisions of your adamant, firm, unqualified commitment to presence of your own creative soul, the child within.

To love responsibility, thereby the echo—the echo of the world that you fear, and have such frustration of— from your past, Lee—this is your work and this will be your greatest prayer meditation of all, this disease at hand.

This is not a passing condition, Lee. This is deep within you, and it's going to take some great prayer on your part—and you are going to manifest this prayer—for your *plan* is to stay in the body, not to leave the body yet.

However, you will have to work hard and prove to your*self*—not to anyone else—your commitment to absolute presence. So we encourage you to go forward with treatment through traditional medical practices, and as well you seek out a holistic healer who understands energy fields, manipulation, and movement of those electromagnetic fields of your self—such as a very skilled acupuncturist, for example, and acquire treatment there as well.

Then, more important than the first two, you will design on paper—yourself and Carol together, Lee—you will design a schedule of meditation beyond anything you imagined would ever be your desire—meditation that is three times a day, and each meditation is at least twenty minutes—preferably thirty or more—and that you have a separate design for each of the three meditations. You must discover this design—the two of you together—of three meditations, so that the first one of every day is the same, the second one of every day is different from the first, but similar, every day—same with third.

The first is a meditation of awakening to the day—a meditation about presence, determination, application, vulnerability.

The second meditation is the relationship between your body and your spirit, and in that meditation you will work with visualization of your spirit and body becoming one. In that meditation you will make contact with these living forces inside of you called leukemia, and understand that this is part of God's universe, Lee, not a failure of the divine universe.

You will make *friends* with these life forces and talk to them. Be their student and ask them to teach you. As one day follows another, and with discipline you apply yourself in this meditation, Lee, they will reveal to you insights about yourself—how they are cooperating with you, not fighting you—and thereby you will become a team. At that point of insight, discovery, and *movement*—healing, in your soul—they will then be willing to follow new orders—new decisions that you make, Lee.

The third is a meditation of commitment to change, and that as you go into your sleep you are dedicated to understanding the power and the love of change within you. More detail you will bring forward in your own design, reverie, reflection for these three meditations, scheduled each and every day, seven days a week.

You will find that these meditations will go far beyond any experience of this life, Lee—except for your meeting of Carol. This experience of meditation will give you an entirely new excitement about life and your presence therein. So be of good cheer. We will come to you, Lee, and we will begin to give you confirmation that you have sought, because of your application—and through your pain and fear, now, you will apply yourself finally, Lee, as never before.

And we look forward to it. I promise you, the desserts will be beautiful to behold.

Your life is not over, my friend.

You've decided to begin anew. God bless you.

CAROL: *(very softly)* Thanks, Dr. Peebles.

It was something of a bombshell, yes, because we had all grown to love Lee and the sparkle in his eyes as he interacted with Spirit. The next time we saw him, which was several weeks later, he had lost about thirty pounds and was looking a bit hollow-eyed. But he was not bowed—and, in fact, there was an even greater sparkle and an even more lovable Lee Chaifetz at the helm now. He lives. And we have become very close friends with this lovely couple. Here is Lee's update, given to us on February 22, 1989:

When I first heard Dr. Peebles on KFOX radio, I had tuned in during the middle of the program and was unaware of what was actually transpiring; that is, a spirit speaking through a trance-medium. I was immediately struck, however, by his wit and humanity.

The first time I actually got to speak with Dr. Peebles, the rush of energy within me was intense. He instantly began to tell me accurate facts about my life. I listened to his comments and answers to questions on the radio and at personal appearances for over a year and was impressed by his consistent insight. Then one day I found myself in the emergency room of a local hospital diagnosed as having leukemia.

At the age of thirty-eight, this news seemed premature. Strangely enough, I had lived with a woman several years earlier who had contracted a completely different type of cancer and had passed away within three months of her diagnosis. I was at the hospital or at home with her each day and became well acquainted with the shortcomings of medical technology in the treatment of such diseases.

As I lay in the hospital, I felt confused but still curious about what Dr. Peebles could tell me about my situation. By coincidence, he was appearing at the Gathering Place on the first day of my hospital stay. My wife, Carol, went to the meeting that night and questioned him on my behalf, then brought me a cassette tape with his reply.

While the doctors spoke of symptoms and percentages, Dr. Peebles addressed my habits and attitudes. Considering my circumstances, I decided there was no reason why I couldn't incorporate all the advice I was being given, both medical and spiritual. I agreed to my doctor's suggestions for treatment and followed Dr. Peebles suggestions of a schedule of meditations and additional holistic treatment [acupuncture].

Taking the advice of Dr. Peebles and my acupuncturist, I have adjusted my eating habits. I have made some definite changes in my style of communicating with others. I have given up much of my anger and fear, and can feel the world moving toward me more than ever before.

As of this writing, seven months after my diagnosis, my

doctor informs me that my blood profile is completely normal, and if I were not to tell a physician examining me about my condition and treatment, he would be hard pressed to diagnose my illness correctly.

Because of the success of my own physical health, I have much gratitude and no doubts about the insights I have gained through this contact with Spirit, and if my faith in our eternal nature had not been renewed by contact with Dr. Peebles, I wonder where I might be right now.

We think it worthy to note that Dr. Peebles advised Lee to seek all possible medical help for his condition, not to rely entirely on a spiritual healing—and we have heard him repeatedly remind others that every manner of healing is a movement of love, as much from God and the spirit as that which we tend to narrowly categorize as spiritual healing.

Not everyone, of course, brings such grim problems to the attention of Dr. Peebles. Never mind, no problem is too small to engage the interest of Spirit—for he tells us over and over again that we are here for growth and that every problem, large or small, is no more and no less than a "delightful opportunity for growth."

Arnette Cookerly can tell you a thing or two about that. Petite, dark-haired, vivacious—Arnette is in management with one of the large Los Angeles advertising agencies, a single mother of two grown daughters and a career woman who feared that her career was going nowhere when she first encountered our good doctor on the radio one day in the spring of 1987. She was successful in finding an open line at the radio station, and this is what transpired:

DR. PEEBLES: Hi, Arnette, God bless your soul.

ARNETTE: God bless you, Dr. Peebles. Recently I'm getting very clear on the fact that I feel I don't belong in the job that I have now and I've been asking to be guided to the work where I will best be able to serve. But I wonder if there is something I should be doing now or looking into now.

DR. PEEBLES: Yes, first we acknowledge you and God acknowledges you, everyone acknowledges you and your desire to serve because we have heard your prayers for not months but for years and it's now important to change your affirmation to how can you best serve self. So you say to yourself, begin today, "How can I serve me? Thank you very much, God. How can I learn to serve me, as well as to serve life—together, hand in hand with each other?"

And only then will you begin to have your clarity. Now, do you feel free to offer the proper name or the formal name of your place of employment?

ARNETTE: I don't feel free, but I can tell you it's in the advertising industry.

DR. PEEBLES: All right, well . . . all right. It's better, all right—when possible, we like to have the proper name. That helps us be more specific for you. Just a moment here. Hmm. Well, this might come as a shock to you, but actually that general field is a field of your talent and of your soul. You are a communicator extraordinaire. You are extremely inventive. You are able to take and see great and unusual alternatives to any traditional problem. You are an inventor. You come forward with unusual points of view. Your challenge is in the process of communication— emotions—where you aren't feeling validated. You aren't feeling acknowledged. You aren't feeling that you get the credit that you deserve. You are tired of politics and collective communications. Well, actually those are the very areas you are here to work on, my dear. So in this case, it is our opinion that it is not to leave a career or even necessarily a job, but to change your perception and change your response. You will have the confidence and the acknowledgment that you want only by putting your hands on your hips and standing with feet apart and saying, "Hi! Here I am, and we're going to work together and these are my ideas and they are correct. I do want to learn from you, but these ideas are worthy of your attention." And, you know, long term you are an independent person. Do you understand?

ARNETTE: Pretty much, I understand. As far as my career, my career is in the business end of that field. Maybe I should be doing something more creative?

DR. PEEBLES: Just a moment here . . . well, the business end is extremely creative. Business more than any other field is localized on communications. Let's see here . . . well, without question your spirits are saying that it's not a time for dramatic change in your outer world. It's in the inner world. So what could you do to dramatically change how you communicate with people?—with people at work. Does anything come to mind for you?

ARNETTE: Yes, maybe I can speak up and be more of myself.

DR. PEEBLES: Exactly. Stand tall, put your hands on your hips, feet apart, and be honest and express yourself with honesty—not what you think is best for everyone, but with honesty. Then you won't need to withdraw from environment. There'd be no reason because you are expressing yourself honestly. You see?

ARNETTE: Yes, I do.

DR. PEEBLES: If you just left this place, you'd re-create the same experience elsewhere, my dear. You really would. So this time—sometimes it's good to change your environment, but not this time—it's to stay present, more than ever, and speak right up and express yourself with great honesty and accept the unknown results as Maxine [a previous caller] was talking about earlier. You understand me?

ARNETTE: Yes, I do.

DR. PEEBLES: Good girl. God bless you.

Arnette comments, nearly two years later: "The next day, *I changed my perception* about my job. Things started to look different to me even before I walked through the door to the building. Immediately, the feeling that I wasn't supposed to be there started to dissolve. I became more enthusiastic and *expressive*. This led to recognition, praise, and joy in my work. Needless to say, I didn't have to work very hard at *changing my response*. I was responding to this change with delight.

"Within eighteen months I had two raises—one quite substantial—mostly because I was being recognized for *expressing my ideas,* which were of great benefit to my company. I was receiving national attention within six months. In addition to all this attention, I was experiencing joy in being of service to my company and that sense of joy is expanding to this day. I feel that I am exactly where I should be, doing what I should be doing. It is satisfying and I am prospering.

"I hope to eventually bring a new way of communicating to an old politically oriented faction of my business—in the area of 'collective communications!'

"I consider this entire process a miracle. Thank you, Dr. Peebles!"

See? Small miracles can be just as dramatic for "growth" as large ones, perhaps more so. Here again we have become good friends with Arnette and have dined together several times. She is delightful, and she is *very expressive*—right, a "communicator extraordinaire."

Another "acquaintance in spirit" who has become a good friend is Summer Michelle Bacon, too modest to characterize herself as a writer (because she has not yet been published) but, as you will see, that could be changing soon. Summer is a shapely slip of a girl who could pass for eighteen if she found a need to, but behind that youthful appearance is a highly educated single mother who is presently working as a director of employee benefits for a local firm, a very talented aspiring writer—and, believe us, a very old soul who is carrying the weight of centuries around inside that lovely head.

With all that—very probably because of all that—Summer has been very troubled for a very long time. She has been a devotee of Dr. Peebles for at least as long as we have, is part of the volunteer staff at the Gathering Place, and is working diligently at getting her inner worlds in order. We asked her to select a particularly meaningful (for her) exchange with Dr. Peebles and to give us her translation of it. She gracefully complied and—give the old soul credit— unhesitatingly "opened her diary" for all of us to read.

SUMMER: Can you say something to me that can make me feel more comfortable with my journey, and to help me with my melancholy?

DR. PEEBLES: Ah, yes. Just a moment here . . . your sense of melancholy is a result of constantly trying to avoid melancholy—of working so hard to avoid what you thought were negative feelings—not just in this life, but in other lifetimes—for you have always concentrated upon the light.

By concentrating upon the light, you did not see the value in the blackness of space. And so the result was, inadvertently, a frequent avoidance of darker colors and of the dark.

That is why in your writing and in your life we ask that you put such great attention upon those lower-frequency colors and the black, for *there* you will find and touch the face of God. You will find that *there* is where fertility begins—where there is space to be filled.

And so you will learn to look at the blackness of yourself, and you do that by choice and as an adventurer. It will no longer be melancholy. Instead, it will be a totally new experience of relationships—to demonstrate their own light as an example.

Right now you feel encumbered. You have felt encumbered for a long time, because of the seeking to know truth and full concepts of truth—which is impossible, for truth is always more than what one can perceive—always.

The universe is in a constant change, and its symbol

is the spiral. So surrender to that journey to your heart instead of resisting it in subtle and beautiful ways. And that is where you will not know melancholy. You will simply know more friends than you've ever had, more lovers than you've ever had, more family than you've ever had—for the life around you, observing you and experiencing your energy, will not feel a requirement to fit in order to play with you.

   Instead, they can be with you and not fit, so to speak. Do you understand me?

SUMMER: Yes *(laughing nervously),* that would be a good lesson for me.

DR. PEEBLES: Yes, well, you'll do it. Understanding heals all things.

Summer's comment:

   So, the object for Summer was to enjoy the winter in her life. Imagine my pain and discomfort at being told that blackness would be where I would "find and touch the face of God!" Imagine my sense of *melancholy* at the possibility of this!

   After all, I had sought the wisdom of Dr. Peebles in order to ease the pain in my life. I had so expected to hear something "New Age" like "surround yourself in white light, Summer," not "look at the blackness." Instead of handing me a prescription to numb the pain, Dr. Peebles was lancing my already deep and festering wounds. His words seemed at first to be like a piece to a puzzle that didn't belong; no matter how I tried to make it fit, somehow it seemed so wrong.

   But something else was happening with me also. Dr. Peebles was doing much more than spewing philosophy; he spoke not to my ears or my mind, but had touched that private place within me, that place that I felt no one really understood.

   It was a bit disconcerting at first, as if someone had read my diary. Yet, with time and understanding there came such a sense of peace inside. It simply felt so good to feel understood from the inside out for once.

   I began to feel greatly relieved because Dr. Peebles had given me the permission I needed to no longer avoid my own melancholy, and I began to fall in love with what I had long considered to be one of my greatest faults. In fact, I realized that I rather enjoyed sitting by a fireplace alone on a rainy night, for instance, with an old bluesy album on the record player, drinking a splash of red wine and reflecting on the darker moments of my life—feeling a bit neglected and lonely, yet somehow deliciously comforted by my melancholy.

I began to see how that same sadness had actually been a wonderful tool in my life—for in reflecting on the often harsh and bitter reality of the life that I had created for myself, I would find some great new insight, some soul-satisfying revelation that would keep me inspired for weeks or months after.

In fact, it breathed life into my creative works. Now, when I feel a surge of sadness erupting from within, I feel confident that it is not the signal that something is wrong with me—as I had previously perceived—but that, to the contrary, it signals that something is about to be very right with me. It is that moment of truth when I allow myself to become vulnerable, where real inner contact is made; the love in my life is magnified and my fear dissipates, and the blackness of my melancholy becomes a warm blanket of hope to be filled with the light of understanding, rather than a black hole where I will be mashed and lose my identity.

Beautiful stuff, Summer. Remember us to your muses, and don't make us wait too long for that splash of Summer in the wintertime.

On such a note we come to Athena Demetrios—and we cannot think of Athena without whispering the prayer, "God bless the child."

Here is her story, exactly as she courageously gave it to us for publication here.

I am the middle child, one of seven children born into a dysfunctional, alcoholic environment. Poverty was a way of life, and I do believe we all lived in a state of mild unspoken panic. When I was six, I was raped, strangled, bound, and threatened into silence by a butcher knife held against my throat by my mother's alcoholic boyfriend, who lived in the root cellar of our basement. I experienced this over a dozen times, and suffered total memory loss, with the exception of one singular incident which I thought was a simple case of molestation, although I couldn't remember anything past a certain point. The memory of it was like watching a television program turn to snow.

As a child I felt a thousand years old, trapped in a little kid's body, and I knew that life was serious business. If I could have spit in the face of God, I would have. I don't know how I knew He even existed, I just knew He did and I hated Him. I was born a soul searcher. Trying to understand why, and who I am, is just part of my nature.

I carried into adulthood deep feelings of despair, anxiety, and depression. I felt powerless, hopeless, extremely separated from life, and suicidal, and I didn't even know why I felt like this. I couldn't feel from my waist down. I couldn't sleep on my back because I felt like I could be stabbed if I did. I didn't know how to have fun, and I didn't know why memories of childhood affected me like being caught in a fog.

A dream of me going down some stairs trying to rescue a little girl out of a basement inspired the following questions to Dr. Peebles.

I asked him, "When I was young and molested . . . did that only happen once?"

Dr. Peebles replied: "No."

"You mean it happened more than once?"

"Yes. And I don't mean less than a dozen times."

"You mean more than a dozen?"

"Yes."

"With the same man?"

"Yes. I can tell you for sure, the same man was more than a dozen times."

"Good Lord! Was I . . . was I under six, can you tell me that?"

"Have you explored this in regression?"

"No . . . no I haven't."

"You need to explore this, with any source that you wish."

"Did he . . . did he physically enter me?"

"Yes, he did."

"God! . . . Was I under six?"

"No . . . no . . . no! That's all we are going to tell you. You see, what will happen, Athena, if we tell you everything and then you go through a regression, you will feel like you are just making it up because Dr. Peebles told you so, but if we tell you just a little and you go through it yourself . . . you won't be able to say that. Will you consider it?"

"Yes . . . I guess so. I want to get this thing resolved once and for all."

"Your teachers here and myself strongly recommend it . . . and it will be wonderful! Wonderful! It will help you understand the healer that you are in this life."

"Was this a blocking?"

"Yes. Definitely. You will experience how and why . . . how and why you created that and the techniques you used to do it. You'll experience them again as well as decisions you made as a child that have had a great impact on your entire life. You'll experience them again, and it will be wonderful! Will you consider it? We believe that you're strong enough and it's timely."

"Well, if I have to then I have to."

"I believe it is even that strong that you have to."

"Yeah, so do I."

I chose hypnotherapy as my tool for exploration and healing. I've learned to walk through fire, so to speak. I've tapped into depths of rage and anger I never knew existed inside of me. I've grieved and cried more than I ever have in my life. I've accepted the loss of what I never had as a child, and I've learned to honor the process of pain and the steps involved in healing.

Prompted by a dream, I returned to the house in Oregon where the rapes took place. I physically went back into the root cellar, and there within the blackness I forgave him and rescued the lost child who had been trapped in that basement for thirty-three years. I took back my power and became my own parent. I love that little girl and she is inside of me now . . . alive, and she was worth all the pain and agony, every bit of it.

Releasing myself from victimhood was not easy. It was hardest to forgive my mother. She died this year and I didn't feel a thing. Not because I've turned off, but because I had already grieved so deeply for what I never had. At her memorial I read, "Mother, I no longer hold you responsible for my experience of sexual abuse. I chose this experience as a soul to grow from. I am not a victim."

The impact of this healing has been dramatic. I can feel from my waist down now. I can sleep on my back. I respect and love my strength and courage. It's good to be alive and to know what self-love is. The deep depression is gone and I know that I am a powerful creator. I'll forever be grateful to Dr. Peebles, Thomas Jacobson, and Dr. Daniel Slavin.

And we are grateful to you, Athena. At the risk of sounding callous to your suffering, which certainly we are not, we would like to suggest that the path of one's life often moves along the most perilous route in order to arrive at the most precious goal. You've arrived, you're there, in everything that we have seen of you, so it would appear to us that the goal has fully justified the journey. Thank you for giving us you.

Of course the journey for each of us is never-ending. We have eternity to look forward to, thus an infinity of goals to be achieved, an eternity of travels along the spiral staircase of being. Sometimes we get confused and lose the way for a moment. But that doesn't change anything. Eternity still beckons us. The path is ever spread before us. Those who seek death as an end to the journey will only awaken to new life and renewed opportunities for growth, a new light upon the pathway.

Which thought brings us to Collin Johnson.

One never quite knows what to expect with Dr. Peebles in public session. The questions from the floor are usually pretty evenly divided between those of a general, philosophical nature and those involving some personal concern. The latter usually have to do with careers and relationships, but often they are intensely personal, quite dramatic, and strongly moving. And these are the moments with our Grand Spirit at his loving and compassionate best, a time when his words and manner become incredibly gentle and soothing. There is a marked change, too, in the general ambience of that room; the atmosphere of love is palpable; one feels it as a living presence.

One such incident occurred at the Gathering Place on the evening of February 25, 1988, when a young woman who identified herself as "Victoria" took the floor microphone and stated to Dr. Peebles: "I have a friend named Collin Johnson who took his life out of this world on February 11, 1988, and I'd like to understand why."

We had never before seen Victoria, nor had we seen the interesting-looking man who sat beside her, but we knew that something special was about to come forward in that room even before Dr. Peebles began to speak. We could feel it coming up; the ambience of the room altered, became downright electrical. Keep in mind here that this interaction occurred two short weeks after Collin's death by his own hand.

Dr. Peebles responded: "Just a moment . . . I can understand why you're confused, for Collin was and is very charismatic . . . much personality and ambition as well, and so how could he possibly want to leave all of a sudden? It doesn't make any sense. Well, you see, all of that was a cover, a camouflage for the confusion inside him that he wouldn't dare to admit to anyone because he wanted to present total togetherness and strength to the world around him, for reasons we won't deal with now. Finally he decided he's not being honest with himself and the world around him, and he wouldn't forgive himself. Period. He just wouldn't forgive himself. And he didn't want to see himself. So, he took himself out of the body instantly and quickly. I might add, with little forethought. He came over here and found that it [leaving the body] didn't work. Here, he is with himself again and still not forgiving himself, and so we've been working with him. He is over here now. He's very active. He's once again becoming the beautiful and very energetic active soul that you knew him as. He is very loved over here. He's surrounded by friends and family. You can be happy for him. It's a different concept of time over here, so there's really no sense of waste. It's just growth, that's all. And he's going to come back into the body and try it again. We're trying to persuade him to come forward as a female, but he's resisting greatly. So . . . yeah—you understand me?"

"Yes. Thank you."

It had already become obvious through her nonverbal responses that Victoria "understood" what Spirit had been telling her about Collin. She seemed a bit overwhelmed and unsure as to how to proceed. Her companion—whom we later learned was Bob Johnson—took the microphone for the follow-up.

"I'm Collin's father. I'd like to know, since Victoria just asked the question that I was going to ask . . . how have we been connected in the past, Collin and I?"

Allow us to interject here some information that we did not have at the time. Collin was twenty-three when he died. Bob does not look old enough to have a son of that age. He is impressively good-looking, tall and lean, very youthful in appearance.

Dr. Peebles immediately replied. "You were brothers. I believe you've dreamed of this, as well—uh, brothers in the distant past and you delighted in going through thick and thin together. You saved each other's lives I don't know how many times!—ah, through thick and thin."

There then followed a large outline of their past lives together as Dr. Peebles elaborated many life cycles in which they began to draw apart and lose this very close friendship—a movement totally related to power issues—"who's in control?" Then both began a cycle of loneliness, seeing others and avoiding them as mere performers in an act rather than as family members—then blaming others for the sense of loneliness—with much anger and frustration. In one interesting series, Collin became Bob's father in the earthly environment and then his son, for a "balancing of the scales," and this brings us into current time.

Dr. Peebles continued: "There was a bit of conflict in this [present] life, but especially you are comrades of the deepest nature as souls who really just want to be strong and provide for the other and prove your love. Do you understand?"

Bob replied, "I do. Thank you. Can I ask you one other question? In some other incarnation, did I take my life?"

Dr. Peebles said, "Well, you probably did if you think you did. Just a moment here. [Pause.] Let me count the ways . . . just a moment here . . . goodness! You drank poison, you slit your wrists—and you did it correctly, there's lots of blood everywhere . . . tried to kill yourself through sex, once . . . that didn't work —you're still trying to, sometimes, and there's a certain someone who wishes you'd stop—no, I tease . . . indirectly, through alcoholism, in another lifetime . . . ah, yes, you have. The answer is yes and you did so with ceremony and ritual. But I would also suggest to all of you, you know, in the long term you always kill yourselves. You bring yourselves over here. Do you understand me?"

Bob quietly replied, "Yes, thank you, and God bless you."

The man was obviously moved by the experience. We had wanted to go over and say something to him when the session ended, but he and Victoria departed before we could get to them.

We saw him again two months later, on April 28, at the Gathering Place, and again he addressed Spirit from the floor: "I was here several weeks ago and I told you that I have a son who took himself from this life. You were very helpful to me in responding to the questions that I had about that. There is still some stuff going on that I'd like you to talk about if you can. Part of it has to do with the fact that even though I know he's fine and doing well on your side, he expressed qualities in this life to me, and to other people who love him, that we miss. Is there any profit in trying to have some contact with him? And, is there a way to do that?"

DR. PEEBLES: His name again?

BOB: Collin.

DR. PEEBLES: Collin? Just a moment here . . .

There is great profit in contact with those who have passed over, relative to the environment in which you in the physical world live your lives. In this case, it is of exceptional merit to reach out to those who have passed on. It is not unusual for spirits to arrive over here who feel some mild confusion as to their ability to communicate with you [back on Earth]. It is not unusual for them to feel confused as to whether the human being—the physical human being—desires contact, for so often that same contact is feared or it is judged, condemned, as not appropriate. So for you to utter that you desire contact is a statement of love, of desire. In this specific case, we encourage you in the strongest terms to reach out for what is already there: Collin. He is a beautiful spirit of great love, wonderful wistful humor, gentle as the wind in the sky, graceful as the dancer of the ballet platform. And he wishes to share with you [the knowledge] that all is well [with him]. He has no confusion. He has no fear. He wants so much to see and experience that you and yours have received his love, his reality. We suggest the following: that you find yourself a seven-day candle, a candle that will burn for twenty-four hours a day for seven days. You choose a place in your home familiar to your child and this is where you will have a ritual. You stand with loved ones and you speak out loud to Collin and you state your desire to have contact and to receive his love. And it is of relevance that all do this with no fear but with excitement in your voices, sincerity in your eyes and hearts. You then light the candle with each and every person gathered holding, touching, this candle as it is lit and put on an altar. This particular place in the room or in the home is left alone throughout the week but twice a day, once in the morning, once in the evening, any of you individually or all of you together gather for at least ten minutes and you speak out and you ask for contact—communication. Each of you have a pad and a pencil or such things in your lap, and you write down your feelings. We would encourage that you consider using a quill with natural fiber paper and natural ink. And, rather than seeking grandiose statements, you seek to capture the wistful nature of one of his beautiful statements. For he was and is able to say so much with a gesture, a movement, a glance as well as a word or two. Although certainly he is quite articulate. So, it is that graceful movement that you will seek to capture through the quill, the paper, and record it as a word or a sentence, a symbol, that is symbolic. And each of you does this individually, then you compare notes afterward. Do this twice a day for seven days. I believe that you will have contact. I would suggest that you personally take a glass of water to the ceremony, clean drinking water, full, and having completed your ceremony you bring that glass of water from the ceremony to your bedside and you ask that this water be touched by Spirit and by your son. You drink it every morning when you awaken. And, as you approach the seventh day, you will have contact through your writing and perhaps in other ways as well. Your son is very talented. I believe he will be able to bridge worlds with you. Please be assured you are not binding him, you are not slowing him down. Quite the contrary! Over here, you know, the spirit comes to us and says, "All right, Collin, time to do a little study!" he says, "I don't want to! I want to talk to my family!" And so it will be a relief for some of us to get this over with. So we encourage you full speed ahead. Do you understand?

Bob softly replied, "I do. Thank you."

But Dr. Peebles was not finished. "Are you aware, Bob, of the beautiful and wistful gestures he's able to communicate so nicely? Extraordinary talent to us over here!"

"Yah, he's recognized even over here for it. God bless you," said Dr. Peebles.

Bob said, "God bless you, and thank you."

Again, we did not find the opportunity to speak to Bob Johnson about the matter, and although we have seen him from time to time since then, the moment had passed and it just did not seem appropriate to approach him on such a sensitive matter. The months slipped by and of course there were never enough hours in any day; we were very busy.

Meanwhile Bob had apparently deepened his involvement with Spirit and had taken classes with Thomas Jacobson. Thomas, of course, is entirely discreet in such matters, never speaking to others about his students, so we did not know of the ongoing work with Bob, and in fact we have not to this day been formally introduced.

When we began working on the final revisions to the manuscript in early 1989, Bob Johnson and his son, Collin, once again occupied our thoughts and we mentioned this to Thomas, who then told us that he could put us in touch, and he did.

It so happened that this came about very near the first anniversary of Collin's death, so again we felt a bit sensitive to Bob's loss and approached him with much circumspection. In a telephone conversation we expressed our feelings that his experience could have considerable meaning for others and told him that we would like to include it in the book.

His response was immediate and warmly cooperative. We wanted some depth of detail, so we arranged it that we would pose four probing questions, in writing, and give him time to thoughtfully develop his response. They were tough questions, and we knew it, in the sense that Bob would be required to reexperience and rehash all the turbulent emotions associated with the untimely passing of his son. But he agreed without equivocation to work on the answers and to give them to us in writing. He did so graciously, with great care and—as you shall see—with great heart.

We have arranged the questions and the responses in interview form, but please understand that this was not a spontaneous exchange and that the answers to the questions posed were arrived at after considerable reflection on Bob's part and with the greatest care to reply fully, as best he could. We are fortunate in having so articulate a correspondent. Here is that "interview:"

Q: Did you "recognize" Collin, or feel that Dr. Peebles actually knew something about him, from the way he was described by Dr. Peebles?

A: Dr. Peebles's first description of Collin in response to Victoria's question was "he is very charismatic with much personality and ambition as well." Yes, Collin was charismatic and his personality was large and friendly. He had a smile a mile wide and twinkling eyes to match. His sense of humor and ability to laugh were irresistible, and they drew people to him like strong magnets. He wasn't always like that—but something in him changed during the last three or four years of his life. Something very good happened to him on the inside. When he walked into a room he lit it up.

The question of his ambition is trickier. He was gifted with considerable intelligence and many talents as well as good looks. Everyone, including himself, knew that he possessed the wherewithal to accomplish whatever he set out to do in life. And when he applied himself, sometimes even halfheartedly, he produced good results and most often excelled. The problem was that despite his accomplishment in any given endeavor, he would stop himself short and suffer the consequence of one incompletion after another. For this he suffered great pain. He knew of his potential—he could feel it on the inside—but he was unable for any length of time to realize it in the outside world. I know that he felt, therefore, that he was a failure.

Dr. Peebles described Collin to me as my brother "in the distant past" and I have a strong sense that this is so. There has always been deep feeling between us, a love as well as a connection that is powerful and lasting. This is so despite the many trials and separations that we experienced as father and son. Looking back to when he was a boy, I remember him fiercely resisting parental authority and trying in any way that he could to be my equal. And it always felt to me that somehow he was. Strangely, it was hard to think of Collin as *just* my son. There was something more to him that I couldn't understand, perhaps it was the unconscious memory of us as brothers in that distant past.

Dr. Peebles's more poetic description of Collin as "a beautiful spirit of great love, wonderful wistful humor, gentle as the wind in the sky, graceful as the dancer on the ballet platform," which he gave on a subsequent evening, is to me a perfect description of Collin's true spiritual nature. I will always treasure these words by Dr. Peebles because they so beautifully reflect who Collin is to me.

Q: Without going into intimately revealing details—in the response to Victoria's question, did you find some resonance (or clue to the death event) in the statement: ". . . Because he wanted to present total togetherness and strength to the world around him, for reasons we won't deal with now."

A: Dr. Peebles's response to Victoria's question confirmed much of what I already knew in my heart to be so. Despite the many encounters that Collin had with various forms of therapy and educational seminars, etcetera, he never admitted to having serious problems with his life. He hated the idea that he was somehow different from everyone else, yet he knew that his life was out of balance and not what he wanted it to be. Still, he resisted strongly the idea of looking *within* in any formal way with professional people who could help him with his life.

As I stated earlier, something changed pretty dramatically during the last three or four years of Collin's life. What I saw was that he stopped "using" people, the way someone might use a drug, and started loving them instead. Whereas before, he would only "take" from people, now he was giving back and it was wonderful to see and experience. Often I would think, "He's turned one corner, he's going to make it. Now all he has to do is reach out for help and everything will be okay."

Q: Did you carry out the "formula" suggested by Dr. Peebles for contact with Collin? Do you feel that it was successful? What was actually experienced?

A: Yes, I did exactly what Dr. Peebles suggested and experienced contact with Collin as a result of this "experiment," as well as in one other way.

The first happened after performing the ritual with the seven-day candle. I created a small shrine that included several pictures of Collin, a couple of personal articles of his, as well as the candle and writing materials that Dr. Peebles indicated. I asked my other son, Aaron, if he would like to join me in the ritual, but he declined, which was okay with me.

After calling upon the "Spirit of Light and Love" to bless the shrine and assist me in making contact with Collin, I lit the candle and followed the procedure outlined by Dr. Peebles. Each morning and evening I would sit with paper and pen in hand and meditate upon my desire to make contact with Collin and I would also speak aloud to him.

The first thing to come through was a strong feeling of warmth and happiness. Without thinking, I drew a picture of the sun. The face on it was bright and open, smiling and happy. I knew at that moment that Collin was fine. It may sound strange, but it was a "knowing" that came from my heart, not my head.

Several other contacts occurred during the ritual. The most direct and positive contact for me was a simple "have fun" that I knew without doubt had come from Collin to me. It wasn't as though I heard his voice or even that I felt his presence, but it was Collin talking to me somehow. He was telling me to have fun, and he was doing so with a smile. His statement came through "loud and clear," and so did his smile.

The only other significant communication that I experienced as a result of this ritual was a powerful feeling that I expressed in the following words: "There is great closeness between us and it will always be there." This came from Collin.

During a course called "Journey to the Heart" conducted by Thomas Jacobson, I felt Collin's presence in the classroom. Thomas had asked me to take paper and pen and write whatever came to me. It was an extremely emotional and powerful experience for me, and I'll never forget it. Writing quickly and without thinking, I put the following on paper: "I'm right here, sort of floating off to your left by the window above Athena. But just because I'm by the light, don't think that I don't also go to dark corners. Go to the dark corners. You can do it, Papa. I'll always be with you. You're doing fine. Now you've got to *fight*. I love you. I'm here. No good-byes."

Q: How has the Dr. Peebles experience helped you to "handle" the death of your son?—and how, do you feel, may it influence your future?

A: My experience with Dr. Peebles, as well as study in other metaphysical areas, has helped me to know that death is a beginning, not an end. Or perhaps a better way to say it is that there really is no "beginning" or "end" but rather an unending spiritual journey expressed through our indestructible soul nature.

Physical life had me hypnotized into thinking that *it* was the only reality. I know now that my greater self could never be expressed by this limited physical picture. Dr. Peebles has patiently and lovingly helped to awaken me to the greater possibilities in life. No longer am I willing to define my life by what I can see, taste, touch, smell, or hear. Given the state of our planet Earth, I feel strongly that each of us must reach out to people and also reach within for guidance from what I will simply call a higher power.

Dr. Peebles is for me one avenue to that power.

To Bob Johnson and to all the others who stood "naked to the world" with such courage and clarity, Linda and I can only say that we love your dance, we love your song, and we love what you represent to the world. God keep. And that goes to Collin too.

13

State of

the Planet

> "Celebrate, celebrate—for you are eternal.
> You cannot fail, and all of the challenges
> of Earth are nothing but schoolbooks in a
> big school called Planet Earth, where you
> are guaranteed graduation . . .
> eventually."
>
> —Dr. Peebles

Whatever, whoever, and wherever Dr. Peebles may be—whether or not *any* human being *could* speak as he speaks—the fact remains that he *does* speak as no other person does in our experience. He delivered a "State of Earth" address at a public gathering in Los Angeles on the evening of June 24, 1986. We present here a transcript of that address and commend it to your close attention, for it speaks to the most basic fears of our planet in this day and time.

Here is our Grand Spirit at his best:

God bless you; Dr. Peebles here. It is a joy and blessing when man and spirit join together in search of the greater truths and awareness. Might I offer encouragement, my dear friends, as you strive to understand the state of Earth. For the state of Earth is one of conflict, it is one of struggle, it is one of confusion; it is, to many points of view, one of isolation and cold.

You are here, my friends, as individual souls—here as students, each and every one—striving to understand the nature of love, the nature of your own divine self, through a study of relationships, yourself and life everywhere—life everywhere students as well, each and every one.

You are here to identify what are temporary illusions of separation—illusions of separation shared by all humanity and by some other life forms as well. To identify these is high fulfillment, and yet not complete; for, as well, you must diminish and dissolve these very same illusions of separation. This *is* your labor of love. It *is* a journey to the heart that will set you free.

The state of Earth is a magnification of each individual. The state of Earth is an amplification of your own self. The state of Earth, this day, focuses on the fear and the threat of total destruction and annihilation of all life through nuclear warfare and the helplessness that is suggested by terrorism.

As you view the news and you listen to the commentaries of your political systems and your communication networks, you are faced with a new scenario each and every day. Your own personal challenge is to find resolution, to understand; for as you view and as you listen to scenarios of the entire planet, it is the same as if it were within your own home.

And so there are those who refuse to listen to the news— it is too threatening and fearful. There are those who seek to understand the news, for there is a challenge to grow and to expand. The state of Earth is now focusing on the threat of nuclear warfare, the threat of terrorism. What is the nature of these two events?

Well, the threat of total annihilation first must be understood as an energy that has been around the planet Earth through all history. It is not a new energy. It is not a new threat. It is not worse now than ever before. Through all history, written and otherwise, there has been a constant threat of annihilation of the local village, of the local state; a total annihilation of family and all loved ones has been a constant threat through all decades of history and all environments.

Even when there were many years of peace and prosperity in some ancient cultures, there still was the talk, there still was the fear, there still was the promulgation of models of defense, so as to maintain that safety. Well, the very creative suggestion of defense thereby invites the experience in your heart of fear, of destruction.

As you live each and every day, then—as in each and

every era of mankind—there is the threat of being overcome, the threat of total oblivion, the threat of annihilation, the threat of helplessness; of not being able to control your own destiny. To understand, then, the global conflicts it is most important that you personalize your perception—that you become intimate with the experience—and you then strive to understand the global conflicts through personal application in your day-to-day life.

As you try to understand the impact, the potential, of nuclear warfare and the threat of retaliation, think of your own life: Is it not true that you have sought to retaliate to people individually? Is it not true that in your life you have sought weapons?—you have sought means through your own psychology, your own mentality, your own systems of communication, to wreak revenge?—more often than not fantasizing that joy that you had in your heart for a moment when you would exact complete revenge on those who have wronged you? And when you wanted that revenge, did you not want complete victory? Did you not want to totally annihilate the point of view of another? Did you not want to have total safety and protection of yourself?

Well, your governments—your governments that represent you nationally—are a reflection of what all of you have asked for and sought. That is a desire for safety. This is shared by all humanity, regardless of nationality, because all human beings have, remember, temporary illusions of separation.

What does that *mean,* temporary illusions of separation? What is the impact of that reality? Well, with separation there is a fear—there is an automatic belief that there are those things that are different from you—otherwise you wouldn't be separate from them, would you?

And if they are different from you, are they compatible? —must you not think about them?—must you not ponder them before you can be intimate?—and in the meantime, until you make that decision to be intimate, must you not protect yourself from possible threat in case they are not comfortable to your energy?

Well, that starts with the illusions of separation, which *is* an illusion, but it is a *lived* reality. It is carried out as a reality in each and every day, and I don't mean Chinese on the other side of the world, I mean you: listening to these words.

The illusions of separation, then, is a personal experience —whether it be in Iran, Russia, Washington, D.C. and the White House, or in the country land of Minnesota. It is a shared phenomenon upon which all governments are built. All governments are built upon religion. All religions are built upon not only the hopes but especially the fears of mankind; which predominantly there is that of survival: to survive, to continue.

This is a natural phenomenon for planet Earth, but it is not a natural phenomenon for the universe, for there is a state of consciousness that goes beyond the instinct for survival. And that greater drive is for intimacy, is for love, is for union. But, you see, the paradox is that when you have union, have you not brought yourself to a threshold where you might lose control for a moment?—for then you must be in union with another point of view and another being who could for a moment dominate you.

So around and around the circle goes, the merry-go-round of growth. It is a magnification of your own personal fears. Nuclear warfare, simply put, is a threat of total destruction—not only to you, but to family and to that consciousness that you love in all life. That has always been present in history. And your feeling of helplessness is equal only to your fear of increased communication.

As you seek to understand what to do regarding nuclear warfare, study yourself this week and in the months to come. Watch how it is that in the most subtle of ways, at times, you will seek revenge—you will seek to have weaponry within yourself, to respond readily so that the other party cannot respond in ways that are not comfortable to you.

This is what your government represents for you, and other governments as well. And so you see the decisions of your governments of late and of the past have been proper, for they have done those things they have been elected for. The bombing of [Libya], for example, by Mr. Reagan, was to an extent a right action, for it is what the people elected him for: protection; indeed, retribution to wrongdoing around the world. And so it was, within that state of time and space, a proper action.

Within your own individual consciousness, what are your alternatives when you are threatened? What are your alternatives when others want you to be helpless and in their power?

How have you communicated in the past? Has it been withdrawn, and when? When have you withdrawn? When have you reacted with great diligence to overcome another point of view?

As you further understand the nature of terrorism, it is

obviously distinct from nuclear warfare. Nuclear warfare is obvious. It is or it isn't. Terrorism seeks to be subtle, seeks to be suggestive. Terrorism seeks to extend fear far beyond the event. Terrorism seeks to own the minds and the psychology. Terrorism seeks to manipulate and control, through fear more so than the actual event.

Terrorism is around you all the time. Each of you in this room in your own way is a terrorist as well as a lover of God. For there is within you illusions of separation. Within all humanity, no matter how great the love in your heart, no matter how sincere your desires, there are moments of anger, of fury, of rage, of retribution, fear of being overcome by others, the desire to protect yourself, to have guns in the house, to eliminate any danger, to teach others lessons.

How often, my friends, have you wanted to teach your friend a lesson—teach another person?—a lover? It's as if the closer you get to each other the more you want to teach each other. How many times have you wanted to teach your mate a lesson?—so they'll *never* do it again.

My friends, that's terrorism, where you did it through threat, implied threat, and direct threat: "You will now do what I say or I'll never talk to you again." That fear and that threat of never being talked to again is equally as violent as a bullet in your head. I say to you it is. For the greater reality of vibration is in your mind—and that does include the physical atmosphere—but as well it includes your mind.

For those beings who are in a silence and dead in their hearts, it's exactly the same as death from the physical body; in fact, it is worse. For when you leave the physical body you are still alive and you can resurrect your emotions. But your emotional death is awesome; your emotional death goes beyond the body.

And so it is that words and wars of words are violent. Now—to be sure, it is a point of debate—to be sure, it is an extraordinary concept. For the blood you can see from the skin; the tears can be hidden in a private room. The pain and the ugliness of life is through the illusions of separation.

How will you then create peace on Earth? It is through peace within yourself. How often have you marched? How often have you written to your senators? How often have you wanted in your mind to increase your communication for greater peace on Earth? How often have you felt indignant at the increased terrorism and the nuclear warfare?

And then someone in ragged clothes the next day walks

by you and asks you for a quarter; and you are offended; and you leave them.

You speak of love by healing the planet Earth; you speak of peace by eliminating weaponry; and then you ignore your brother next door. To understand the nature of terrorism, to understand the nature of nuclear war, do not look to Washington, D.C.; do not look to Moscow; look within your own heart.

Understand *your* weaponry, understand *your* fears, so that you can empathize with Moscow and you can empathize with Washington, D.C., instead of the massive illusions of separation. For only with the empathy can there begin to be union.

But then there's a new problem. How do you define union? Union is *not* collective agreement. Union is allowance —indeed, fascination—with *dis*agreement. Lack of allowance of disagreement, and the force to create agreement, is lack of union.

These are your thoughts to help you create a new day. For you have the right for joy, you have the right for prosperity, you have the right for freedom.

No one denies you freedom ever, no matter what part of the globe you are in, no matter what concentration camp you are in; you deny yourself that freedom only through your fear of increased communication.

And when others radically increase their communications too quickly, it can feel violent. The more you increase yours, the more present you will know the pleasures of Earth.

Earth is not a cold place. It is warm; it does have peace. In fact, heaven *is* on Earth. It is through a major retranslation and reevaluation of the nature of things, beginning with the study of the illusions of separation.

Your political processes are a macrocosm of your own being. Your government is not different from you. Other governments are not different from you. Understand this, then you will be able to make a difference in your life—and yes, in other people's lives.

You *will* be able to make a difference on the planet Earth, for there must be greater love; and there will be—but only through responsibility, a diminishing of the illusions of separation within self. Don't try to do it in others; within self. *There* is the healing.

You can then offer opportunities, communication, ideas, for others to transform their self. But you see it is that rapturous desire by all communities of the Earth to change other communities—always for the higher good, is it not?—that leads to conflict; a lack of allowance for the different points of view.

All of you gathered this day, all of you hearing these words, are spiritual beings who have lived long upon the planet Earth—and, for many of you, beyond the planet Earth. In your own ways of thought, please consider: you often equate peace with low noise levels, but if you would have peace then you must equate peace as a fascination, a curiosity, an excitement, a joy at different points of view, rather than a fear of them.

For all points of view, in a moment, have some truth and are part of God. Anger, fury, and rage are part of God as well. For you cannot be in a rage unless you cared so much about being understood, accepted, and ultimately loved. You could not be in a rage of God unless you cared so much about your point of view.

And so, as you come forward into your day tomorrow, in your country of the United States, your world, look at the news and understand that your interaction with the news is valid and worthy of your attention. What are your solutions?

And when you become confused—which you will—personalize it. Personalize it to your own life, to your next phone call, to your spouse, to your friend, to your enemy, and understand yourself.

Then the words of wisdom will flow through you and—more important—people will want to listen for the first time. For they will feel your intimacy, your responsibility; that you are not above, or below, but instead present as a student.

There will *not* be nuclear destruction of the planet Earth. There *will* be some further nuclear accidents. One of these accidents will be within a military context—not a plant of energy, vibrating energy—but within weaponry, and it will be within this century.

However, it will be anticipated, slightly—and controlled . . . slightly. But you need not fear loss of life, for loss of life cannot be avoided.

Each of you in this room, hear me well, is gonna die; and I promise you it will be one of the most magical moments of your life. For you *will* be alive—to your amazement—you *will* be conscious, and you *will* be victorious.

The goal is not to avoid life, it is to avoid withdrawal; it is to avoid the fear of retribution, the desire to give retribution;

to be present as never before. Life is an opportunity; it is here right now.

Understand how you wish you had a nuclear bomb at times. Understand how you have wanted to terrorize in revenge, so that others would lose authority over you, and you will understand the planet Earth. *All* share the same illusions.

This is not a prophecy of doom; it is a reality of responsibility. The life on Earth has been a challenge all along. The fear of annihilation has always been a fear; and now, are you going to live in that fear of tomorrow?—or will you live in presence today?

Celebrate, celebrate—for you are eternal. You cannot fail, and all the challenges of Earth are nothing but schoolbooks in a big school—a big classroom—called planet Earth, where you are guaranteed graduation, eventually—sometimes rather *slowly* for a few of us—us *elderly* souls of the planet Earth— wise but still reincarnating, aren't we. Yes, uh . . .

God bless you, my friends. Would you have questions or comments?

QUESTION *(from audience)*: Many teachers have said that there is going to be a major shift of the planet, and I wonder when that might be coming—and will it be a physical shift or a spiritual shift?

DR. PEEBLES: Yes, well, those thoughts were predicated, most of them, upon a shift of the axis of the physical planet Earth, which was still a possibility years ago; however, it no longer is . . . a movement of the polar ice caps that in their stupendous weight would create enough imbalance for a change in the rotation of the planet and would shift the poles. However, human science and technology—and the nature of things—will, uh, this will be anticipated and it will be dispelled and dispersed and it will not take place.

On inner levels, however, there is a shift, to be sure, in the consciousness of mankind. The age that you have lived in now for two thousand years has been that of the individual, the age of the Piscean. Now you are entering into the age of the Aquarius.

The age of the Aquarius is the age of the collective. Fundamentally, the shift is from the individual to the collective. You are now on that threshold of change. The old habit for all of you, then, is to want to emphasize individuality, but the new curiosity and mild drives is the collective. However, of course it is a new energy on Earth so there are fears of the collective, of being lost in the ambiguity of it all.

But, you see, as you embrace the collective in your own personal being, you do not lose yourselves, my friends. You gain a larger self. You become larger in your self-image. So the shift is from the individual to the community, to the many rather than to the few. You are then advised to consider projects that involve others, and not just yourself, to consider relationships that lean toward family, rather than isolation, and so forth.

The shift in the heart fundamentally is to be present, now, to be boldly honest and present with the heart, and not just the mind.

This Aquarian Age that is at hand is a time of truth-seeking. So there will still be bias on the Earth, but it will be a new manner of bias. The priorities will become seeking truth. The illusion will be that truth is only in one area, and falsehood lies in another. Ultimately truth is everywhere all the time, as it enlarges its scope and its reality.

So this shift that is taking place is increased communication, because there is an increased attitude of community in the collective. Thereby your media, your communications systems and technology, are participating—of your own creation. There is increased communication internationally, increased community concerns and debates internationally.

This will continue to grow, and as it grows it will also magnify the differences of opinion, won't it? So there will be violence, there will be disagreements. However, these confrontations will serve as lessons. It will not equal massive death upon the planet Earth physically. It will equal episodes that are rather colorful, to say the least.

But they are opportunities for growth. You are to learn from then, not to avoid them, but to be present with your heart, to take life on, hand in hand, as a lover.

Does that help you?

RESPONSE: Yes, thank you. As a second part to that question, will there be tremendous earthquakes and—?

DR. PEEBLES: Yes. In the eyes of history, looking back on the time, it will seem like many took place in a short period. But in the eyes of your day-to-day life—remember, personalize it—there will be lots of gaps. It's not like you're going to wake up every morning with a new earthquake,

you see. You will have time to adjust, to move around
. . . oh, for some people to die in that way, in that manner. Sounds terrible, doesn't it? You're all going to die—
when will you learn that? God bless you, quit trying to
avoid it.

So, you're going to have—the weather patterns are
going to change. Over all the Earth it's going to become
hotter—and I do mean soon, sooner than later. The
weather patterns, winter as well as summer, will become
warmer. In the midst of that process you will also have
extraordinary opposites of what should be at times.
Records will be broken at both ends of the spectrum; it's
already begun, it will continue.

You will find more and more fires, more and more
hot spells, dry spells . . . you'll find volcanoes, earthquakes, rather consistently . . . there'll be a tidal wave
or two thrown in, and a dash of hurricane. It's going to be
wonderful—how boring if you didn't have all that. It's
going to be growth, it's going to be—it's positive, it's a
transformation, a cleansing, not negative. It is transformation. Look within your own heart. Open your own heart.
Create some volcanoes in *you*. If you would allow an
earthquake or two to take place in you, you might enjoy it.
As you open up, and you create a crevice, you create new
space, you see.

Again, personalize it—new weather patterns inside
you. Do you want to keep acting the way you've been
acting? No one in this room does! No one does, or you
wouldn't still be in the body. You'd be dead and enlightened. You understand me. You know, you can avoid an
earthquake and have an auto accident. You can avoid an
auto accident and your own biological stroke will take
place. You're going to leave when you're supposed to
leave. You can bet on it. God bless you.

QUESTION: Are these physical changes you mention a result of
the collective mass consciousness?—forming, and changing all of that?

DR. PEEBLES: The changes, literally speaking, are based on
solar and universal systems of energy and physics. The
free will of the human being is involved to the extent that
you choose to be here now, that you look down and you
say, "Oh, it looks like there's gonna be lots of volcanoes
and earthquakes. I think I'd like to be born *then*, that will
stimulate me and challenge me to reevaluate," you see, to

confront some issues." Now, that is dominant. Secondary to that, yes, the collective communications of humans through history, the diversity, the conflict, the illusions of separation, the desires to change others—without permission and so forth—has created stresses within the vibration of the planet Earth that the planet is incorporating, is channeling.

But that is secondary to the natural motions of the universe. You understand me.

QUESTION: My question is about Jimmy Carter. When he was in office as president, it was my perception that he was ahead of his time, that he was too honest, almost embarrassingly honest to most of us, and that he wished more for a sense of cooperation and sharing in the world. We voted him in and yet we booted him right out again. And I'm wondering what is the significance of that moment in history.

DR. PEEBLES: God bless you. There is great truth in what you say. It's also true that he was a little *behind* the times in some ways. He was ahead of his time in that he did seek increased communication, he did seek to receive other points of view rather than to deny them or control them. He did seek unity.

Now, his moments of confusion at times were that he unconsciously defined union as agreement rather than allowance of disagreement. As well, he had understandable concern about violence. His definition of peace, unconsciously—referencing our earlier statement—leaned toward less noise rather than an amplification or a coloration of new communications.

So on the one hand he was seeking increased communication, and yet on the other there was a certain avoidance of conflict that was justified as a desire for peace. Very understandable. But yet it's not complete. Not just Jimmy Carter, but the nation of people. It is a collective view regarding peace that we speak of. And he did incorporate that.

Yes, overall I would say he was more *ahead* of his time than *of* his time or behind. He had his own lessons, but he was a vision of the future in many ways. I agree. The lesson of history, at that time, was to reevaluate the nature of peace. He stimulated people through suggestion, indirectly, to continue thinking about what does peace mean—what do we really want?—what is our true motivation? For his ongoing rhetoric and honesty was to have peace—but what does that mean, for goodness gracious sake? There's only five letters in the word—what does it *mean?*

And so the lesson of history will look back and see that here was a peacemaker who inadvertently was inspiring people to reevaluate the *nature* of peace, and how that quantifies with increased and decreased communication, honesty and dishonesty. Yes, he was a leader. As history looks back, it will see this gentleman as someone who was underestimated. You understand me.

RESPONSE: Yes, I do. But how was his being elected a reflection of our collective consciousness? We elected him and then voted him out again.

DR. PEEBLES: Yes, all right . . . the collective consciousness of that time in the late sixties and into the seventies was priority of seeking peace—remember? Peace, peace, peace. No matter what the cost, almost . . . peace. If you think about it, it was a rather amazing assumption, collectively, of what peace means. Do you remember very many debates about what peace means? In the media?—or on talk shows or in the political systems, or at parties you attended? There was some, but few.

Instead, everyone seemed to believe that what others thought was peace was what *they* thought was peace. Which equaled—and I am exaggerating slightly, by intent —tended to equal lack of noise, lower volume of noise. You know: keep the volume down so I can have some peace around here. That's what peace meant. Turn the volume down on the planet Earth. So—now, again, this is semiconsciously, inadvertently—so this energy is what brought this gentleman into office. He reflected that same study. More peace, but yet a certain abstinence from— now, that's a qualified abstinence—from depth perception, depth definition of the nature of peace.

To be sure, in Mr. Carter's private moments in office, he was thinking about it all the time. It was a shocking reevaluation that gave him great pain, but he was in the midst of study rather than answers, and he was not prepared to bring that painful study of new concepts of peace to a public view. It was too threatening to those who supported him, and he felt that he had obligations to them.

He left office as humans imagined and visualized greater peace in their lives and they began to feel a little bored. They wanted some increased communication, some increased interaction and presence, some increased clarity. So this is one of the lessons throughout history. It's the seeking of peace and then just when people get it, what do they do? They say, "I've changed my mind, I think that's not as much fun as I thought! I want something else! How about a little disagreement?" And then the other person disagrees in a way different from how you wanted them to. And you are furious.

So then you have to create borderlines or annihilate the other person before they drive you crazy. That's been going on throughout history, over and over. See it as a personal experience and you will see the lessons of history.

So, in your pursuing this thought, as you think of Mr. Carter, think of yourself. Imagine yourself in office at that time, and your vibration, and you will understand.

QUESTION: I want to know why so many wars throughout the history of the world have been fought in the name of religion, which has as its base the teachings of love—

DR. PEEBLES: It bothers me too! When you know the answer, let me know. I would love to hear it.

QUESTION: . . . I don't understand how that happens.

DR. PEEBLES: Well, if you would indulge a slight redundancy on my part here, I would say it is because first and foremost—please listen with all your hearts and souls and minds—and you can disagree later, but listen fully now . . . *All* humans—that includes Jesus when he was on the planet, and others . . . *all* humans, for the moment of living, have lesser or greater illusions of separation. Even when they are lesser, they are illusions of separation. For a moment. That is what the school of Earth is all about.

Now . . . with the illusion—let's pretend that your own illusion of separation grows in this room right now, my dear—all of you. Imagine that you feel not an illusion but the reality, that you are separate from some others in this room. Take a look around you. It should be very easy for you to pretend that because you do feel that way, by the way, and you feel a little more separate from some other people.

Well, try to feel those people sitting behind you and next to you, that you don't know very well and you think you might not want to know, and feel that feeling of separation that they are not really the same as you, not the same vibration. Well, how are you going to protect your-self when they want to come talk to you?

Here he comes! And you know you don't want him to talk to you! What you gonna do?—I think I'll have some coffee over here on the other side of the room! And you try to avoid his advance. And he sees you do that, so he feels rejected, or feels like you're gonna leave. Because he loves you, he wants to come close to you . . . so he walks faster.

Now, how are you feeling as he walks faster? My goodness!—what's he doing? Are you not beginning to feel attacked?

Well, here comes an attack!

Now, because all humans are networked and vibra-tionally part of each other, he can *feel* what you are feel-ing. He sees you over there getting coffee and sees your eyes growing as big as saucers, and it seems to have some-thing to do with him coming toward you.

How's he feeling? He's feeling, "What's going on here? I'm a nice person. She's looking at me like I'm a monster or something."

So. What's he going to want? He's going to withdraw, or he's going to want revenge. As you are going to with-draw or want revenge. You're going to want to protect yourself from him or her, because of the illusions of sepa-ration. Well . . . and there are so many examples.

So, it takes place all day long. In the most subtle and consistent of ways—do you hear me? And it is these illu-sions of separation that take place first and foremost. With that feeling that you don't have safety from attack, from that someone bothering you, from someone that doesn't feel like you—how are you going to protect yourself?

So there's a feeling of insecurity. With a feeling of insecurity, there's a feeling of reaching out to know higher truth, to know a sense to it all, what seems like chaos. This gives birth to religion, the natural drive to go to a higher understanding, to know and to touch the face of God—and this is a pure thought, but remember that the pure thought is based on an illusion, based on an activity that is an illusion. That activity is communication predi-cated on illusions of separation.

So no matter how loving, no matter how well in-tended, no matter how structured and objective and fair the religion seeks to be, it is based on a fundamental error.

And that is the belief that there are significant and long-term differences between beings. Thereby it is your need, as a student of religion, to identify those who are evil—very separate, from a point of view—of the leader of the religion, usually—and those who are good, which means they agree with the leader of the religion.

This gives birth to a constant need for protection and a constant, guaranteed violence. *You* don't like to be protected against, do you? How do you feel when others want to protect themselves against you? You want to bang their walls down, don't you? Or you want to never speak to them again, no matter what happens.

Well, this is the birth of religion. And of course religion *is* well intended. Its disciples *do* want to create love on Earth. But how can you do that when you are constantly having to try to identify what is evil and what is good? And when one is evil, you are an eternity in hell. Silly, silly, silly! *All* things are part of God. *All* things have rage for a moment. Have you not been in a rage, each of you in this room? But did you not eventually become forgiving? Did you not have a smile on your face eventually, you see?

So, yes, it is a puzzle. To many it is a very great paradox. And it is one that will be addressed in the new age. Religions are going to change dramatically. But don't hold your breath for a perfect environment in your terms! Because it will be translated from different points of view, won't it? Look around your metaphysical community now. Who's seeking to create new religions, new ways of praising God and understanding enlightenment? Look at all the different points of view!

You see. And look at all the fear of negativity again. The new religions based on the metaphysical community are no different from the old religions. They as well—*you*—are teaching people to surround themselves with white light so that negativity cannot enter their being—eh?—and you can think only *positive* thoughts, and ignore *negative* thoughts what*ever* you do!

Now, what are negative thoughts?

Well, they're something that other people have. And on and on it goes, around and around, it's the same thing as the religions that have been there all along, it's no different. The new religions are different from some religions in that they do promulgate reincarnation, and karma, cause and effect . . . but many religions of the past and in other parts of the world do that as well. So it's not as different as you might like to think it is.

Why isn't it different? Because you, my friends, are not different from those who founded religion. See how you want to see yourself as different? You are different now, aren't you, from those who founded those silly religions. You've grown, you're more mature.

Well, you have grown. So have they grown, but you still have illusions of separation. Please do not be frustrated by that. Instead, try to create a new thanksgiving. When you wake up every morning, you go, "Ah, here I am awake! And I'm in the body again—I must have something to learn! Hallelujah! I have something new to learn!" There is the rapture of life! "I never want to stop learning about *me* and my relationship with life everywhere! What a glorious thing to behold!" You are then on the threshold of masterhood.

So just—you know, it's all silly, but enjoy the silliness, it's all based on legitimate sincere desires for love. And that is based on real and temporary illusions of separation that are quite similar to your own, my friends. God bless you.

Don't resist that. Be in glory of it, that you are *conscious* in your learning.

My friends, I must leave the body soon. A final brief question, perhaps . . . ?

QUESTION: When you say definitively that there is not going to be a global nuclear war in our near future, could you share the process that you go through to arrive at that conclusion?

DR. PEEBLES: God bless you. As I look at the vibrational spirals of human thought collectively, I am able to see color patterns, shifts and changes, intensities from pale to dark —these represent intentions. As we look at these, we see beyond time and space, we see beyond what you are thinking this moment, but also what you are planning for tomorrow and forevermore.

We do not see that in concrete terms for an individual, but for collectives, where it is a multiconcept of many thoughts and intentions, it becomes clearer. So, there was a major decision in the early seventies, from the experience of Vietnam, that affected the entire globe, unconsciously. And that was to quiet down a little bit, to communicate, to see that the governments of the world are not divided into white hats and black hats, but there are many shades of gray.

And so a little bit of air was taken out of the balloons. A little bit of indignation was identified and released. So now there is a significant new degree of . . . a little more communication, little more hesitation before there is confrontation.

This can be viewed; it is seen. It is similar, my friend, to decisions that you make before you come into your body, that embrace your whole life on Earth, and yet in your free will you can make them sooner or you can make them later, you can even change them a little bit, but there is predestination of things that must take place, that will take place in the family of mankind and in the mind of the individual. But your free will can make it sooner or later, according to your growth, according to your change and your shift. You see.

I must leave. My friends, go your ways in peace, love, and harmony. Life is a joy. You always are the creator, never the victim. Personalize all experience of your international world and you will understand truth, you will empathize, thereby you will give yourself permission to speak and to be counted. This is the joy of life, to see how people will respond to you, so you *can* identify your bias rather than pretend otherwise. *There* is the rapture and the joy you seek, the freedom beyond freedom beyond your wildest dreams and imaginations.

My friends, it is *our* thanksgiving that *you* have shared with *us* this night, for I have grown and *we* have grown—from your love, from your insight, and from your faith.

Certainly, as you see the pain of your every day, see as well the humor, the growth, the new opportunity; for the sun rises again each and every day. As you seek your enlightenment, then, do not resist disagreement but instead *learn* from disagreement, within you as well as others.

You are light. You are also shadow. And both are God.

God bless you each and every one.

14

End Notes

*"Understand that each of you is your own
higher self, as you are right now, and
doing the best you can."*

—Dr. Peebles

We realize that we have barely scratched the surface of the phenomenon here—and indeed it has been our major intent to merely call attention to it and invite further interest.

As Dr. Paul Weisberg suggested (see Chapter Four), many of us "don't get to the point of having a satisfactory and gratifying existence," so further interest in the multidimensional experience would seem warranted. Wherever you may live in the world today, chances are you will find spiritual explorers nearby who are involved in "an enterprise devoted to major change" and who would love to share their discoveries with you. Many, such as Thomas Jacobson, are devoting their full time and energies as teachers and counselors. Look around; you will find them.

Thomas himself conducts intensive workshops in transformational spirituality and spiritual psychology and has dedicated his life to helping others find their own paths. If you cannot find a teacher or study group in your vicinity, you may contact Thomas directly at the address given on page 261.

We do intend to spend more direct time with Spirit, to fill in some of the blanks that you may have noted herein, and to extend the depth of our understanding. We could not and would not presume to contain it all within a single book.

So, yes, this book is at its close (and we are a bit sad about that) but the adventure is far from ended.

Someone may ask: What is the good of knowing all this if you cannot put it to use in your own life?

Indeed.

We even had a problem trying to understand why successive lives on the planet are necessary if we already *knew* it all in heaven. But, you see, there's the rub—and the rub is the answer to both questions.

Knowing is not *doing.*

Spirit tells us that repeatedly. People who have the rare privilege of a direct consultation with Spirit, even though blown away and amazed and enraptured by what they *learn* through the experience, may still go straight back to their confined, conventional, and pained little lives just as though the experience had never happened —or as though it were something to be experienced theoretically and then dropped.

We have noted this (and *that* is the *real* phenomenon) to greater and lesser degrees in checking back with some who have been touched by Spirit. It seems that, for many people, it is more natural to simply play with this stuff as a pleasant (or even engrossing, for a moment) diversion—or perhaps it is just that it is "safer" and less demanding on our comfort with self-image to keep it all at arm's length.

But that is okay, too, if that is where you are. At least you are *theorizing* reality in a new and different way, so that couldn't be all bad. So, yes, you can put it to practical use, if that is your desire— but even if you do not, you are better off from the exposure alone if that is where you prefer to keep it for now. It is "okay to be skeptical"—as Karen pointed out, as long as you do not allow your skepticism to keep you away from the dance.

Early in our interviews with Spirit, it became clear to us that Dr. Peebles did not wish to dwell upon details of his former life on Earth, as though it would be a waste of precious time better spent on more important considerations—but also, we felt, because he seemed to feel a bit uncomfortable discussing his own accomplishments during that lifetime.

We respected his feelings in the matter because we felt, too, that time was of the essence and also because we understood that he had traveled far since those brief moments in Earth time—far enough, in fact, that he will be visiting Earth again soon (relatively—give or take a century or two) in another body but as a fully realized being—but we feel no sense of violation in reporting that he seems to have been last born on Earth as James Martin Peebles in Vermont on March 23, 1822.

This Peebles was from a family that originated in Scotland, settled in Northern Ireland in about 1670, then emigrated to Massachusetts in 1718. He was a leader in the Spiritualist movement in this country and abroad, authored about a dozen books, served briefly as consul to Turkey, had a friendship with Samuel L. Clemens (Mark Twain), and was regarded as an eloquent and persuasive orator.

Apparently he outlived his own biographers; we have learned that he died on February 15, 1922, just short of his 100th birthday, and was very active to the end.

We have been trying to locate a very elderly man who attended one of Thomas's appearances at a church in Los Angeles recently and who is reported to have said that he once attended a lecture by this Dr. Peebles, adding, ". . . and he hasn't changed a bit."

So apparently this is our man.

We had the privilege of leafing through a book titled *Immortality* and authored by this Peebles in 1879, first published in 1880 by Colby and Rich, Boston. The copy we saw was a fifteenth edition, published in 1907, so it was obviously widely read. It sure reads like our Doc Peebles. Here is a brief quote from that book (compare with the tutorial on "will" in Chapter Ten herein):

> The theory that force is an attribute of matter is disproved by the fact of inertia. It cannot change its state. It will ultimately be shown, I believe, that *inertia* is the sole attribute of matter, while the other properties usually ascribed to it are simply secondary qualities which inertia involves. Force, therefore, is the antithesis of matter, not simply one of its attributes. *Will* is the single attribute of force, and will is self-determining; not motion, but the antecedent of motion, and the antithesis of inertia.

And perhaps he would not mind if we gave you a description found in a biography, *The Spiritual Pilgrim*, by J. O. Barrett, published in 1872 (when Peebles was fifty years of age). The following is attributed to a Mrs. H.F.M. Brown:

Mr. Peebles's leading characteristic is, perhaps, *individuality*. He is independent in thought and speech; condemns cowardice and jealousies without stint: he commends where he can, never looking to see which way the tide is setting, or waits public approval. But he is quite willing that others should live their lives, if principles are not compromised. He is orderly, generous, social, mirthful, and a great lover of the beautiful. In personal appearance, he is tall, straight, of slender form, brown hair, blue eyes: his face is of Roman mold: his teeth faultless. He dresses with great care, avoiding alike the dandy and the sloven. He is tall and slim as a May-pole; as fair and frail as a delicate woman. Consumption looks him in the face occasionally; but, by sailing the world half round, he has eluded the unwelcome phantom. But, after all, the mistake might have been in putting the right soul into the wrong body. Spiritwise, Mr. Peebles is a mountaineer. He is calm in a storm, laughs at the lightning, and listens to the thunder as friend to friend. His thoughts, like mountain-streams, gush forth with freshness, music, and originality. If he is a thought-borrower, his benefactions are the ferns, the dewy mosses, the wild-flowers, the cloud-crowned hills, and green valleys of his native state. I said to my soul, while listening to him, Emerson had this very man in his mind when he said, "In your heart are birds and sunshine: in your thoughts the brooklets flow."

I can understand, though, why Doc would not want a lot of attention on that past life; it must seem almost irrelevant to him now. Like maybe how you would feel if the whole world became fascinated with your adventures in kindergarten instead of focusing on your adult accomplishments.

"You're all gonna die," he tells us with that mischievous twinkle in the voice, "so you'll have your proofs soon enough." In the flash, yeah, of an angel's eye. We're reading you, Doc.

The proofs are in the puddings themselves, of course, and each life is its own pudding. And as I have already mentioned, Linda knew the truth about Doc Peebles before I knew it. But, of course, Linda is more spiritually advanced than I am. I had always tended toward the intellectual examination of reality. I am learning that this is not necessarily the best way to acquire understanding.

Linda, for example, already knew that our adventure did not *begin* with Dr. Peebles. It actually began several years earlier, when our eyes sparked truth across a crowded room, a truth that inspired her to write the moving verse which I give you here in closing, and which she says sustained her through those early years of turmoil.

THE EDGE OF FOREVER

Across the infinite expanses of the universe,
through the swirling mysteries of the cosmos,
my soul awakened, recognizing its place.
At the edge of forever,
spinning through time and space,
the spark of acknowledgment flashed,
ignited, exploded, convulsed,
bringing to an immediate halt
all semblance of time.
Reaching out, pulling to my breast
all that encompasses infinity;
standing at the brink,
discovering the uniqueness of my self,
I drew in to me all there was to absorb.
At the edge of forever,
recognizing the magnetic force,
the enormous cosmic implication of another soul
merging, fusing,
harmonizing with mine.
Through the cosmic evolution,
two souls,
each with its own uniqueness,
accelerating through the universal vastness:
two souls in unison
from the edge of forever and beyond.

It is not ended, right. We are dancing the dance of angels . . .
and the adventure continues.

Afterword

A NEW HOPE

A new human life can be conceived in the flash of an eye, but it still takes nine months to deliver the child into the world for all to see and experience. This book was created in forty days of intensely concentrated activity, and here we are many months later, at its delivery into the world.

Much has happened to reach this point. We have maintained a close relationship with Thomas and Dr. Peebles, and we have experienced another seventy-five or so public appearances by the good doctor. We've met many beautiful people along the way, engendered lasting friendships, witnessed incredible magic, deepened our own convictions, expanded our lives in ways never dreamed of two years ago. Our adventure has indeed become our lives, and we want you to know that.

Now we'd like to share with you Dr. Peebles's latest message of hope, delivered in February 1989:

Yes . . . welcome, my friends, we have gathered here to-day to respond to your quest for insights for public dissemination. It is our excitement to share our points of view, and we say to you and to all that the coming years shall be prosperous for all.

For years now the general public of North America—all countries therein—have harbored increasing fears of financial failure and upheaval, as only part of upheaval around the world. Please be assured that you will find early signals that will absolutely contradict much of this prediction.

Yes, you still will have some response and some responsibility, you will still be paying for some collective social political decisions of yesteryear, but overall you will see signals that the changes that are at hand will be ever so much more a blessing. Why?—because in the world in general and in the societies of North America you are going to find a greater faith and hope, a greater hope of happiness, a greater desire for relationships and love in the world. You are going to find that various political leaders will increase their cooperation, the desire for community—and in that community of the world, of course, it is most important that one and all love the differences rather than trying to change the same. And that is where you will discover peace on Earth, in collective terms.

In personal terms you will find that same peace, as you recognize yourself as student—a student of magic, a student of manifestation, a student of will, all of which are from God, the divine within. To understand this transformation of self, you must embrace change rather than fear the same. To become the pilot, looking forward to greater locomotion and mobility —an opportunity to create a sound, and from that sound an echo, and from that echo an opportunity to learn yet again of thine own divine self.

Look forward to change, and you will know happiness. Resist the same, and you will know pain. Understand each and every event of each and every day as no more and no less than a delightful opportunity for growth.

God bless you, and welcome. Would you have questions or comment?"

DON: Yes, thank you so much. In your opening statement you spoke to us about the bright prospects in the years just ahead . . . and of course we here in the United States have recently had a change of presidents. Ronald Reagan was one of our most popular presidents, I think, ever . . .

could you speak just a little bit about what you feel is the mark that Reagan's presidency has left on history, and also as a second part of that question, I'm sure you are familiar with what is called the twenty-year cycle of tragedy for American presidents who are elected in the first year of even-numbered decades. Reagan was elected in 1980 and managed to live through his eight years as president. If there was anything to this so-called cycle of tragedy or presidential curse, what did Reagan do to beat that?

DR. PEEBLES: Yes, all right. To understand President Reagan is first to consider the probable future, that at the turn of the century you are upon a new age. There is no need for anyone to feel disconcerted or offended by that concept, but instead to celebrate the new with awareness that the new always incorporates the old, without exception but with a new twist, a new slant, another review.

And so it is that in the next century, the beginning of your new age, there is going to be greater fellowship than ever before. It's just the plan for Earth that there will be continued studies of the illusions of separation, but it will be a much more direct and honest one, the result of which will find people tending to reach out and hold each other in their study, a greater allowance rather than condemnation of error or even sin as some would call it, and thereby a greater ability and attribute to remain present with each other and to discover greater intimacy therein.

Well, so moving backward through the decade of the nineties and the latter part of the eighties, you are going to experience signals from leaders of various countries and movements and individuals in your local town and within yourself, regarding a greater desire for all of the above stated. To remain increasingly present, to try with a little more honesty and to try harder, and to be more honest and aware of judgment, and to embrace failures and failing as a measuring stick for reevaluation and growth rather than a signal of destitution or lack.

So collectively and individually you are in the beginning of a new hope in the world, and this will have direct ramifications in politics, in your monetary systems, and so forth. Simultaneously you will be suffering the residue of that old priority of safety, sanctuary, and survival of many decades past, of two thousand years past. Safety, sanctuary, and survival have been for nineteen hundred and eighty-eight years the priority. You are now within ten years of changing that priority to a collective dance of consciousness —not losing the individual or camouflaging the same, but through that collective movement discovering a larger self, a larger individual, a larger passion and permission to live life.

Well . . . Reagan was the end of a lineage. With great heart and sincerity he was determined to provide the statement of love, a safe and secure environment, and saw that as his dominant responsibility. Properly so, for this was the platform desired and supported by the majority who elected him.

President Bush is the cusp, the moment of change into the new priorities. You will find that each administration through the decade of the nineties will be more and more directly concerned with cooperation, more so than protection, and President Bush is moving in that direction.

Regarding the twenty-year cycle, there was no curse. The decades of the American presidents and the synchronicities of tragedy in office were seen by some as destiny over a long term, but these were local events and should be seen as a symbol of the collapse of will within community, the events made manifest to confront and to confound the priority of safety and sanctuary at the very moment when you thought it was guaranteed. This was an act of consciousness that was channeled, brought forward, by the presidents of the time, beginning with William Harrison and culminating with John Kennedy, without regard for personalities or individual destinies and all for a very positive purpose.

Reagan, as the end of an era representing nineteen hundred eighty-eight years, remained within the body as a statement of life for the new pattern that is at hand, a pattern that he has greeted and helped to make manifest. You understand.

DON: So this is almost like a living testament that the old is giving way to the new.

DR. PEEBLES: Yes, there is not now the need for shock to confront the priority of safety and sanctuary, but instead there's a grace now. For your society is very much on the verge of major change of priorities.

DON: And you see this as a global pattern.

DR. PEEBLES: Yes.

DON: This would also explain the new movements inside Russia and the recent movements within the Middle East—this is all part of a global pattern, isn't it?

DR. PEEBLES: Yes, and you will find that with the great changes that are at hand, as you embrace those changes you will find prosperity in the world. As you look forward to collective states of consciousness and acts of life, you will find fulfillment. As you concentrate on resistance to the above, you will find isolation and pain.

Yes, it is worldwide. There will be acts of sabotage, there will be acts of terrorism, of course, there will be acts of revenge. These are statements that are creating dramatic symbols representing a massive period of time—nineteen hundred eighty-eight years—where survival was the priority. Now, the terrorism represents the past, not the future. It will be all but gone by the turn of the century. It will be gone.

DON: Does this same pattern have something to do, Dr. Peebles, with what is seen as the breakdown of family patterns—divorce, working mothers, alienation of the young, street crime, addictions, and so forth?—and, if so, how will we resolve all this confusion?

DR. PEEBLES: Yes, it is linked, and that is why you will find in the very near future, through the end of this century and into the next century, that there will be a return of family values, community values, collective values. The collective, the community, has been an implied paradox for the seeker, for it represented safety and sanctuary, but it also represented a very large echo, or threat, to any resistance to change on the part of souls who fear self-responsibility. The collective increases the sense of responsibility, for it imposes standards of behavior that could be seen as burdensome and threatening to those who just want their way all the time.

According to individual karma and perception, choices have been made between the desire for intimacy and the perceived need for a resistance to change. But there will be—there is such a force in the world now, Don, that is coming forward for the transformation of the entire planet, that more and more cooperation will be at hand for unification that will, this time, feel fragrant—smell fragrant—for it will be not for security, it will be for exercise of love. What is now a concentration on fitness of the body is quickly going to become a fitness regimen for the soul—through family, collective activities, and so forth. You see?

DON: So the whole planet is sort of starting to move together. We are literally becoming a small world.

DR. PEEBLES: Yes.

DON: Well, I believe that about covers . . .

DR. PEEBLES: How are you, Linda! Are you ready for all this creativity that's going to come out of you?

LINDA: I'm fine. Yes, I'm ready.

DR. PEEBLES: I'm glad to hear it.

DON: Linda has been hot on the tracks of your terrestrial life. She's been coming up with some amazing information. And I might say that we are both so tremendously impressed with your life on Earth and what a great inspiration it could be to everyone, your great devotion and dedication over so many years—you were such a busy, busy man.

DR. PEEBLES: Thank you, it was a very fulfilling life for me. I have some great delight of my life, but also I was a bit of the proselytizer. I played the open mind sometimes and lived otherwise, so it's, uh—your words are very generous and, uh, and somewhat true, I might add. So, thank you—and, Linda, your creativity is going to—is guaranteed, for as you have worked to research, to understand myself—and what great honor you have paid me—you are going to understand yourself. You will find it unavoidable to research yourself, Linda, as much as you've researched me. You might call it a personal curse on yourself!

In fact, you have guaranteed that the world can research you now, with as much directness as you've researched me. Tricky, aren't we? It's all part of divine plan. And you'll find all that brilliance spilling out of you. You won't be able to camouflage it anymore. God bless you.

LINDA: Thank you.

DON: Thank you, Dr. Peebles, thank you so very much for coming.

DR. PEEBLES: God bless you, God bless you all. Go your ways in peace, love, and harmony—for life is a joy and you can know harmony as you love the differences within yourself as well as the world around you. It has been our delight, a dance of the angels to be sure. God bless you each and every one.

Bibliography

and Suggested Reading

Barrett, Joseph O. *The Spiritual Pilgrim, A biography of James M. Peebles*, Boston: W. White & Co., 1872.

Campbell, Joseph, with Bill Moyers, *The Power of Myth*. New York: Doubleday, 1988.

Gibran, Kahlil. *The Prophet*. New York: Alfred A. Knopf, 1923.

Griffin, John H. *Black Like Me*. Boston: Houghton Mifflin, 1977.

Head, Joseph, and S. L. Cranston. *Reincarnation: The Phoenix Fire Mystery*. New York: Julian Press, 1977.

Jung, C. G. *Collected Works of C. G. Jung*. Princeton, N.J.: Princeton University Press, 1969.

Kubler-Ross, Elisabeth, M.D. *On Children and Death*. New York: Macmillan, 1983.

—— *On Death and Dying*. New York: Macmillan, 1969.

Longfellow, Henry Wadsworth. "The Song of Hiawatha," *Favorite Poems of Henry Wadsworth Longfellow*. New York: Doubleday, 1947.

Meek, George W. *After We Die, What Then?* Franklin, N.C.: MetaScience Foundation, 1980.

Moody, Raymond A. M.D. *Life After Life*. New York: Bantam Books, 1976.

Murphet, Howard. *Hammer on the Mountain, The Life of Henry Steel Olcott*. Wheaton, Ill.: Theosophical Publishing House, 1972.

Peebles, James M., M.D. *Immortality*. Boston: Colby and Rich, 1880.

—— *Seers of the Ages*. Boston: W. White & Co., 1869.

Pendleton, Don. *Eye to Eye*. New York: Popular Library, 1986.

—— *Life to Life*. New York: Popular Library, 1987.

Sherman, Harold. *You Live After Death*. New York: Ballantine Books, 1984.

Stevenson, Ian, M.D. *Twenty Cases Suggestive of Reincarnation*. Charlottesville, Va.: University of Virginia Press, 1974.

Stromberg, Gustaf. *The Soul of the Universe*. New York: David McKay, 1940.

Sugrue, Thomas. *There Is a River*. New York: Henry Holt, 1943; Virginia Beach, Va.: A.R.E. Press, 1973.

Van Dyke, Henry. *The Story of the Other Wise Man.* New York: Harper and Brothers, 1895.

Viscott, David, M.D. *The Language of Feelings.* New York: Arbor House, 1976; New York: Pocket Books, 1977.

—— *The Viscott Method.* Boston: Houghton Mifflin, 1984.

Weiss, Brian L., M.D. *Many Lives, Many Masters.* New York: Simon & Schuster, 1988.

Whipple, Edward. *A Biography of James M. Peebles, M.D., A.M.* Battle Creek, Mich.: self-published, 1901.

Wilson, Colin. *Afterlife.* New York: Doubleday, 1987.

—— *The Occult, a History.* New York: Random House, 1971.

Letters to the authors may be addressed c/o the publisher:
Don and Linda Pendleton
c/o Zebra Books
475 Park Avenue South
New York, NY 10016

For direct contact with Thomas Jacobson, mail should be addressed:
Thomas Jacobson
13428 Maxella Avenue
Suite 506
Marina Del Rey, CA 90292

Index